Achieving Health Equity

Achieving Health Equity

The Role of Law and Policy

Y. Tony Yang
George Washington University
Washington DC, USA

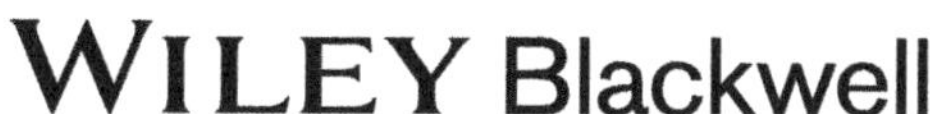

This edition first published 2025
© 2025 by John Wiley & Sons Ltd

Registered Offices
John Wiley & Sons, Inc., 111 River Street, Hoboken, NJ 07030, USA
John Wiley & Sons Ltd, The Atrium, Southern Gate, Chichester, West Sussex, PO19 8SQ, UK
Wiley-VCH GmbH, Boschstr. 12, 69469 Weinheim, Germany
John Wiley & Sons Singapore Pte. Ltd, 134 Jurong Gateway Road, #04-307H, Singapore 600134

For details of our global editorial offices, customer services, and more information about Wiley products visit us at www.wiley.com.

Wiley also publishes its books in a variety of electronic formats and by print-on-demand. Some content that appears in standard print versions of this book may not be available in other formats.

Library of Congress Cataloging-in-Publication Data applied for:

Paperback ISBN: 9781394263721

Cover Design: Wiley
Cover Image: © Jobalou/Getty Images

Set in 9.5/12.5pt STIXTwoText by Straive, Pondicherry, India

Contents

Foreword

As a public health leader who has spent my career working to advance health equity, particularly for racial and ethnic minoritized people and people living in medically under-resourced communities, I am deeply encouraged by this vital and timely book. *Achieving Health Equity: The Role of Law and Policy* provides an essential roadmap for addressing one of the most pressing moral and public health imperatives of our time – eliminating unjust and avoidable differences in health outcomes that stem from systemic racism and discrimination.

My experiences serving as the health director in the Nation's Capital for nearly a decade, during some of the most challenging times in public health including the COVID-19 pandemic, drove home just how critical it is that we transform the legal and policy frameworks that shape health outcomes. The pandemic, in particular, laid bare in stark terms the deadly consequences of long-standing health inequities, as communities of color experienced dramatically higher rates of infection, hospitalization, and mortality. At the same time, the national reckoning on racial justice in the wake of high-profile police murders of George Floyd and Breonna Taylor increased public recognition of racism as a public health crisis.

As we emerge from the acute phase of the pandemic, there is growing awareness that we cannot simply return to a pre-pandemic "normal" that was plagued by pervasive and growing health inequities rooted in systemic injustice. We have a once-in-a-generation opportunity – and obligation – to build a more equitable and resilient public health system and society. This book provides an invaluable guide for seizing that opportunity.

By taking an ecosystem approach to examining how laws and policies across sectors intersect to shape health equity, this volume illuminates the powerful role that legal and policy frameworks play in perpetuating or dismantling health inequities. It offers a comprehensive look at key policy levers across the major domains that determine health outcomes – from healthcare access and quality, to health behaviors, social and economic factors, and the physical environment.

Importantly, this book goes beyond simply describing problems to offer concrete policy strategies, case studies, and tools for enacting laws and policies that can dismantle structural drivers of health inequity. It provides a practical blueprint for policymakers, public health practitioners, healthcare and social service providers, community advocates, and other stakeholders committed to advancing policies that give everyone a fair and just opportunity to live their healthiest life.

As someone who has been met with the responsibility for translating health equity principles into practice, I appreciate how this volume consolidates complex concepts into an accessible format for a wide readership. Whether you are a student, health system administrator, public health official, policy-maker, or researcher, you will find valuable insights to inform your work.

The path to achieving health equity requires transformative changes to laws and policies that center racial justice and equity, as well as collective action from health and equity allies across all sectors and levels of government. This book accelerates those efforts by equipping advocates with both an understanding of how law and policy created – and can help dismantle - health inequities, along with practical tools and strategies for driving policy change.

The health equity movement stands at an inflection point, facing unprecedented challenges but also new possibilities. This volume serves as both a call to action and a roadmap for the critical work ahead to build a more just, equitable, and healthy future for all. I hope it will inspire and empower a new generation of leaders to take up this vital cause.

LaQuandra S. Nesbitt, MD, MPH
Former Director, the Washington, D.C. Department of Health (2015-2022)
Executive Director, GW SMHS Center for Population Health Sciences and Health Equity
Senior Associate Dean for Population Health and Health Equity
Bicentennial Endowed Professor of Medicine and Health Sciences
The George Washington University School of Medicine and Health Science

Acknowledgment

This book is the product of the collective wisdom, guidance, and support of many individuals and organizations, to whom I owe my deepest gratitude.

First and foremost, I express my heartfelt appreciation to my dedicated community health partners, whose tireless work in advancing health equity has been a constant source of inspiration. Supported through various federal grants, these remarkable organizations—including the Health Betterment Initiative-DC, Emerson Diversity Health Foundation, Alliance of Concerned Men, SDM-1 STOP Clinic, American Diversity Group, Arlington Free Clinic, and Social Capital Solutions—are instrumental in shaping healthier, more equitable communities. Your unwavering commitment is at the heart of this book.

I am also profoundly grateful to the many esteemed scholars and colleagues who have influenced my thinking and contributed to my understanding of the intricate role of law and policy in health equity. While it is impossible to mention everyone, I particularly acknowledge Sara Rosenbaum, Michelle Mello, David Studdert, Scott Burris, Wendy Parmet, Ross Silverman, Dorit Reiss, and William Sage. Your contributions to the field continue to inspire my work.

The support from my institutional colleagues has been invaluable throughout this journey. I offer special thanks to my coauthors over the years who have shaped my perspectives on health equity and policy: Carla Berg, Sawali Sudarshan, Jana Shaw, Robert Olick, Sarah Schaffer DeRoo, Paul Delamater, and Brian Chen. Your collaboration has been deeply enriching, and I am grateful for the insights we have shared.

Lastly, I owe an immeasurable debt of gratitude to my family, whose encouragement has been my constant source of strength. To my wife, Katie Yang, thank you for your unwavering support and invaluable contributions to our shared mission of promoting health equity. This book would not have been possible without you.

1

Empowering Marginalized Communities: Legal and Policy Levers for Health Equity

Abstract

This chapter introduces "Achieving Health Equity: The Role of Law and Policy," a comprehensive guide exploring how legal and policy frameworks shape health outcomes of marginalized populations, especially racial minorities in the United States. It establishes the purpose and importance of examining health equity through law and policy, defining key concepts like health equity, social determinants of health, marginalized populations, and structural discrimination. The chapter outlines the book's ecosystem approach, organized around four key health-determining domains: healthcare access and quality, health behaviors, social and economic factors, and physical environment. It highlights cross-cutting themes and policy levers, such as resource investment, community engagement, safety net strengthening, civil rights protections, and data disaggregation. Underscoring the COVID-19 pandemic's illumination of deep-rooted health inequities and racism as a public health crisis, the chapter frames the book as an urgent call to action. It positions the guide as a roadmap for equitable policy change, offering concrete strategies and tools to dismantle structural drivers of health inequity. The chapter concludes by identifying the book's wide-reaching intended audience, including students, healthcare administrators, public health officials, regulators, and researchers, emphasizing its potential for advancing the critical work of building a more just, equitable, and healthy future for all.

Keywords *health equity; legal frameworks; policy levers; marginalized populations; social determinants of health; structural discrimination; COVID-19 pandemic; racial justice*

1.1   Navigating Law, Policy, and Health Inequities

In the United States, many individuals face a multitude of challenges that can have detrimental effects on their health and well-being. Discrimination, social exclusion, poverty, disenfranchisement, and unequal access to opportunities are just a few of the obstacles that marginalized populations encounter on a daily basis. Communities of color, low-income populations, those with low education levels, and other underserved groups continue to experience dramatically poorer health outcomes compared to their more privileged counterparts.

Achieving Health Equity: The Role of Law and Policy, First Edition. Y. Tony Yang.
© 2025 John Wiley & Sons Ltd. Published 2025 by John Wiley & Sons Ltd.

"Achieving Health Equity: The Role of Law and Policy" is an extensive exploration of how legal and policy frameworks influence the health outcomes of marginalized populations, with a particular focus on racial minorities in the United States. While primarily centered on US law and policy, the insights and lessons presented in this book have global relevance, as the United States serves as an influential model worldwide, including in how it has relied on systemic racism to shape healthcare, public health, and access.

This book primarily caters to learners in health-related disciplines and professionals in health fields exploring the confluence of health, race, law, and policy [1]. While its foundation is academic, there's a significant crossover potential, reaching audiences not only across various disciplines but also beyond academia, particularly among activists and professionals in racial justice and health equity domains.

The primary goal of this book is to enhance understanding of the critical role that law and policy play in achieving health equity. The content is informed by research indicating that health is determined by a complex interplay of factors, with healthcare accounting for 20%, health behaviors for 30%, social and economic factors for 40%, and the physical environment for 10% [2]. By breaking down these determinants, the book demonstrates how law and policy can be leveraged to promote more equitable health outcomes.

This accessible guide is tailored for nonlegal audiences who are keen on grasping the key aspects of health equity law and policy. It fills a notable gap in the literature by consolidating health equity principles in an approachable format for a wide readership, including health system administrators implementing diversity, equity, and inclusion initiatives, public health officials, regulators, researchers, and more [3]. The COVID-19 pandemic has only heightened interest in and the urgency of addressing health inequities, making this book a timely and essential resource.

1.2 The Purpose and Importance of Examining Health Equity Through Law and Policy

The most powerful determinants of health are the laws and policies that have perpetuated legacies of racism, discrimination, and segregation [4]. Unjust laws and practices embedded in our political, economic, and social systems have shaped unhealthy physical environments, limited economic and educational opportunities, and created barriers to accessing quality healthcare for marginalized groups over many generations [5].

As a result of these systemic inequities, low-income communities and communities of color experience higher rates of chronic diseases, maternal mortality, infant mortality, and premature death compared to wealthier, predominantly white communities [6]. These health inequities are deeply entrenched and, in many cases, growing wider despite overall public health gains [7].

Attempting to reduce health inequities requires different strategies than efforts to improve public health overall [8]. Rather than a "rising tide lifts all boats" approach, a combination of targeted and universal interventions is needed to redistribute key health determinants, such as healthy environments, economic resources, power, and opportunities.

Law and policy are essential tools for this paradigm shift because they have the power to express societal values against bias, unfairness, and injustice [9, 10]. They influence how money, power, and opportunities are distributed and can transform unjust structures and systems that have perpetuated health inequities [11]. Law and policy enable widespread, population-level change by focusing on structural determinants rather than individual behaviors [12]. They guide and coordinate multisector actions to improve health equity and sustain positive changes over the long term.

Enacting more equitable laws and policies requires policymakers, public health practitioners, healthcare and social service providers, community advocates, and other stakeholders to work together in new ways [13, 14]. It requires examining how every policy decision, across sectors, will affect health equity [15]. And it requires authentic community engagement to center solutions on the lived experiences and priorities of marginalized groups [16].

This book provides a practical blueprint for advocates committed to advancing policies that give everyone a fair and just opportunity to live their healthiest lives. It offers concrete policy strategies, case studies, and tools for enacting laws and policies that dismantle structural drivers of health inequity.

1.3 Key Concepts and Definitions

To lay the foundation for delving into health equity law and policy, it's important to establish shared language around core concepts. Health is defined as a state of complete physical, mental, spiritual, cultural, and social well-being, not merely the absence of disease or infirmity [17]. Health equity refers to a state in which everyone has the opportunity to attain their full health potential, and no one is disadvantaged in achieving this potential because of social position or any other socially defined circumstance [18].

Social determinants of health are the conditions in the environments where people are born, live, learn, work, play, worship, and age that affect a wide range of health, functioning, and quality-of-life outcomes and risks [19]. Key domains include healthcare access and quality, education access and quality, social and community context, economic stability, and neighborhood and built environment [20].

Marginalized populations are groups that have been systematically excluded from accessing resources and opportunities that enable health and well-being [21]. These groups include communities of color, low-income populations, LGBTQ+ people, immigrants, people with disabilities, and those living in rural communities, among others.

Structural discrimination, or structural racism, refers to a system of structuring opportunity and assigning value based on race or other socially defined characteristics that perpetuate unfair disadvantages for some and unearned advantages for others, across multiple systems and institutions [22]. Structural drivers of inequity are created and maintained by mutually reinforcing systems of stigma, stereotypes, and bias; discriminatory practices and policies; uneven distribution of resources and opportunities; and imbalanced power [23].

While often used interchangeably, this book makes a distinction between law and policy: policy refers to a written statement of a public agency's or organization's position, decision, or a course of action. The law refers specifically to the codification and institutionalization of a policy by a government in the form of an ordinance, statute, or regulation. Thus, all laws are policies, but not all policies are laws.

1.4 An Ecosystem Approach to Health Equity Law and Policy

This book takes an ecosystem approach to examining how laws and policies across sectors intersect to shape health equity. While healthcare is an important determinant, access to quality housing, education, jobs, transportation, and other social and economic resources are equally vital [24].

The book is organized around four key domains that determine health and health equity: healthcare access and quality (20% of health), health behaviors (30% of health), social and economic factors (40% of health), and physical environment (10% of health).

In the healthcare access and quality domain, which accounts for 20% of health outcomes, the book explores a range of critical policy issues and levers. It examines how the Affordable Care Act and Medicaid expansion have helped to narrow health access disparities [25], and discusses initiatives by state and federal governments to cap insulin costs, making this life-saving medication more affordable for those who need it. The book also delves into the importance of ensuring language access in healthcare settings, as well as policy measures to address the stark disparities in maternal health outcomes experienced by Black women [26]. Other key topics in this section include legal approaches to combat algorithmic bias in healthcare decision-making [27, 28], efforts to promote equity in organ transplantation and blood donation policies, and the FDA's plan to drive diversity in clinical trials. The healthcare chapter also explores policy reforms to strengthen the social safety net and mitigate health inequities in the wake of the Dobbs decision, which overturned Roe v. Wade, as well as strategies to advance mental health equity.

The health behaviors section, which accounts for 30% of health outcomes, focuses on policies and laws that facilitate equitable access to resources and environments that promote healthy behaviors [29]. This includes strategies to promote physical activity in underserved communities, such as investing in safe parks, sidewalks, and bike lanes. The book also examines regulatory measures to reduce sugary beverage consumption, a key driver of obesity and related chronic diseases that disproportionately impact marginalized populations [30]. Other important topics in this section include policies to promote health equity through tobacco control, strategies to achieve equity in drug overdose response and prevention, and efforts to confront the ongoing HIV/AIDS epidemic, which continues to take a heavy toll on marginalized communities.

In the social and economic factors section, which accounts for 40% of health outcomes, the book takes a deep dive into the policies and laws that shape the social determinants of health [31]. It examines the growing movement to declare racism a public health crisis and explores the potential of reparations to address the health harms of historical and ongoing systemic racism [32]. The book also looks at legal measures to address food insecurity during the COVID-19 pandemic and beyond, as well as anti-racist early care and education policies that can help promote lifelong health and well-being [33]. Other key topics in this section include paid family and medical leave policies, which are critical for promoting health equity [34], as well as strategies to advance rural, remote, and tribal health equity. The book also explores potential reforms to address the crushing burden of medical debt on marginalized communities [35], efforts to reform exclusionary zoning and promote inclusive communities, and strategies to preserve diversity in healthcare and higher education in the wake of legal challenges to affirmative action. Additionally, the social and economic factors section examines public charge rule reforms to advance immigrant health equity [36], the promise of Health in All Policies approaches to embed health and equity across sectors, the role of repealing state preemption laws in promoting local health equity innovation, and the importance of promoting vaccine equity and data equity to address disparities illuminated by the pandemic.

Finally, the physical environment section, which accounts for 10% of health outcomes, examines the policies and laws that shape the places where people live, work, play, and learn. This includes a deep dive into housing policies that can promote health equity, such as affordable housing development, tenant protections, and eviction prevention. The book also looks at transportation policies that can promote healthy, equitable communities, such as transit-oriented development and Complete Streets approaches. Other key topics in this section include policies to ensure equitable access to clean water and air, as well as strategies to address the disproportionate impact of climate change on marginalized communities through resilient community design and planning [37].

Several crosscutting themes and policy levers emerge across these domains. These include investing resources proportionate to need in underserved communities, meaningfully engaging impacted communities in policy development and implementation, strengthening social and economic safety nets, improving the availability and affordability of health-promoting resources, mitigating exposure to health risks, enhancing civil rights protections and anti-discrimination enforcement, repealing preemptive laws that limit local innovations, leveraging governance levers like Health in All Policies to embed health and equity in decision-making, and disaggregating data to make inequities visible and guide targeted interventions.

1.5 An Urgent Imperative

The COVID-19 pandemic laid bare the deadly consequences of long-standing health inequities, with communities of color experiencing infection, hospitalization, and mortality rates significantly higher than white populations across the United States [38]. The national reckoning on racism in the wake of high-profile police killings of Black Americans also increased public awareness of racism as a public health crisis.

There is a growing recognition that returning to a pre-pandemic "normal" is not enough, as normal was plagued with pervasive and growing health inequities rooted in systemic injustice [39]. The path forward requires transformative laws and policies that center health equity and racial justice, as well as collective action from health and equity allies across all sectors and all levels of government [40].

This book aims to accelerate those efforts by equipping advocates with an understanding of how law and policy are created and can help dismantle health inequities, along with practical tools and strategies for policy change. The health equity movement is at an inflection point, with unprecedented challenges and new possibilities on the horizon. The chapters ahead are a call to action and a roadmap for the work ahead to build a more just, equitable, and healthy future for all.

1.6 Conclusion: A Roadmap for Equitable Policy Change

"Achieving Health Equity: The Role of Law and Policy" provides a comprehensive and accessible examination of how legal and policy frameworks shape the health outcomes of marginalized populations, particularly racial minorities in the United States. By breaking down the complex interplay of factors that determine health, the book demonstrates how law and policy can be leveraged to promote more equitable health outcomes.

The book fills a notable gap in the literature by consolidating health equity principles in an approachable format for a wide readership, including health system administrators, public health officials, regulators, researchers, and more. It offers concrete policy strategies, case studies, and tools for enacting laws and policies that dismantle structural drivers of health inequity.

The COVID-19 pandemic and the national reckoning on racism have underscored the urgent need to address long-standing health inequities rooted in systemic injustice. This book aims to accelerate efforts to build a more just, equitable, and healthy future for all by equipping advocates with an understanding of how law and policy are created and can help dismantle health inequities, along with practical tools and strategies for policy change.

"Achieving Health Equity: The Role of Law and Policy" is a valuable resource for students pursuing studies in health-related disciplines who are interested in gaining a comprehensive understanding of health equity. The book is suitable for both major and nonmajor students at the undergraduate and graduate levels. It is structured and written based on robust scholarly research, making it an excellent resource for mastering the subject area.

Furthermore, this book is useful for healthcare professionals involved in developing and implementing diversity, equity, and inclusion policies, as well as public health officials, regulators, and scientific researchers interested in health equity. The book can reach its intended audience through targeted advertisements in related scholarly journals, promotional campaigns via professional associations, and a strong presence on relevant social media platforms. To ensure accessibility, the book should be available in academic libraries and both physical and online bookstores frequented by professionals in these fields.

The chapters ahead provide a roadmap for the work ahead, exploring specific policy issues and levers across four key domains that determine health and health equity: healthcare access and quality, health behaviors, social and economic factors, and physical environment. By taking an ecosystem approach and examining cross-cutting themes and policy levers, the book offers a comprehensive blueprint for advancing health equity through law and policy.

References

1 Dawes, D.E. (2020). *The Political Determinants of Health*. Johns Hopkins University Press.

2 Hood, C.M., Gennuso, K.P., Swain, G.R., and Catlin, B.B. (2016). County health rankings: relationships between determinant factors and health outcomes. *American Journal of Preventive Medicine* 50 (2): 129–135. https://doi.org/10.1016/j.amepre.2015.08.024.

3 Michener, J. (2022). Equity in and through public health law. *The Journal of Law, Medicine & Ethics* 50 (2): 183–191. https://doi.org/10.1017/jme.2022.34.

4 Yearby, R. (2020). Structural racism and health disparities: reconfiguring the social determinants of health framework to include the root cause. *The Journal of Law, Medicine & Ethics* 48 (3): 518–526. https://doi.org/10.1177/1073110520958876.

5 Phelan, J.C. and Link, B.G. (2015). Is racism a fundamental cause of inequalities in health? *Annual Review of Sociology* 41: 311–330. https://doi.org/10.1146/annurev-soc-073014-112305.

6 Adler, N.E., Glymour, M.M., and Fielding, J. (2016). Addressing social determinants of health and health inequalities. *JAMA* 316 (16): 1641–1642. https://doi.org/10.1001/jama. 2016.14058.

7 Arcaya, M.C., Arcaya, A.L., and Subramanian, S.V. (2015). Inequalities in health: definitions, concepts, and theories. *Global Health Action* 8 (1): 27106. https://doi.org/10.3402/gha.v8.27106.

8 Frieden, T.R. (2010). A framework for public health action: the health impact pyramid. *American Journal of Public Health* 100 (4): 590–595. https://doi.org/10.2105/AJPH.2009.185652.

9 Wiley, L.F. (2021). Structural racism in the COVID-19 pandemic: moving forward. *American Journal of Bioethics* 21 (3): 56–74. https://doi.org/10.1080/15265161.2020.1851808.

10 Benfer, E.A., Mohapatra, S., Wiley, L.F., and Yearby, R. (2021). Health justice strategies to combat the pandemic: eliminating discrimination, poverty, and health inequity during and after COVID-19. *Yale Journal of Health Policy, Law, and Ethics* 19 (3): 122–171. https://digitalcommons.law.yale.edu/yjhple/vol19/iss3/3.

11 Gostin, L.O., Monahan, J.T., Kaldor, J. et al. (2020). The legal determinants of health: harnessing the power of law for global health and sustainable development. *The Lancet* 393 (10183): 1857–1910. https://doi.org/10.1016/S0140-6736(19)30233-8.

12 Goldberg, D.S. and Kotagal, M. (2022). Health equity through crisis and beyond: investing in community health infrastructure. *The Milbank Quarterly* Advance online publication. https://doi.org/10.1111/1468-0009.12573.

13 Buchanan, E. (2022). Advancing health equity through a health in all policies approach. *Journal of Public Health Management and Practice* 28 (1): E1–E5. https://doi.org/10.1097/PHH.0000000000001428.

14 Burris, S., Ashe, M., Levin, D. et al. (2016). A transdisciplinary approach to public health law: the emerging practice of legal epidemiology. *Annual Review of Public Health* 37: 135–148. https://doi.org/10.1146/annurev-publhealth-032315-021841.

15 Blacksher, E. and Valles, S.A. (2021). White privilege, white poverty: reckoning with class and race in America. *Hastings Center Report* 51 (S1): S51–S57. https://doi.org/10.1002/hast.1226.

16 Smith, M., Thompson, A., and Upshur, R.E. (2022). Public health as social justice? A qualitative study of public health policy-makers' perspectives. *BMC Public Health* 22 (1): 1–11. https://doi.org/10.1186/s12889-022-13030-1.

17 World Health Organization (2021). Constitution of the World Health Organization. https://www.who.int/about/governance/constitution (accessed 23 August 2024).

18 Braveman, P., Kumanyika, S., Fielding, J. et al. (2011). Health disparities and health equity: the issue is justice. *American Journal of Public Health* 101 (S1): S149–S155. https://doi.org/10.2105/AJPH.2010.300062.

19 Marmot, M., Friel, S., Bell, R. et al. (2008). Closing the gap in a generation: health equity through action on the social determinants of health. *The Lancet* 372 (9650): 1661–1669. https://doi.org/10.1016/S0140-6736(08)61690-6.

20 Healthy People 2030 (2023). *Social Determinants of Health*. U.S. Department of Health and Human Services, Office of Disease Prevention and Health Promotion. https://health.gov/healthypeople/priority-areas/social-determinants-health (retrieved 12 April 2023).

21 Williams, D.R., Lawrence, J.A., and Davis, B.A. (2019). Racism and health: evidence and needed research. *Annual Review of Public Health* 40: 105–125. https://doi.org/10.1146/annurev-publhealth-040218-043750.

22 Bailey, Z.D., Krieger, N., Agénor, M. et al. (2017). Structural racism and health inequities in the USA: evidence and interventions. *The Lancet* 389 (10077): 1453–1463. https://doi.org/10.1016/S0140-6736(17)30569-X.

23 Artiga, S. and Hinton, E. (2018). *Beyond Health Care: The Role of Social Determinants in Promoting Health and Health Equity*. Kaiser Family Foundation. https://www.kff.org/racial-equity-and-health-policy/issue-brief/beyond-health-care-the-role-of-social-determinants-in-promoting-health-and-health-equity/.

24 Institute of Medicine (2003). *Unequal Treatment: Confronting Racial and Ethnic Disparities in Health Care*. The National Academies Press. https://doi.org/10.17226/12875.

25 Sommers, B.D., Gawande, A.A., and Baicker, K. (2017). Health insurance coverage and health – what the recent evidence tells us. *The New England Journal of Medicine* 377 (6): 586–593. https://doi.org/10.1056/NEJMsb1706645.

26 Mullan, F. (2017). Social mission in health professions education: beyond Flexner. *JAMA* 318 (2): 122–123. https://doi.org/10.1001/jama.2017.7286.

27 Hall, M.A. and Carlson, J.L. (2022). Health equity, privacy, and artificial intelligence in medicine. *The Journal of Law, Medicine & Ethics* 50 (2): 220–227. https://doi.org/10.1017/jme.2022.38.

28 Obermeyer, Z., Powers, B., Vogeli, C., and Mullainathan, S. (2019). Dissecting racial bias in an algorithm used to manage the health of populations. *Science* 366 (6464): 447–453. https://doi.org/10.1126/science.aax2342.

29 Salhi, B.A., Zahnd, W.E., Rahman, A., and Molina, Y. (2021). Policy interventions to address health disparities in cancer. *JAMA Network Open* 4 (9): e2125498. https://doi.org/10.1001/jamanetworkopen.2021.25498.

30 Krieger, N., Waterman, P.D., Kosheleva, A. et al. (2020). Not just smoking and high-tech medicine: socioeconomic inequities in U.S. mortality rates, overall and by race/ethnicity, 1960–2015. *International Journal of Health Services* 50 (2): 213–235. https://doi.org/10.1177/0020731420902564.

31 Tobin-Tyler, E. and Teitelbaum, J.B. (2019). *Essentials of Health Justice: A Primer*. Jones & Bartlett Learning.

32 Darity, W.A., Hamilton, D., Paul, M. et al. (2022). COVID-19 and the case for reparations. *The Review of Black Political Economy* 49 (2): 79–104. https://doi.org/10.1177/00346446221084005.

33 Hahn, R.A., Barnett, W.S., Knopf, J.A. et al. (2016). Early childhood education to promote health equity: a community guide systematic review. *Journal of Public Health Management and Practice* 22 (5): E1–E8. https://doi.org/10.1097/PHH.0000000000000378.

34 Gee, G.C. and Ford, C.L. (2011). Structural racism and health inequities: old issues, new directions. *Du Bois Review: Social Science Research on Race* 8 (1): 115–132. https://doi.org/10.1017/S1742058X11000130.

35 Himmelstein, G., Lawless, R.M., Thorne, D. et al. (2019). Medical bankruptcy: still common despite the Affordable Care Act. *American Journal of Public Health* 109 (3): 431–433. https://doi.org/10.2105/AJPH.2018.304901.

36 Taylor, J. (2018). *Racism, inequality, and health care for African Americans*. The Century Foundation https://tcf.org/content/report/racism-inequality-health-care-african-americans/.

37 Ransom, M.M., Winn, L.M., Ayele, R.A. et al. (2021). The global pandemic of environmental racism and the role of healthcare organizations in addressing environmental health inequities. *Journal of Public Health Policy* 42: 434–453. https://doi.org/10.1057/s41271-021-00298-7.

38 Yearby, R. and Mohapatra, S. (2021). Law, structural racism, and the COVID-19 pandemic. *Journal of Law and the Biosciences* 7 (1): lsaa036. https://doi.org/10.1093/jlb/lsaa036.

39 Platt, J., Raj, M., and Kardia, S.L. (2021). The public health crisis of underinvestment in racial and ethnic minority health. *Journal of Public Health Management and Practice* 27 (2): 114–117. https://doi.org/10.1097/PHH.0000000000001289.

40 Hardeman, R.R., Medina, E.M., and Boyd, R.W. (2021). Stolen breaths. *The New England Journal of Medicine* 383 (3): 197–199. https://doi.org/10.1056/NEJMp2021072.

Part I

Health Care: Examining Access and Quality

This part explores critical issues and policies aimed at improving access and quality of healthcare, particularly for marginalized communities. Chapter 2 discusses how the Affordable Care Act and Medicaid expansion have narrowed health access disparities, enhancing coverage for millions. Chapter 3 examines initiatives to cap insulin costs, addressing affordability through state and federal measures. Chapter 4 focuses on ensuring language access in healthcare, highlighting the importance of interpretation services for Limited English proficiency (LEP) populations. Chapter 5 addresses Black maternal health disparities, emphasizing policy measures to reduce mortality and improve outcomes. Chapter 6 tackles algorithmic bias in healthcare, presenting legal approaches and case studies to mitigate discriminatory practices. Chapter 7 promotes equity in organ transplantation policies, examining barriers and recommending inclusive strategies. Chapter 8 advocates for easing blood donation restrictions, discussing legal and scientific perspectives to enhance donor diversity. Chapter 9 highlights the FDA's diversity plan for clinical trials, aiming to drive health equity through inclusive research practices. Chapter 10 analyzes the impact of the Dobbs decision on reproductive health, emphasizing the need to strengthen the safety net for vulnerable populations. Chapter 11 advances mental health equity, proposing policies to address disparities and improve access to mental health services. Together, these chapters provide a comprehensive roadmap for achieving equitable healthcare access and quality.

Achieving Health Equity: The Role of Law and Policy, First Edition. Y. Tony Yang.
© 2025 John Wiley & Sons Ltd. Published 2025 by John Wiley & Sons Ltd.

2

Narrowing Health Access Disparities: The Affordable Care Act and Medicaid Expansion

Abstract

This chapter examines the impact of the Affordable Care Act (ACA) on narrowing health access disparities in the United States, particularly among racial and ethnic minority populations. It begins by providing an overview of the historical context of health disparities and insurance coverage in America, highlighting the persistent gaps in life expectancy and disease rates between white Americans and minority groups. The primary barrier to accessing quality healthcare is identified as the lack of insurance coverage, which disproportionately affects people of color and low-income households. The societal and economic costs of these disparities are also discussed. The focus then shifts to the ACA, exploring its mechanisms for increasing health insurance coverage, such as Medicaid expansion and the establishment of health insurance marketplaces. The ACA's effectiveness in reducing uninsured rates and narrowing disparities in healthcare access, particularly for black Americans and Hispanics, is assessed. The challenges faced by the ACA, including political opposition and attempts to repeal the law, are also acknowledged. The potential ramifications of an ACA repeal are examined, projecting increases in the number of uninsured individuals and the erosion of progress made in closing health insurance coverage gaps for people of color. In conclusion, the ACA's crucial role in reducing healthcare disparities and increasing access to care for millions of Americans, particularly those from minority communities, is emphasized. Policymakers, advocates, and the public are called upon to recognize the importance of the ACA and work to protect and strengthen its provisions for the benefit of all Americans.

Keywords   *Affordable Care Act (ACA); Medicaid expansion; health disparities; insurance coverage; racial and ethnic minorities; health equity; uninsured rates; policy impact*

> *John, a 55-year-old black American, had been putting off a routine colonoscopy for years due to the high cost of the procedure. Without health insurance, he feared the financial burden would be too much for his family to bear. When he finally underwent the screening after gaining coverage through the Affordable Care Act (ACA), doctors discovered early-stage colorectal cancer, which could have turned fatal if left undetected.*

> *Sarah, a single mother working two part-time jobs, struggled to make ends meet for her family. Neither of her employers offered health insurance, and she couldn't afford private coverage. When her daughter developed a severe ear infection, Sarah had to choose between paying for the doctor's visit and antibiotics or putting food on the table. The ACA's Medicaid expansion provided Sarah with the coverage she needed to get her daughter the care she required without sacrificing other essentials.*

2.1 Health Disparities and Insurance Coverage in America: A Century of Change

Between 1900 and 2018, the average American life expectancy increased dramatically from 47.3 to 78.7 years, largely due to scientific and medical advancements that have enhanced the quality of life for many individuals [1]. Despite these improvements, significant health disparities persist among certain subsets of the American population, with black Americans experiencing a life expectancy of 3.8 years lower than white Americans and many minority groups facing higher rates of diseases such as cardiovascular disease and HIV/AIDS [2]. Experts attribute these disparities to a complex interplay of historical and contemporary social, cultural, economic, political, medical, and legal factors.

The primary barrier to accessing quality healthcare in the United States is not the availability of services, but rather the lack of insurance coverage. Uninsured adults are more likely to forgo necessary medical care and experience poorer health outcomes compared to their insured counterparts, particularly when managing chronic conditions like cancer and heart disease. The US healthcare system has long been plagued by significant disparities in health insurance coverage along racial and ethnic lines, with people of color more likely to live in low-income households and lack access to affordable insurance options, even when employed full-time. In the mid-2000s, approximately 47 million Americans (16% of the population) were uninsured, with minority populations, especially black Americans and Hispanics, experiencing significantly higher uninsured rates than whites [3].

The consequences of lacking health insurance extend beyond individual health, imposing significant societal and economic costs. Uninsured individuals often rely on emergency rooms as their primary source of care, straining medical facilities and resulting in billions of dollars in unpaid services. Moreover, uninsured individuals receive an estimated $100 billion in annual healthcare services for conditions that could have been treated more cost-effectively if diagnosed earlier [4]. Between 2003 and 2006, $229.4 billion (30%) of medical expenditures for black Americans, Asians, and Hispanics were excess costs attributable to health inequalities [5]. Reducing exposure to substantial medical expenses has been shown to improve credit scores and decrease the risk of bankruptcy, highlighting the potential for addressing health insurance disparities to mitigate economic inequality.

The ACA, signed into law by President Barack Obama on March 23, 2010, was designed to reduce health inequities based on race and ethnicity, with the original text containing 34 references to the term "disparities" [6]. The ACA expanded health insurance options for uninsured individuals in low- and middle-income households, which are disproportionately represented by black Americans and Hispanics [7]. Since its implementation, the ACA has led to significant coverage gains among people of color, helping to narrow health coverage disparities. However, the ACA has faced persistent opposition from Republicans and conservatives, with numerous attempts to repeal the law and three Supreme Court challenges (2012, 2015, and 2020) [8]. Despite these challenges, the ACA has largely survived, but it is crucial to understand the potential consequences of its repeal. The following sections of this chapter will examine the ACA's mechanisms for addressing health coverage inequities, evidence of its successes, and the implications for public health policies should the law be repealed.

2.2 The ACA's Mechanics and Effectiveness

The ACA was designed to address gaps in health insurance coverage through a combination of private and public sector provisions targeting states, insurance companies, employers, and individuals. This section explores the various methods employed by the ACA to expand coverage and assesses the law's effectiveness in achieving its goals.

2.2.1 How Did the ACA Increase Health Insurance Coverage?

The ACA increased health insurance coverage through two primary mechanisms. First, it expanded state-run Medicaid programs. Prior to the ACA, Medicaid eligibility was limited to unemployed parents with income below 37% of the federal poverty level (FPL) and employed parents with income below 63% of the FPL, with the FPL being determined annually by the Department of Health and Human Services. Most states denied Medicaid benefits to adults without dependent children, regardless of income [9]. The ACA required states to expand Medicaid coverage to all non-Medicare eligible individuals under 65 with household income up to 133% of the FPL, threatening to withhold federal Medicaid funds from states that refused to comply.

However, in the 2012 case, National Federation of Independent Business (NFIB) v. Sebelius, the Supreme Court ruled that the ACA's Medicaid expansion was unconstitutionally coercive. Chief Justice John Roberts determined that when the federal government conditions grants of federal funds (in this case, for state Medicaid programs), it must provide states with a "genuine choice" in accepting the conditions [10]. In this instance, states lacked a genuine choice because refusing to accept the federal government's conditions would result in the loss of existing Medicaid funds. While the Court's decision ultimately retained the ACA's provisions, it effectively made Medicaid expansion optional for states. States that choose not to expand Medicaid coverage will forgo federal funds related to the expansion but cannot lose funds for existing Medicaid programs.

The second major way the ACA sought to increase health insurance coverage was through the establishment of health insurance marketplaces. These marketplaces provide access to insurance for individuals who cannot obtain coverage through employer-sponsored plans. Although the ACA instructed states to set up their own exchanges, the vast majority opted to join the federal exchange (accessed at http://HealthCare.gov). Lower-income families participating in these marketplaces can qualify for additional savings through premium tax credits and cost-sharing reductions.

2.2.2 The ACA's Effectiveness

The ACA yielded immediate increases in health insurance coverage. In 2013, just before the ACA's main provisions took effect, 20.4% of working-age adults in the United States were uninsured [11]. By 2018, that figure had dropped to 12.4%. Prior to 2013, black American and Hispanic adults reported significantly higher rates of cost-related barriers to healthcare compared to white adults. Following the ACA's enactment, these populations experienced the largest overall improvements in healthcare access, narrowing the disparities between whites and black Americans/Hispanics in cost-related access problems. For black Americans, the disparity fell from 8.1% to 4.7%, while for Hispanics, it dropped from 12.7% to 8.3% between 2013 and 2018.

The ACA's passage led to the most significant improvements in healthcare access for black Americans and Hispanics. In 2013, 23% of black American adults reported avoiding healthcare due to costs, which decreased to 17.6% after the ACA's implementation. Similarly, the percentage of Hispanics avoiding care due to costs dropped from 27.8% to 21.2%. In comparison, the percentage of whites avoiding care due to costs only decreased from 15.1% to 12.9%. The data is even more encouraging for residents of states that have opted to expand Medicaid.

Studies indicate that black American adults living in states with Medicaid expansion are less likely to be uninsured than white adults in states without the expansion [12]. Although Hispanic adults in both expansion and non-expansion states reported lower uninsured rates, the healthcare access gains were more substantial in expansion states. Black Americans in expansion states are nearly as likely as white adults in those states to have a usual source of care. A comparison between Louisiana (an expansion state) and Georgia (a non-expansion state) is particularly revealing. Between 2013 and 2015, white and black adults in both states with incomes under 200% of the FPL experienced health insurance access gains [13]. However, when Louisiana expanded Medicaid in 2016, uninsured rates for white and black adults dropped an additional 12.2%, while uninsured rates for white and black adults in Georgia remained unchanged.

Despite the significant coverage gains made between 2013 and 2016, progress has stalled and even eroded for black Americans, Hispanics, and all Americans in recent years. Between 2016 and 2020, the uninsured rate for black Americans increased by 0.7%, while whites experienced a 0.5% increase over the same period [14]. Experts suggest that several factors may be responsible for this stagnation in progress, including rollbacks of enrollment efforts for ACA coverage, changes to Medicaid renewal processes, and the elimination of the individual mandate penalty for health coverage.

> *"The Affordable Care Act upholds a fundamental truth: that in America, healthcare is not a privilege for the fortunate few, but a right for all."*
>
> Former President Barack Obama

2.3 Ramifications of an ACA Repeal

The ACA has survived three Supreme Court challenges: (i) NFIB v. Sebelius in 2012; (ii) King v. Burwell in 2015; and (iii) California v. Texas in 2021 [15]. Despite congressional Republicans' electoral promises to repeal the ACA over the past decade, the law has remained intact. However, the ACA's current security does not guarantee its future. This section explores the potential consequences of an ACA repeal.

Between 2013 and 2017, the ACA's provisions led to the coverage of 15 million previously uninsured individuals. A repeal of the ACA would leave these 15 million people "in the lurch." Some repeal proposals have even suggested funding Medicaid below pre-ACA levels, potentially causing even more than 15 million people to become uninsured and eroding support for long-term care for people with disabilities, a key function of Medicaid.

Other studies and commentators estimate that repealing the ACA would increase the number of uninsured people by 20 million, primarily due to the elimination of Medicaid expansion for low-income adults and premium tax credits for low- and middle-income individuals purchasing insurance on the health insurance marketplace [16]. While most people obtain insurance through their employers, the COVID-19 pandemic has led to historic levels of job loss. One estimate suggests that 27 million people are at risk of losing employer-sponsored health coverage after losing a job [17]. Currently, many of these individuals are able to retain healthcare coverage through expanded Medicaid or more affordable marketplace plans. However, an ACA repeal could subject these people to dire consequences.

Moreover, repealing the ACA would undo progress made in closing health insurance coverage gaps, particularly for black Americans and Hispanics. If Medicaid expansion is lost as part of an ACA repeal, states would lose access to the federal funding required to offer Medicaid to those not previously eligible. This would make it difficult for states to maintain coverage for low-income families with children and likely eliminate coverage for childless adults, regardless of their income level. Additionally, individuals who rely on tax credits and subsidies in health insurance marketplaces might lose their ability to pay for health insurance coverage.

As of 2020, approximately 33% of non-elderly black Americans, Hispanics, and American Indian and Alaska Natives are covered by Medicaid, compared to less than half that percentage (15%) for whites [18]. The statistics presented in Part IIB demonstrate the ACA's effectiveness in increasing healthcare coverage for people of color in the United States. Consequently, logic dictates that an ACA repeal would disproportionately impact these communities, reversing the health coverage gains for people of color who already face significant disadvantages in numerous facets of life.

2.4   Conclusion: The ACA's Impact on Health Equity Amid Ongoing Challenges

Despite the controversy and fervor surrounding the ACA's passage, the law has undeniably led to a significant progress in addressing healthcare inequities for people of color [19]. Large portions of the population who previously lacked access to proper care due to cost barriers now have the opportunity to receive the care they deserve. The ACA increased healthcare coverage through two primary mechanisms. First, states have the option to expand Medicaid, which increases the number of low- and middle-income individuals who can obtain healthcare coverage that they otherwise would not have had. Second, the establishment of health insurance marketplaces allows low-income individuals to receive tax credits and subsidies to purchase health insurance.

Although the ACA's successes are undeniable, the law has faced constant political threats since its passage. The ACA has been subject to three challenges before the Supreme Court. While the Court required certain adjustments to the law, specifically allowing states to opt-in to Medicaid expansion, the ACA has ultimately survived all challenges. Moreover, there appears to be no current appetite within the Republican party to mount another charge against the ACA.

However, there are no guarantees in life, and defenders and supporters of the ACA must remain vigilant and understand the consequences of a potential repeal. If the ACA were to be repealed, the number of uninsured individuals would increase exponentially, with this trend being particularly detrimental to people of color. Any progress made in addressing healthcare coverage inequities would be lost. Therefore, ACA supporters must work to ensure that the law remains intact.

In conclusion, the ACA has proven to be a crucial tool in reducing healthcare disparities and increasing access to care for millions of Americans, particularly those from minority communities. While the law has faced numerous challenges and threats, it has demonstrated resilience and effectiveness in achieving its goals. As the nation continues to grapple with issues of healthcare access and equity, it is essential that policymakers, advocates, and the public recognize the importance of the ACA and work to protect and strengthen its provisions for the benefit of all Americans.

ACA's Impact on Health Equity: Key Policies and Provisions

Category	Topic	Details
ACA Provisions and Goals	ACA Provisions for Equity	The ACA includes multiple provisions specific to race, ethnicity, and language, impacting diverse populations
	Expansion of Coverage	The ACA expands coverage through Medicaid expansion, marketplaces, and subsidies, reducing racial and ethnic disparities
Delivery Systems and Care Models	Access Points and Networks	Patient-centered medical homes, community health centers, and rural health centers form "medical villages" to share resources and best practices
	Service and Payment Reforms	Reforms like Accountable Care Organizations (ACOs) and value-based purchasing improve care quality and reduce costs for underserved populations
	Primary Care Focus	Emphasizes primary care as the healthcare foundation, with programs like the Primary Care Extension Program enhancing comprehensive care
	Equity-Focused Models	Links insurers, educational services, health homes, and social services to improve health equity by ensuring continuous coverage and addressing social determinants of health
Partnerships and Collaboration	Public–Private Partnerships	Encourages collaborations between public and private sectors to enhance health equity efforts
Safety Net and Support Systems	Challenges and Strengthening	Safety net providers like Federally Qualified Health Centers (FQHCs) remain crucial despite expanded coverage, with increased demand requiring strengthened support
Affordability and Coverage	Affordability and Continuous Coverage	Affordable insurance is a key to continuous coverage, preventing care gaps and addressing unmet needs, especially for low-income and minority populations
	Parental Coverage Impact	Parents' insurance status significantly impacts children's coverage, with gaps leading to worse health outcomes
Technology and Innovation	Technology and Innovation	Information technology, like Electronic Health Records (EHRs), helps share information among insurers, educational services,medical homes, and social services to improve coverage and outcomes

References

1 Arias, E. and Xu, J. (2020). United States life tables, 2018. National vital statistics reports: from the Centers for Disease Control and Prevention, National Center for Health Statistics. *National Vital Statistics System* 69 (12): 1–45.

2 Kochanek, K.D., Arias, E., and Anderson, R.N. (2013). How did cause of death contribute to racial differences in life expectancy in the United States in 2010? *NCHS Data Brief* 125: 1–8.

3 Davis, K. (2007). Uninsured in America: problems and possible solutions. *BMJ (Clinical Research ed.)* 334 (7589): 346–348. https://doi.org/10.1136/bmj.39091.493588.BE.

4 Coughlin, T. A. (2014). Uncompensated Care for the Uninsured in 2013: A Detailed Examination. https://www.kff.org/uninsured/report/uncompensated-care-for-the-uninsured-in-2013-a-detailed-examination/.

5 Xin, H. (2017). Editorial: health disparities – an important public health policy concern. *Frontiers in Public Health* 5: 99. https://doi.org/10.3389/fpubh.2017.00099.

6 Serakos, M. and Wolfe, B. (2016). The ACA: impacts on health, access, and employment. *Forum for Health Economics & Policy* 19 (2): 201–259. https://doi.org/10.1515/fhep-2015-0027.

7 Buchmueller, T.C., Levinson, Z.M., Levy, H.G., and Wolfe, B.L. (2016). Effect of the Affordable Care Act on racial and ethnic disparities in health insurance coverage. *American Journal of Public Health* 106 (8): 1416–1421. https://doi.org/10.2105/AJPH.2016.303155.

8 Jost, T.S. and Keith, K. (2020). The ACA and the courts: litigation's effects on the law's implementation and beyond. *Health Affairs (Project Hope)* 39 (3): 479–486. https://doi.org/10.1377/hlthaff.2019.01324.

9 Lin, Y., Monnette, A., and Shi, L. (2021). Effects of Medicaid expansion on poverty disparities in health insurance coverage. *International Journal for Equity in Health* 20: 1–11.

10 Weeks, E., Chirba, M.A., and Noble, A.A. (2023). National Federation of Independent Business v. Sebelius, 567 US 519 (2012).

11 Baumgartner, J.C., Collins, S.R., Radley, D.C., and Hayes, S.L. (2020). How the Affordable Care Act has narrowed racial and ethnic disparities in access to health care. *The Commonwealth Fund.* https://doi.org/10.26099/kx4k-y932.

12 Akinyemiju, T., Jha, M., Moore, J.X., and Pisu, M. (2016). Disparities in the prevalence of comorbidities among US adults by state Medicaid expansion status. *Preventive Medicine* 88: 196–202.

13 Selden, T.M., Lipton, B.J., and Decker, S.L. (2017). Medicaid expansion and marketplace eligibility both increased coverage, with trade-offs in access, affordability. *Health Affairs* 36 (12): 2069–2077.

14 Lee, H. and Porell, F.W. (2020). The effect of the Affordable Care Act Medicaid expansion on disparities in access to care and health status. *Medical Care Research and Review* 77 (5): 461–473.

15 Béland, D., Rocco, P., and Waddan, A. (2023). *Obamacare Wars: Federalism, State Politics, and the Affordable Care Act.* University Press of Kansas.

16 Banthin, J., Blumberg, L.J., Buettgens, M. et al. (2019, December). *Implications of the Fifth Circuit Court decision in Texas v. United States.* Urban Institute. https://www.urban.org/sites/default/files/publication/101361/implications_of_the_fifth_circuit_court_decision_in_texas_v_united_states_final_121919_v2.pdf.

17 Fronstin, P., and Woodbury, S. A. (2020). How Many Americans Have Lost Jobs with Employer Health Coverage During the Pandemic?. https://www.ebri.org/docs/default-source/pbriefs/ebri_ib_esicovidloss-8oct20.pdf?sfvrsn=f0763a2f_6.

18 Donohue, J.M., Cole, E.S., James, C.V. et al. (2022). The US Medicaid program: coverage, financing, reforms, and implications for health equity. *JAMA* 328 (11): 1085–1099.

19 Kominski, G.F., Nonzee, N.J., and Sorensen, A. (2017). The Affordable Care Act's impacts on access to insurance and health care for low-income populations. *Annual Review of Public Health* 38: 489–505. https://doi.org/10.1146/annurev-publhealth-031816-044555.

3

Tackling Insulin Affordability: Addressing Systemic Failures and Policy Solutions

Abstract

This chapter explores the complex issue of insulin affordability in the United States, highlighting recent progress, disparities, and the need for systemic change. It begins by discussing the financial burden of insulin costs on individuals with diabetes, particularly those from marginalized communities, and the impact of recent initiatives by Medicare, states, and drug manufacturers to cap monthly insulin costs. The chapter then delves into various state-level initiatives aimed at addressing insulin affordability, including mandated insurance coverage for diabetes supplies, copay caps, patient assistance programs, and efforts to promote biosimilar insulin. It examines the benefits and limitations of these policies. The chapter also analyzes federal efforts to tackle insulin affordability, focusing on the Inflation Reduction Act of 2022 and its provisions for capping out-of-pocket insulin costs for Medicare beneficiaries and allowing Medicare Part D to negotiate prescription drug prices. It discusses the limitations of these measures, particularly their failure to extend protections to the uninsured and those with commercial insurance plans. Building on this analysis, the chapter presents policy recommendations to improve insulin affordability and access. The chapter concludes by emphasizing that future interventions should focus on prevention, target social determinants of health, and implement comprehensive policies that extend beyond short-term price caps to create a more equitable healthcare system that ensures access to affordable insulin for all who need it.

Keywords *insulin affordability; systemic failures; policy solutions; Medicaid expansion; uninsured patients; price caps; diabetes management; health equity*

> *Sarah, a single mother with type 1 diabetes, works two part-time jobs to make ends meet. Despite her best efforts, she often struggles to afford her monthly insulin supply. With no insurance coverage and limited access to assistance programs, Sarah is forced to ration her insulin, jeopardizing her health and well-being. She fears for her future and her ability to provide for her young daughter.*
>
> *James, a 65-year-old retiree on Medicare, recently discovered that his out-of-pocket insulin costs would be capped at $35 per month under the Inflation Reduction Act. While this news brought*

some relief, James couldn't help but think about his son, Michael, who has type 1 diabetes but is uninsured. Michael continues to struggle with the high cost of insulin, often skipping doses to make his supply last longer.

Ayana, a young African American woman, was excited to start her new job. However, she soon realized that her employer-sponsored health insurance plan had a high deductible, leaving her to pay hundreds of dollars each month for her insulin. Ayana's dreams of financial stability and career growth were overshadowed by the constant worry of affording her life-sustaining medication.

3.1 Insulin Affordability: Progress, Disparities, and the Need for Systemic Change

Recent initiatives by Medicare, some states, and drug manufacturers have led to a decrease in insulin prices for some of the estimated 8.4 million Americans who rely on the medication to survive [1]. These efforts have capped monthly costs at $35 for qualifying patients. However, not all patients are eligible for this assistance, and the level of help an individual receives depends on factors such as the specific drug, insurance coverage, deductible amount, and, in some cases, income.

Insulin remains a significant financial burden for people with diabetes in the United States. A staggering 14% of insulin users spend at least 40% of their post-subsistence income – the money available after paying for food and housing – on this life-saving medication [2]. Consequently, one in four people with diabetes has resorted to "insulin rationing" or taking the medication in ways other than prescribed to stretch their supply and reduce monthly costs [3]. Despite these hardships, insulin prices continue to rise in the United States.

From 2002 to 2013, the prices of the most popular insulin products tripled, and between 2012 and 2016, the average price paid by patients with type 1 diabetes nearly doubled [4]. Payers are also facing drastic increases, with Medicaid reimbursements for insulin products increasing at near-exponential rates from 1991 to 2014 [5]. In 2015, the second-largest expenditure of Medicare Part D was for Sanofi's top insulin product, Lantus [6].

The affordability and quality of insulin prescriptions vary significantly based on insurance, coverage type, and income [7]. While privately insured individuals make up nearly half of all insulin-using people with diabetes aged 18–64, they constitute only 4% of those who paid full price for a standardized insulin formulation with a total reimbursed cost of at least $500 [8]. Most privately insured patients incur out-of-pocket costs between 0% and 20% of the total cost of their prescriptions, with the majority paying less than $100. Medicaid patients typically face similar out-of-pocket costs. However, people with high-deductible plans, including those obtained through the Affordable Care Act (ACA) state marketplaces, could face thousands of dollars in out-of-pocket costs before reaching their deductibles.

In contrast, uninsured people and those with gaps in coverage, who represent 17% of the insulin-using population with diabetes, constituted 80% of those who paid full price for an insulin prescription with a total reimbursed cost greater than $500 at some point during a year [2]. Uninsured people also tend to use older forms of insulin, which may have increased risks and less predictability for glycemic control [9]. About 47% of prescriptions filled by uninsured patients were paid for fully out-of-pocket, while only 21% had no out-of-pocket costs [9]. This socioeconomic disparity creates a situation where people who are unemployed or employed but uninsured tend to underuse insulin.

High insulin prices disproportionately affect Native Americans, Black Americans, and Hispanic Americans due to the higher prevalence of diabetes in their communities and their lower likelihood of having insurance [10]. According to a Centers for Disease Control and Prevention (CDC) study analyzing data from 2017 and 2018, the prevalence of diagnosed diabetes was highest among American Indians/Alaska Natives (14.7%), people of Hispanic origin (12.5%), and non-Hispanic blacks (11.7%), followed by Asians (9.2%) and non-Hispanic whites (7.5%) [11]. Moreover, minority children are more likely to develop type 2 than type 1 diabetes, which has significant economic, public health, and healthcare system implications for these young individuals who develop a chronic condition at such an early age. Minorities in the United States are more likely to develop microvascular complications of diabetes and lower limb amputations, which can contribute to disability [12]. These complications are exacerbated because these communities are more likely to lack insurance and pay out-of-pocket for their healthcare costs. Nearly 20% of African Americans and 17% of Hispanics with diabetes use insulin either alone or with other medications, and poverty rates for these demographics are higher than the general population, leading to a lower likelihood of being able to access necessary care [5].

Traditionally, insulin access has been addressed mainly through assistance programs, manufacturer and pharmacy discounts, and diabetes organizations and charities, rather than policy initiatives [13]. However, these solutions perpetuate structural problems in the healthcare system and fail to address the underlying cost issues. The recent increase in public scrutiny of prescription drug prices has led insulin manufacturers and pharmacies to pledge to limit the costs that consumers pay for insulin [14]. Yet, these changes merely lead to cost-shifting elsewhere in the system and rely on private companies to adjust their own prices, rather than instituting a regulatory scheme that ensures continued access [15].

> *"Unaffordable insulin is a symptom of a system that keeps out competition, empowers drug corporations to set higher and higher prices, and has failed patients and communities. We demand sweeping and structural change that makes all medications more affordable."*
>
> Shaina Kasper, Policy & Advocacy Director of T1International

3.2　State Initiatives on Insulin Affordability: An Overview

States have taken various steps to address the issue of insulin affordability and access for their residents. While federal action has been limited, state legislatures have implemented a range of policies aimed at reducing out-of-pocket costs for insulin and ensuring that individuals with diabetes have access to this life-saving medication. These state-level initiatives include mandated insurance coverage for diabetes supplies, copay caps, patient assistance programs, and efforts to promote the use of biosimilar insulin. However, the effectiveness and reach of these policies vary, and they often face limitations due to factors such as federal preemption and the inability to address underlying price inflation. This section explores some of the key state initiatives related to insulin affordability and access, highlighting their benefits and limitations.

3.2.1 State-Mandated Diabetes Coverage: Benefits and Limitations

States can include increased coverage requirements in their essential health benefits plans for ACA marketplace plans [16]. For example, Virginia covers medical supplies, including insulin pumps and glucose monitors. Delaware requires all group and blanket health insurance policies, contracts, or certificates in the state to provide coverage for a medically necessary insulin pump at no cost to a covered individual, including deductible payments and cost-sharing amounts. Similarly, in addition to capping cost sharing at $100 a month, West Virginia has mandated coverage for blood glucose monitors, supplies, insulin, injection aids, syringes, insulin infusion devices, and other diabetes equipment and supplies in its public employee's insurance act [17].

Both of these initiatives are helpful for cutting costs once people are covered and requiring insurance companies to provide the supplies and equipment at a low cost. However, they do not reach uninsured populations. Furthermore, the populations that could access these benefits are limited: West Virginia's initiative only applies to its own state employee plans, and Delaware's does not apply to the Employee Retirement Income Security Act (ERISA) plans, which are self-funded employer-sponsored health plans that are exempt from state insurance regulations [17].

3.2.2 State Copay Caps: Limited Impact and Scope

As of 2024, approximately half of all states and Washington, DC, have instituted copay caps ranging from $35 to $100 per insulin prescription, making them the most common policy intervention at the state level [18]. While state lawmakers tout these policies, the restrictions have limited impact for several reasons.

First, copay caps remove the high sticker cost from the attention of a large bloc of voters without addressing the underlying price inflation problem. These caps only target the sticker price that insured patients see at the pharmacy, but they are unlikely to change the underlying cost of an insulin prescription. Because these caps only impact a relatively small group of patients, distributors may even shift costs by increasing prices for other patients who are not subject to copay limits to compensate for the lost profits.

Second, state-level copay caps impact a limited population of individuals who are insured through state plans. Uninsured populations that need insulin pay the full price of the prescription without any copay and will be subject to the final cost. Additionally, most insurance plans are not subject to many states' insurance laws. States only have regulatory power over state insurance plans, which include state marketplace plans. Most employee group plans are self-funded and governed by federal law (ERISA), which preempts state policies with the purpose of encouraging nationwide uniformity and predictability of plans.

3.2.3 State Insulin Safety Net Program: A Limited Solution

In 2019, Minnesota passed a law creating the "Insulin Safety Net Program," which requires insulin manufacturers to establish procedures to make insulin available to eligible individuals who are in urgent need of insulin or who are in need of access to an affordable insulin supply. This program is designed for individuals with less than a seven-day supply of insulin who need it to avoid the likelihood of suffering significant health consequences. Eligible individuals can receive a 30-day "urgent need supply of insulin" through the program once per year if they are Minnesota residents, not enrolled in medical assistance or MinnesotaCare, and not enrolled in a prescription drug coverage that limits the total amount of cost sharing that the enrollee is required to pay for a 30-day supply of insulin to $75 or less.

While this law serves as an example of a policy that states could implement to protect their un- and underinsured populations with high-cost burdens, it has limitations. The policy reflects the coupon system already prevalent in the pharmaceutical industry and does little to address the underlying costs that individual patients pay. Given the socioeconomic demographics of populations who do not qualify for Medicaid but are also not in an employer plan, it is likely that individuals who have less than a 7-day supply of insulin once will face the same situation again within a 12-month period. Moreover, waiting until a person's situation becomes urgent before providing assistance fails to create long-term structural changes that promote good health or address their ability to pay.

3.2.4   Biosimilar Insulin: Interchangeability, State Initiatives, and Challenges

Insulin is considered a biosimilar, which means it is a highly similar version of an approved biologic product. An interchangeable biosimilar is a product that a pharmacist can substitute without needing to contact the prescribing healthcare professionals. Like biosimilars, interchangeable biosimilars undergo a rigorous FDA approval process to ensure safety and effectiveness. Interchangeable biosimilar insulin may be more cost-effective for some individuals.

Most states allow biosimilar substitution when the product is FDA approved as interchangeable [19]. In California, lawmakers have allocated funding to launch a generic insulin drug label, aiming to make affordable insulin available to Californians through pharmacies, retail stores, and mail orders [19].

This policy carries high upfront costs and significant risks. Some lawmakers are skeptical that the drug could be produced at a lower cost in a smaller supply than what the three major companies currently offer [20]. However, Governor Newsom has stated that the market in California is large enough to ensure lower prices. This approach is likely not replicable at a state level for most other states due to their smaller market sizes. A similar initiative has been proposed at the federal level, but its passage is considered unlikely.

3.3   Federal Efforts and the Inflation Reduction Act for Insulin Affordability

Insulin costs have received significant attention at the federal level, though much of the dialogue neglects the impact that insulin costs have on marginalized communities. In January 2019, Congress held hearings on insulin prices with top executives from insulin companies and launched a bipartisan probe in February 2019. Several members of Congress introduced proposals to address insulin pricing specifically [21]. In late 2018, Senator Warren suggested the federal government could create its own generic manufacturing plant, with insulin put forth as one product of focus [22]. In July 2019, a group of legislators filed proposed legislation aimed at creating a "new insulin pricing model" predominantly focused on regulating insulin rebates from pharmacy benefit managers (PBMs) [22]. In February 2019, Representatives Peter Welch (D-VT) and Francis Rooney (R-FL) submitted a bill to allow the importation of affordable insulin from Canada and possibly other countries [22].

The Inflation Reduction Act, which President Biden signed in 2022, introduced significant changes to insulin pricing and affordability. The Act caps out-of-pocket insulin costs at $35 a month for Medicare enrollees, with the cap taking effect in 2023. In response to this legislation, three leading insulin manufacturers (Sanofi, Eli Lilly, and Novo Nordisk) have reduced the price of insulin to $35 through price caps or savings programs.

The Act also allows Medicare Part D to negotiate prescription drug prices. This requires the Department of Health and Human Services (HHS) to identify Medicare's 100 most expensive drugs and choose 10 for price negotiations beginning in 2023, with prices to take effect in 2026. A second provision penalizes drug companies that raise prices faster than inflation by forcing them to pay a rebate on their Medicare sales.

While the $35 insulin copay cap for Medicare patients is a good step toward making the final consumer prices of insulin more affordable, it mirrors issues in the state copay caps because it does not protect the uninsured or individuals with commercial plans. The Medicare Part D cap resembles a voluntary savings model that CMS announced and piloted beginning in 2020, which had a maximum $35 copay per 30-day supply of insulin.

Provisions in the original bills and proposed compromises that would have made some of the changes applicable to the private market were removed to ensure the legislation's passage in both chambers [23]. The Senate parliamentarian also struck down any extension to the commercial insurance market. Critics warn that failing to extend the measures to the private sector will create a situation similar to the broad healthcare system, where Medicare pays below the cost of treating patients, leading to providers charging private insurance plans more [24]. Others caution that this legislation may cause drug companies to launch new drugs at higher prices to compensate for the future negotiated prices and the inflation cap [25].

3.4 Policy Recommendations

Pass Federal Legislation Capping Copays and Expanding Price Caps to the Commercial Sector: Recent developments in insulin pricing, with Medicare, certain states, and drug manufacturers capping monthly costs at $35 for millions of Americans relying on insulin, underscore the need for broader federal legislation. The most pressing recommendation is to expand these price caps to the commercial sector. Currently, not all patients qualify for these caps, and the level of assistance varies based on factors like the specific drug, insurance coverage, deductible amount, and income. Expanding these measures would offer more comprehensive relief. While this legislation is underway, it requires careful crafting to secure bipartisan support and pass through the Senate's budget reconciliation process. Notably, many senators who opposed the initial policy in the Inflation Reduction Act represent regions with high diabetes and insulin use rates.

Expand Medicaid and Mandatory Coverage for Marketplace Plans: Expanding Medicaid coverage and mandatory coverage for marketplace plans would significantly protect people with diabetes from high out-of-pocket costs for insulin and other essential care. Medicaid provides low-income families with coverage, and states have the option to expand eligibility to adults with income at or below 133% of the federal poverty level. However, many states have not opted for this expansion. For most Medicaid recipients, prescribed insulin is covered. Expanding Medicaid eligibility would increase this coverage and subject prescriptions to CMS-negotiated rates under the Inflation Adjustment Act [26]. This expansion would further address equity issues, as many people struggling to afford insulin lack insurance or have high-deductible plans [27]. By expanding Medicaid, individuals who fall into the gap between current low-income eligibility and more expensive coverage would gain reliable access to necessary care.

Improve Competition in the Insulin Market: Congress should encourage competition in the insulin market through two primary strategies: (i) promoting the development of generic or biosimilar insulins to increase supply and consumer choice and (ii) allowing reciprocal approval of insulin products from other countries. Congress should support the development of generic or biosimilar insulins [28]. A law passed on March 23, 2020, allowed insulin to be regulated by the FDA as biologics, paving the way for biosimilar insulins to be approved. This would enable companies to develop biosimilar versions of current insulins. A generic insulin is expected to enter the market in 2024. However, so far, no generic or biosimilar insulins have been approved in the United States, except for the authorized generics fast-tracked by brand-name manufacturers. While patents for insulin compounds are nearing expiration, patents on delivery devices like pens and pumps remain, delaying competition [29]. Also, Congress should permit the reciprocal approval of insulin products used in other countries. Currently, only three companies – Novo Nordisk, Sanofi, and Eli Lilly – supply insulin in the United States, although there are about 34 insulin manufacturers globally. These manufacturers represent only about 10% of the global market and none supply insulin to the United States. Increased competition could compel the existing manufacturers to lower prices or introduce their own generic versions.

Key Policy Interventions and Equity Considerations for Insulin Affordability

Policy Intervention	Barrier Addressed	Details
Copay Caps	High out-of-pocket costs	State-level and Medicare Part D/B cap insulin costs at $35 monthly. Limited to insured patients, not addressing uninsured individuals. Costs may shift to insurance premiums.
PBM Rebate Transparency	Hidden, negotiated rebates	Legislation in several states and proposed federal laws to increase transparency in PBM practices. Aims to uncover rebate systems that incentivize list price increases.
Drug Manufacturer Rebates	Rising prices beyond inflation rates	Inflation Reduction Act mandates rebates for price hikes beyond inflation for Medicare. Medicaid cap removal on rebates could lead manufacturers to pay Medicaid to use their drugs.
Drug Pricing Negotiation	High list prices	Inflation Reduction Act allows Medicare to negotiate prices for select drugs, including some insulins. Does not address high launch prices of new medications.
Public Production	High list prices, lack of competition	California's CalRx program aims to produce generic insulin at reduced prices. Public manufacturing bill proposed to create an Office of Drug Manufacturing for select generics to increase competition and ensure access.
Reducing Barriers to Competition	Anticompetitive practices, delayed biosimilar entry	Proposed bills like the Affordable Prescriptions for Patients Act and the Biosimilar Red Tape Elimination Act to curb product hopping and simplify biosimilar interchangeability to encourage competition and lower prices.
List Price Caps	High list prices	Proposed Insulin for All Act to cap insulin at $20 per 1000 units. Broader proposals like the Elijah E. Cummings Lower Drug Costs Now Act aimed at setting drug prices using international reference standards.

3.5 Conclusion: Addressing Systematic Failures for Equitable Insulin Access

Recent developments in insulin pricing have brought some relief to many Americans who rely on this life-saving medication. Medicare, some states, and drug manufacturers have moved to cap monthly insulin costs at $35. However, not all patients qualify for this assistance, and the level of help an individual receives depends on various factors. While the vast majority of people qualify for some assistance, the current interventions fail to address the systematic failures in the healthcare system that have led to dramatic price increases, making insulin inaccessible to many patients.

Insulin serves as a stark example of the numerous systematic failures in the healthcare system that have resulted in dramatic price increases, rendering life-saving drugs inaccessible to patients. Although current interventions ensure access for some, they neglect the un- and underinsured individuals, as well as those with high-cost sharing burdens. Ultimately, capping drug prices and other proposed policy solutions to address the high insulin cost merely mirror other pricing issues in our healthcare system. To truly address equity problems and ensure access to consistent care, more systematic level interventions are needed.

Future interventions should focus on prevention and target areas of social determinants of health that improve population-level diabetes treatment for underserved and minority populations [30]. By addressing the root causes of health disparities and implementing comprehensive policies that extend beyond short-term price caps, we can work toward a more equitable healthcare system that ensures access to affordable, life-saving medications like insulin for all who need them [31].

References

1 CDC (2020). National Diabetes Statistics Report. Atlanta, GA: Centers for Disease Control and Prevention, U.S. Dept of Health and Human Services.

2 Herkert, D., Vijayakumar, P., Luo, J. et al. (2019). Cost-related insulin underuse among patients with diabetes. *JAMA Internal Medicine* 179 (1): 112–114.

3 Gucciardi, E., Vahabi, M., Norris, N. et al. (2014). The intersection between food insecurity and diabetes: a review. *Current Nutrition Reports* 3 (4): 324–332.

4 Hua, X., Carvalho, N., Tew, M. et al. (2016). Expenditures and prices of antihyperglycemic medications in the United States: 2002-2013. *JAMA* 315 (13): 1400–1402.

5 Luo, J., Avorn, J., and Kesselheim, A.S. (2015). Trends in Medicaid reimbursements for insulin from 1991 through 2014. *JAMA Internal Medicine* 175 (10): 1681–1686. https://doi.org/10.1001/jamainternmed. 2015.4338.

6 Cubanski, J., Neuman, T., True, S., and Damico, A. (2019). *How Much Does Medicare Spend on Insulin?* Kaiser Family Foundation https://files.kff.org/attachment/Data-Note-How-Much-Does-Medicare-Spend-on-Insulin.

7 Myerson, R., Lu, T., Tonnu-Mihara, I., and Huang, E.S. (2019). Medicaid eligibility expansions may address gaps in access to diabetes medications. *Health Affairs* 38 (8): 1200–1207.

8 Cefalu, W.T., Dawes, D.E., Gavlak, G. et al. (2018). Insulin access and affordability working group: conclusions and recommendations. *Diabetes Care* 41 (6): 1299–1311.

9 Glied, S.A. and Zhu, B. (2020). *Not So Sweet: Insulin Affordability Over Time*. The Commonwealth Fund https://www.commonwealthfund.org/publications/issue-briefs/2020/sep/not-so-sweet-insulin-affordability-over-time.

10 Spanakis, E.K. and Golden, S.H. (2013). Race/ethnic difference in diabetes and diabetic complications. *Current Diabetes Reports* 13 (6): 814–823.

11 Centers for Disease Control and Prevention. (2020). *National Diabetes Statistics Report 2020: Estimates of Diabetes and Its Burden in the United States*. U.S. Department of Health and Human Services. https://diabetesresearch.org/wp-content/uploads/2022/05/national-diabetes-statistics-report-2020.pdf.

12 Peek, M.E., Cargill, A., and Huang, E.S. (2007). Diabetes health disparities: a systematic review of health care interventions. *Medical Care Research and Review* 64 (5_suppl): 101S–156S.

13 Beran, D., Hirsch, I.B., and Yudkin, J.S. (2018). Why are we failing to address the issue of access to insulin? A national and global perspective. *Diabetes Care* 41 (6): 1125–1131.

14 Rajkumar, S.V. (2020). The high cost of insulin in the United States: an urgent call to action. *Mayo Clinic Proceedings* 95 (1): 22–28.

15 Chua, K.P., Lee, J.M., and Conti, R.M. (2020). Potential change in insulin out-of-pocket spending under cost-sharing caps among pediatric patients with type 1 diabetes. *JAMA Pediatrics* 174 (5): 410–418.

16 Fung, V., Graetz, I., Galbraith, A. et al. (2014). Financial barriers to care among low-income children with asthma: health care reform implications. *JAMA Pediatrics* 168 (7): 649–656.

17 National Conference of State Legislatures (2023). *Diabetes State Mandates and Insulin Copayment Caps*. NCSL https://www.ncsl.org/health/diabetes-state-mandates-and-insulin-copayment-caps.

18 Chua, K.P., Lee, J.M., and Conti, R.M. (2021). Prevalence of state-level insulin copayment caps and effect on out-of-pocket spending among patients with private insurance coverage. *JAMA Network Open* 4 (4): e218304–e218304.

19 Humphreys, S. (2023). Understanding interchangeable biosimilars at the federal and state levels. *The American Journal of Managed Care* 29 (7 Spec): SP545–SP548.

20 Rome, B.N. and Kesselheim, A.S. (2020). Transferrable market exclusivity extensions to promote antibiotic development: an economic analysis. *Clinical Infectious Diseases* 71 (7): 1671–1675.

21 Cefalu, W.T. and Lipska, K.J. (2019). The rising cost of insulin in the United States: an urgent call to action. *Diabetes Care* 42 (4): 564–566.

22 Knox, R. (2020). Insulin insulated: barriers to competition and affordability in the United States insulin market. *Journal of Law and the Biosciences* 7 (1): lsaa061. https://doi.org/10.1093/jlb/lsaa061.

23 Chua, K.P. and Conti, R.M. (2019). Policy implications of the Affordable Care Act's coverage expansion for insulin. *JAMA Internal Medicine* 179 (3): 429–430.

24 Kesselheim, A.S., Avorn, J., and Sarpatwari, A. (2016). The high cost of prescription drugs in the United States: origins and prospects for reform. *JAMA* 316 (8): 858–871.

25 Gellad, W.F., Schneeweiss, S., Brawarsky, P. et al. (2008). What if the federal government negotiated pharmaceutical prices for seniors? An estimate of national savings. *Journal of General Internal Medicine* 23 (9): 1435–1440.

26 Sommers, B.D., Maylone, B., Blendon, R.J. et al. (2017). Three-year impacts of the Affordable Care Act: improved medical care and health among low-income adults. *Health Affairs* 36 (6): 1119–1128.

27 Galvani, A.P., Parpia, A.S., Pandey, A. et al. (2020). The imperative for universal healthcare to curtail the COVID-19 outbreak in the USA. *eClinicalMedicine* 23: 100380.

28 Luo, J., Kesselheim, A.S., and Sarpatwari, A. (2020). Insulin access and affordability in the USA: anticipating the first interchangeable insulin product. *The Lancet Diabetes & Endocrinology* 8 (5): 360–362.

29 Beall, R.F., Nickerson, J.W., Kaplan, W.A., and Attaran, A. (2016). Is patent "evergreening" restricting access to medicine/device combination products? *PLoS One* 11 (2): e0148939.

30 Hill-Briggs, F., Adler, N.E., Berkowitz, S.A. et al. (2020). Social determinants of health and diabetes: a scientific review. *Diabetes Care* 44 (1): 258–279.

31 Wilkinson, R.G. and Pickett, K.E. (2006). Income inequality and population health: a review and explanation of the evidence. *Social Science & Medicine* 62 (7): 1768–1784.

4

Ensuring Equitable Healthcare: Overcoming Language Barriers Through Policies

Abstract

Language barriers in healthcare are an important issue in the pursuit of health equity. The COVID-19 pandemic placed this challenge front and center. For many Americans, the ever-changing landscape of COVID-19, marked by evolving expert understanding, healthcare measures, and shifting policies, had proven challenging to follow and comprehend. As the grasp of the virus, its variants, and effective preventive strategies such as masking, social distancing, testing, and vaccination progressed, so too had the guidelines, often resulting in widespread confusion. This predicament became even more grave for individuals with limited English proficiency, exacerbating the existing disparities in healthcare access and quality due to language barriers. Language constraints pose significant hurdles in navigating the healthcare system. Non-English speakers often struggle to access critical information and services in the United States, while healthcare providers may find it difficult to communicate effectively when interpretation services are inadequate. In situations where conveying symptoms and treatment plans accurately can be a matter of life or death, these barriers become even more impactful. This chapter delves into the legal aspects of language access within healthcare settings. It portrays the challenges encountered by those with limited English proficiency within the healthcare system, and provides an overview of the federal and state laws regulating language access and language discrimination. Further, it discusses the recent advancements and practical hurdles in implementing changes to language access in healthcare environments. Finally, it proposes long- and short-term solutions to enhance language access, thereby bridging the existing healthcare gap.

Keywords *language barriers; health equity; interpretation services; limited English proficiency (LEP); federal laws; Affordable Care Act (ACA); cultural competency; healthcare access*

> *Maria, a Hispanic woman in her late 40s, rushed her asthmatic son to the emergency room. As her son struggled to breathe, Maria felt helpless, unable to clearly explain the severity of her son's condition. The hospital didn't have a Spanish interpreter readily available. Maria's distress multiplied as she saw her son's condition worsen while she scrambled to make herself understood.*

> *Dr. Lee, a Korean-American surgeon in California, often found himself acting as an impromptu translator for his Korean patients. He saw firsthand how language barriers could hamper the delivery of care. He remembers an elderly patient, Mrs. Kim, who almost underwent an unnecessary procedure due to a simple linguistic misunderstanding.*
>
> *Sofia, a 10-year-old, often found herself translating medical jargon for her Romanian grandparents. She vividly recalls the anxiety of translating her grandmother's cancer diagnosis, fearing she'd get something wrong.*

4.1 Challenges and Implications of Language Barriers in Healthcare

In the United States, over 25 million individuals grapple with limited English proficiency, spanning across more than 350 languages [1–3]. Unfortunately, the existing number of bi- or multilingual healthcare providers falls short of meeting these diverse linguistic needs. Not only are there cost constraints and resource scarcity in providing these types of services (i.e. interpreters), but a lack of diversity in the medical profession has left bi-lingual providers with disproportionate work loads in providing care [4]. However, seamless communication between patients and providers is paramount for successful health outcomes [5].

There is much that is taken for granted when addressing patients with limited English proficiency. Language barriers can hinder one's ability to obtain, process, and understand health information, from booking appointments to comprehending treatment options for informed consent [6]. Research indicates a substantial link between disparities in health status, access to healthcare, and delivery of health services with race, ethnicity, and primary language. Effective communication with patients in their preferred language can dramatically enhance healthcare quality and outcomes. In contrast, language barriers can breed miscommunications and misunderstandings, potentially deterring patients with limited English proficiency from seeking timely medical attention and preventive care. Misunderstandings due to language discrepancies can breed distrust in the healthcare system and reduced rapport between the patient and healthcare provider, particularly when each party assumes the other should overcome language barriers [7].

Additionally, when there is a deficit of language access services, many institutions utilize makeshift services. Families and friends are usually utilized asked to fill in this gap, even though experts generally discourage this approach due to the high risk of misinterpretation of critical healthcare information. Furthermore, enlisting minor children to translate for family members not only incurs the same risk of misinterpretation, but also can place an undue emotional burden on them. Cultural differences, including nonverbal communication, tone, and social cues, can further complicate communication and impact the quality of healthcare [8]. Providers unfamiliar with these differences might inadvertently offend, confuse, or discomfort patients. As a consequence, patients with limited English proficiency are less likely to establish a regular source of medical care, access preventive services, and adhere to medication regimens [9]. Language barriers obstruct patients from fully understanding their diagnoses, treatment plans, and the necessary follow-up care. Implementing interpretation services and other language access initiatives can improve patient access to preventive and primary care. Healthcare institutions can collaborate with certified language service providers or employ in-house interpreters to ensure real-time communication assistance. Furthermore, leveraging digital platforms for translation and interpretation can provide instantaneous support, especially in emergency situations or for less commonly spoken languages.

4.2 Federal Laws Addressing Language Needs in Healthcare

Experts have continually pushed for improvements in language access to rectify disparities in healthcare quality affecting certain populations, an issue that has become even more pertinent amidst recent public health emergencies. Despite existing laws to improve language access in healthcare settings, enforcement remains inadequate and resources for providers to comply with the law are often lacking [10].

4.2.1 Federal Authority and Related Standards and Guidance

Key among federal legislation in this area is Title VI of the 1964 Civil Rights Act [11]. This law prevents any healthcare program, activity, or institution receiving federal financial assistance from discriminating based on national origin. An additional authority underpinning these rights are Section 504 of the Rehabilitation Act of 1973 and the Americans with Disabilities Act of 1990 [12]. This ensures individuals with limited English proficiency have comparable language access to English speakers in various settings, including employment, public accommodations, and healthcare [13]. But unfortunately, the reality often falls short.

> *"No person in the United States shall, on the ground of race, color, or national origin, be excluded from participation in, be denied the benefits of, or be subjected to discrimination under any program or activity receiving Federal financial assistance."*
>
> Title VI of the Civil Rights Act of 1964

Beyond Title VI, other federal initiatives aim to address language barriers in healthcare [14]. Notably, President Clinton's Executive Order 13166, "Improving Access to Services for Persons with Limited English Proficiency," and the subsequent Department of Health and Human Services (HHS) guidance issued in August 2000 aim to aid healthcare providers in their obligation to reduce language barriers [15]. Following this, the federal government established the National Standards for Culturally and Linguistically Appropriate Services, featuring four standards specifically addressing language access [16]. These standards mandate cost-free language assistance services, the provision of notices informing patients of their right to such services, the assurance of language assistance competency, and the availability of easily comprehensible patient-related materials and signage.

While these standards serve as valuable guidelines, they are not legally binding and are primarily used by organizations as a template to meet legal requirements. The early 2000s saw the Bush administration uphold and modify the policies outlined in Executive Order 13166, providing four criteria to assess the type and extent of language assistance required by providers. The federal government has the power to investigate complaints, ensure compliance, and withhold federal funds from noncompliant organizations under Title VI of the Civil Rights Act of 1964. And yet healthcare providers often find challenges in consistently ensuring the provision of adequate language assistance as required under Title VI. Accountability for language access is also highly dependent on individual litigation and enforcement – which can be daunting for individuals who lack English proficiency [17]. This results in patients with limited English proficiency often being unaware of their rights or how to access services.

The Department of Justice provided additional resources to help organizations meet federal language accessibility requirements [18]. However, despite these resources, many providers fail to comply with federal law. This is often attributed to a lack of awareness about their obligation to provide language access, compounded by the scarcity of resources allocated to address language barriers.

4.2.2 The Affordable Care Act

The Affordable Care Act (ACA), while predominantly known for addressing healthcare coverage, has also been instrumental in improving language access in healthcare settings [19]. The ACA expands the civil rights protections outlined in Title VI to encompass any health program or activity receiving federal financial assistance, executive agency-administered programs, and state exchanges.

One of the critical requirements of the ACA is that group health plans and health insurance providers furnish a summary of benefits and coverage, alongside notices about available internal and external appeals processes, in a "culturally and linguistically appropriate manner" [20]. This requirement underscores the importance of delivering information in a language that the intended audience can understand easily.

Furthermore, the ACA includes provisions for funding and reimbursement plans that incentivize activities aimed at reducing healthcare disparities, including language services. Other components of the law mandate the federal government to formulate standards for collecting language data for quality measurement purposes. These incentives and standards catalyze improvements to language access in both the short and long term.

In 2020, a new final rule introduced modifications to ACA regulations. Section 1557 of the ACA, which prohibits discrimination based on race, color, national origin, sex, age, or disability in health programs and activities, underwent changes [21].

The changes introduced in 2020 were motivated by a desire to reduce administrative and fiscal burdens on healthcare providers and to align with statutory mandates. The proponents of the changes argued that the earlier requirements were too onerous for providers and that some of the mandates exceeded the scope of the original legislation.

The previous implementation rule mandated covered entities to issue a notice of nondiscrimination, outlining how an individual can file a complaint in case of discrimination, and details about the availability of nondiscrimination assistance services.

While the 2020 rule still compels covered practices to "take reasonable steps to provide meaningful access to each individual with limited English proficiency," it has removed the requirement to post these taglines in the top 15 non-English languages spoken by limited English proficiency individuals in the region where the entity operates.

Moreover, the 2020 rule repealed the obligations for grievance procedures, such as designating a compliance coordinator and setting up grievance procedures for prompt and fair resolution of complaints.

Although this modification eases some of the burden on providers trying to adhere to federal law, it could potentially exacerbate language barriers for patients with limited English proficiency.

It is important to critically evaluate these changes to understand their impact on language accessibility. The removal of certain requirements might ease administrative pressures, but it raises concerns regarding the potential dilution of language access services and the resultant impact on healthcare equity.

4.2.3 Additional Federal Laws and Funding

Apart from the key federal laws discussed earlier, language access is further supported through other legal underpinnings, legislative instruments, and funding mechanisms. For example, legal theories of informed consent greatly inform rights to language services. Patients can only make informed medical decisions if they can understand them. Given this right, language access becomes required by legal duty [22]. Another example is of the Hill-Burton Act, providing funds to hospitals, explicitly prohibiting these hospitals from discriminatory practices in service delivery [23]. To facilitate language access, the Act necessitates that hospitals display notices in English, Spanish, and any other language spoken by at least 10% of the households in the service area.

Furthermore, the federal government leverages additional funding mechanisms to provide matching funds to states [24]. These funds cater to services rendered to Medicaid and CHP+ enrollees and can be deployed to cover administrative costs such as reimbursements for language services. In addition, other federal laws, such as the Americans with Disabilities Act (ADA), may indirectly influence language accessibility, especially when the effective execution of the law's provisions hinges on clear communication with patients who have limited English proficiency. However, it's crucial to acknowledge that while these federal laws bolster language access, many of these funding programs are optional. For instance, the State Plan Home and Community-based Services (HCBS) 1915(i) program is one such optional Medicaid benefit that states can choose to provide or not. Moreover, enforcement of other anti-discrimination stipulations is often inadequate. The existing laws and standards lay a robust foundation for language access, but for meaningful impact, providers need to be informed of their responsibilities, encouraged to utilize available funding opportunities, and held accountable for adherence to anti-discrimination laws.

4.3 State Initiatives

While all states must comply with federal laws on language access, they can also introduce supplementary measures to bolster these federal laws [25]. Every state, including the District of Columbia, has implemented measures to address language barriers in healthcare settings. These measures span mandatory continuing education for health professionals, certification for healthcare interpreters, and reimbursement for language services for Medicaid/SCHIP enrollees. In fact, each state has at least three laws pertaining to language access.

Some states have enacted laws mandating language assistance services or necessitating such services as a licensure condition for providers and facilities. Such laws aim to foster adherence to language accessibility requirements. Additionally, certain states require health professionals to undertake continuing education that includes training on language access and cultural competency, thus heightening awareness and potentially boosting the provision of language services. Several states have enacted laws addressing language services for specific populations, such as women, children, and people with disabilities. These laws stipulate appropriate language accessibility services, ensuring that patients understand essential information about their care and treatment.

The scope of language accessibility laws varies significantly across states. However, despite these strides, only a handful of states have introduced comprehensive cultural and linguistic requirements. California stands out with the broadest and most comprehensive language accessibility laws, boasting 257 distinct laws. These laws impose linguistic requirements for diverse services, mandate multilingual notices in healthcare settings, require private insurance providers to provide language assistance services, and much more.

However, despite these additional protections provided by state laws, states grapple with similar challenges as the federal government. These include lack of funding, difficulties recruiting interpreters, and a knowledge gap regarding existing laws and patient rights. These challenges can hamper providers' ability to enhance the quality of care for patients with limited English proficiency. In the absence of federal standards for interpreter competency, some states regulate and require certification for interpreters. This regulation is a double-edged sword; although it aims to mitigate risks associated with incorrect information and patient confidentiality, it could exacerbate the existing shortage of interpreters by creating an additional barrier to service provision.

4.4   Recent Developments and Practical Challenges

It is widely accepted among experts that prioritizing competent language services is critical for ensuring equal quality of care across patients, irrespective of their language proficiency [26]. By assessing existing services and committing resources to their enhancement, healthcare providers can not only comply with federal law but also address health disparities faced by individuals with limited English proficiency. Recent advancements in language accessibility in healthcare, spurred by the COVID-19 pandemic, have highlighted practical challenges that require attention [27].

The onset of the COVID-19 pandemic exacerbated language access issues in healthcare, hampering individuals with limited English proficiency from obtaining vital information about vaccines, treatments, and testing [28]. Additionally, the pandemic-induced transition to telemedicine exposed the inadequacy of current technologies in providing video and audio interpreting services, thereby compounding language accessibility problems. This lack of preparedness rendered individuals with limited English proficiency particularly vulnerable to the virus.

Long-term solutions proposed by experts, such as translations, multi-language notices, oral assistance (interpreters), outreach, education, and data analysis, were difficult to implement swiftly during the pandemic. Additionally, recommendations to enhance future physicians' multilingual abilities and provide training on best practices for treating patients with limited English proficiency, although valuable, offer limited immediate relief.

In 2021, the Language Access for Medicare Beneficiaries Act was introduced into the House of Representatives, aimed at enhancing language access at community health centers and for Medicare

Beneficiaries were proposed. This legislation planned to provide grants to these centers to recruit and hire professionals fluent in non-English languages. However, as of now, no COVID-era federal legislation regarding language access has been passed.

Addressing language access barriers requires time, resources, and prioritization. Organizations are advised to conduct a needs analysis to identify weaknesses in their current approaches to oral and written language needs. Following this, they can channel resources to improve language accessibility, develop and disseminate language access policies, hold staff accountable for implementation, and provide regular training. Periodic policy reviews are also recommended to ensure ongoing compliance with accessibility standards.

However, the cost of providing language access services can be prohibitive, and it's often challenging to find staff with the requisite language competency. Numerous hospitals report difficulties in meeting federal requirements for language access, pointing to a need for a long-term strategy involving thorough assessment, training, and recruitment to effectively address these issues [29].

4.5 Conclusion: Charting a Path to Linguistically Inclusive Healthcare

Addressing language accessibility is crucial in ensuring equitable healthcare, although it is often seen as a costly endeavor. Limited funding can obstruct efforts to bridge language gaps, thereby compromising the quality of care among distinct linguistic groups. Nevertheless, the urgency to surmount these barriers is paramount and demands a multi-faceted approach involving various stakeholders.

Healthcare systems confront an array of challenges in enhancing language accessibility. These include the assessment of existing services, strategic allocation of resources, recruitment of proficient staff, and rigorous training on policies pertaining to limited English proficiency assistance. Overcoming these challenges necessitates a thorough reassessment and an overhaul of the present systems, which is undoubtedly a time-consuming process.

To provide more clarity on the actionable steps and the entities responsible for implementing them, it is vital to identify strategies at federal, state, local, and organizational levels. Federal agencies can initiate nationwide policies to standardize language accessibility across states. They can allocate specific funds for language services and encourage research and development of cost-effective language assistance tools. State and local governments should identify the unique linguistic needs of their communities. Tailored policies can be enacted to ensure that healthcare providers in the region are equipped with the necessary resources and training to meet these needs. Regular audits can be conducted to ensure compliance and efficacy of language assistance programs. On an organizational level, healthcare providers need to act swiftly and strategically. Immediate steps, such as displaying notices in multiple languages and recruiting interpreters or bilingual staff, can provide short-term relief. Simultaneously, healthcare institutions should conduct comprehensive assessments to understand their specific language service requirements better. Private stakeholders, including NGOs and community organizations, can collaborate to augment language services through funding, advocacy, and community outreach.

In essence, a synergistic effort involving stakeholders at various levels is essential. While immediate measures can alleviate existing disparities, a long-term and sustained approach is required for holistic improvement. By leveraging funding opportunities and strategically deploying resources, federal, state, and local authorities, along with private entities, can work cohesively to champion language accessibility. This cohesive approach will ensure the delivery of equitable healthcare services across linguistic communities.

Key Policy Areas and Equity Considerations for Language Access in Health Care

Category	Policy Area	Details
Federal Legal Requirements	Title VI of the 1964 Civil Rights Act	Prohibits discrimination based on national origin in programs receiving federal financial assistance, requiring health organizations to provide language services to LEP individuals.
	Executive Order 13166	Issued in 2000 to improve access for LEP individuals, supported by HHS guidance for health care providers.
	ACA Section 1557	Extends civil rights protections to health programs receiving federal financial assistance.
Language Access Standards	ACA Section 1001	Mandates culturally and linguistically appropriate communication of benefits and appeals.
	National CLAS Standards	Standards 4–7 require health organizations to provide language assistance services, inform patients of their rights, ensure interpreter competence, and make patient materials accessible.
Financial Assistance and Incentives	Federal Matching Funds	States can receive a 50% federal match for Medicaid language services, including written translation and interpretation.
	Incentives for Bilingual Professionals	Financial assistance for providers offering language services and incentives for bilingual individuals to enter health professions.
State-Level Policies	Colorado Laws	Colo. Rev. Stat. 10-16-704(9)(e) requires managed care plans to address LEP needs. Colo. Rev. Stat. 12-38.1-202(2)(b) promotes outreach to non-English speakers in health professions.
Patient Support	ACA Patient Navigators	Authorized to guide patients through health care systems, providing culturally and linguistically appropriate information.
Data Collection and Analysis	ACA Section 4302	Requires standards for collecting and analyzing language data to monitor health disparities, aiding in the development of targeted health policies.

References

1 Flores, G. (2006). Language barriers to health care in the United States. *The New England Journal of Medicine* 355 (3): 229–231.

2 Chang, P.H. and Fortier, J.P. (1998). Language barriers to health care: an overview. *Journal of Health Care for the Poor and Underserved* 9 (Supplement): S5–S20. Johns Hopkins University Press. https://doi.org/10.1353/hpu.2010.0706.

3 Das, L.T., Kutscher, E.J., and Gonzalez, C.J. (2020). Addressing barriers to care for patients with limited English proficiency during the COVID-19 pandemic. *Health Affairs Blog* https://doi.org/10.1377/hblog20200724.76821.

4 Li, C., Son, N., Abdulkerim, A. et al. (2017). Overcoming communication barriers to healthcare for culturally and linguistically diverse patients. *NAJ Medical Sciences* 10 (3): 103–109. Steinberg, E.M. et al. (2016). The "Battle" of managing language barriers in health care. *Clinical Pediatrics (Phila.)* 55:1318.

5 Meuter, R.F., Gallois, C., Segalowitz, N.S. et al. (2015). Overcoming language barriers in healthcare: a protocol for investigating safe and effective communication when patients or clinicians use a second language. *BMC Health Services Research* 15: 371.

6 Schenker, Y., Wang, F., Selig, S.J. et al. (2007). The impact of language barriers on documentation of informed consent at a hospital with on-site interpreter services. *Journal of General Internal Medicine* 22 (Suppl 2): 294–299.

7 Alpers, L.M. (2018). Distrust and patients in intercultural healthcare: a qualitative interview study. *Nursing Ethics* 25 (3): 313–323.

8 Schyve, P.M. (2007). Language differences as a barrier to quality and safety in health care: the joint commission perspective. *Journal of General Internal Medicine* 22 (Suppl 2): 360–361.

9 Shi, L., Lebrun, L.A., and Tsai, J. (2009). The influence of English proficiency on access to care. *Ethnicity & Health* 14 (6): 625–642.

10 Youdelman, M.K. (2008). The medical tongue: U.S. laws and policies on language access. *Health Affairs (Project Hope)* 27 (2): 424–433.

11 Chen, A.H., Youdelman, M.K., and Brooks, J. (2007). The legal framework for language access in healthcare settings: title VI and beyond. *Journal of General Internal Medicine* 22 (Suppl 2): 362–367.

12 Teitelbaum, J., Cartwright-Smith, L., and Rosenbaum, S. (2012). Translating rights into access: language access and the Affordable Care Act. *American Journal of Law & Medicine* 38: 348.

13 Gonzales Rose, J. (2014). Race inequity fifty years later: language rights under the civil rights act of 1964. *Alabama Civil Rights and Civil Liberties Law Review* 6: 167.

14 Snowden, L.R., Masland, M., and Guerrero, R. (2007). Federal civil rights policy and mental health treatment access for persons with limited English proficiency. *The American Psychologist* 62 (2): 109–117.

15 Executive Order No. 13166 (2000). Improving access to services for persons with limited English proficiency. *Federal Register* (11 August).

16 Estrada, R.D. and Messias, D.K. (2015). A scoping review of the literature: content, focus, conceptualization and application of the National Standards for culturally and linguistically appropriate services in health care. *Journal of Health Care for the Poor and Underserved* 26 (4): 1089–1109.

17 Teitelbaum, J., Cartwright-Smith, L., and Rosenbaum, S. (2012). Translating rights into access: language access and the Affordable Care Act. *American Journal of Law & Medicine* 38: 348.

18 Department of Justice (2023). Language access plan. https://www.justice.gov/atj/department-justice-language-access-plan (accessed 4 September 2024).

19 Applebaum, B. and Robbins, S. (2016). Language access and health equity: changes under the affordable care act. *Journal of Health Care for the Poor and Underserved* 27 (2): 416–426.

20 Lu, T. and Myerson, R. (2020). Disparities in health insurance coverage and access to care by English language proficiency in the USA, 2006-2016. *Journal of General Internal Medicine* 35 (5): 1490–1497.

21 Office for Civil Rights (2010). Section 1557 of the Patient Protection and Affordable Care Act. 42 U.S.C. § 18116.

22 Teitelbaum, J., Cartwright-Smith, L., and Rosenbaum, S., Canterbury v. Spence, 464 F.2d 772 (D.C. Cir. 1972).

23 Largent, E.A. (2018). Public health, racism, and the lasting impact of hospital segregation. *Public Health Reports (Washington, D.C.: 1974)* 133 (6): 715–720.

24 Youdelman, M. (2007). *Medicaid and SCHIP Reimbursement Models for Language Services.* National Health Law Program https://healthlaw.org/wp-content/uploads/2017/02/Medicaid-CHIP-LEP-models-FINAL.pdf.

25 Youdelman, M. (2019). *Summary of State Law Requirements Addressing Language Needs in Health Care.* National Health Law Program https://healthlaw.org/wp-content/uploads/2019/04/Language-Access-NHeLP-50StateSurvey.pdf.

26 Yang, C., Prokop, L., and Barwise, A. (2023). Strategies used by healthcare systems to communicate with hospitalized patients and families with limited English proficiency during the COVID-19 pandemic: a narrative review. *Journal of Immigrant and Minority Health* 1–9. Advance online publication. https://doi.org/10.1007/s10903-023-01453-w.

27 Ortega, P., Martínez, G., and Diamond, L. (2020). Language and health equity during COVID-19: lessons and opportunities. *Journal of Health Care for the Poor and Underserved* 31 (4): 1530–1535.

28 Knuesel, S., Chuang, W., Olson, E., and Betancourt, J. (2021). Language barriers, equity, and COVID-19: the impact of a novel Spanish language care group. *Journal of Hospital Medicine* 16 (2): 109–111.

29 Squires, A. (2018). Strategies for overcoming language barriers in healthcare. *Nursing Management* 49 (4): 20–27.

5

Confronting the US Maternal Mortality Crisis: Addressing Racial Disparities

Abstract

This chapter focuses on the persistent racial disparities that intensify the maternal mortality crisis in the United States, particularly affecting Black women. It examines the underlying causes linked to systemic racism and socioeconomic factors that lead to significantly higher risks of mortality and morbidity for Black mothers compared to their white counterparts. The analysis extends to the inefficiencies within healthcare access and quality, exacerbated by structural inequities and racial bias in medical treatment. The chapter further delves into the legislative and policy frameworks that have been introduced to mitigate these disparities. It discusses the role of federal initiatives aimed at enhancing maternity care and reducing preventable deaths through funding, education, and the implementation of evidence-based practices. State-level responses, particularly the expansion of Medicaid and the establishment of Maternal Mortality Review Committees, are highlighted as critical measures to improve maternal health outcomes. Moreover, the chapter underscores the importance of community-based interventions and the need for comprehensive, culturally sensitive approaches that address both medical and social determinants of health. It concludes with recommendations for future policies and practices that prioritize equity and access to quality healthcare, aiming to create a more inclusive and effective maternal healthcare system.

Keywords   *maternal mortality; racial disparities; systemic racism; Medicaid expansion; healthcare access; federal initiatives; community-based interventions; social determinants of health*

> *Jasmine, a 28-year-old Black woman, was excited to welcome her first child. Despite having a college degree and a stable income, Jasmine faced numerous hurdles in accessing quality prenatal care. Her concerns were often dismissed by healthcare providers, and she felt her pain was not taken seriously. Tragically, Jasmine died from preventable complications shortly after giving birth, leaving behind a devastated family and a motherless child.*
>
> *Samantha, a Native American woman living in a rural area, was determined to have a healthy pregnancy. However, limited access to transportation and the lack of nearby obstetric services*

Achieving Health Equity: The Role of Law and Policy, First Edition. Y. Tony Yang.
© 2025 John Wiley & Sons Ltd. Published 2025 by John Wiley & Sons Ltd.

> *made it difficult for her to attend regular prenatal checkups. When complications arose during her pregnancy, Samantha struggled to find the specialized care she needed, putting both her life and her baby's life at risk.*
>
> *Emily, a white woman from a low-income background, knew something was wrong when she experienced severe abdominal pain and bleeding during her second trimester. Despite her concerns, her doctor assured her that everything was fine and sent her home without further investigation. It wasn't until Emily advocated for herself and sought a second opinion that she received the life-saving treatment she needed, narrowly escaping becoming another maternal mortality statistic.*

5.1   Racial Disparities Fuel US Maternal Mortality Crisis

The United States faces a dire maternal mortality crisis, with rates more than double those of similarly developed countries like Canada, France, and Sweden. Despite being a highly developed nation, the United States ranks 33rd out of 35 countries in the Organization for Economic Cooperation and Development, with 17.4 maternal deaths per 100,000 births in 2018 [1]. Between 700 and 900 American women die annually due to pregnancy-related complications, a figure that has risen over the past two decades [2]. The COVID-19 pandemic further exacerbated these issues, contributing to 25% of all maternal deaths in 2020 and 2021, and disproportionately affecting women of color by limiting access to transportation and childcare [3].

The root cause of the US's high maternal mortality rate lies in the stark maternal and infant health inequalities that persist along racial lines. Black women face a three to four times higher risk of dying in childbirth or during the immediate post-partum period compared to white women,[1] while Black infants have a mortality rate 2.4 times higher than white infants [4]. Shockingly, this racial disparity persists even as socioeconomic status and education levels increase, with high-income Black women facing a higher likelihood of death or serious injury during birth than low-income white women [5]. A study found that women at both ends of the income distribution have the highest rates of complications, although those with higher incomes have better access to care [6]. The pregnancy-related mortality rate for college-educated Black women is 5.2 times higher than that of their white counterparts and 1.6 times higher than that of white women with less than a high school diploma [7].

While disparities in health insurance coverage and access to care contribute to worse maternal and infant health outcomes for people of color, the primary drivers are inequities in broader social and economic factors, as well as structural and systemic racism and discrimination. Studies suggest that Black women are more likely to receive lower-quality obstetric care in hospitals compared to white women [8]. Other factors include supply-side barriers within the healthcare system, such as insurance coverage and access to long-term healthcare providers, and demand-side barriers rooted in a long history of racism, including policy-induced segregation, disparities in exposure to chemicals and

---

1 Black women are dying in childbirth or during the immediate postpartum period at rates three to four times higher.

pollutants, and toxic stress [9]. Toxic stress, resulting from race-related aggressions and insults, has been shown to have a physical effect on the body, causing premature aging.[2]

> *"Black women have a 53% increased risk of dying in the hospital during childbirth, no matter their income level, type of insurance, or other social determinants of health."*
>
> American Society of Anesthesiologists

5.2 Preventable Deaths: Addressing Systemic Barriers via Policy

Recent studies reveal that a staggering 80% of pregnancy-related deaths in the United States are preventable [10]. These deaths may be attributed to clinical errors or a lack of established protocols for addressing complications that arise during pregnancy or childbirth. Moreover, social determinants of health play a significant role in preventing many women from accessing the necessary quality interventions to address their health challenges, whether due to financial, geographic, or other barriers. Before the passage of the American Rescue Plan Act during the COVID-19 pandemic, women lost access to Medicaid coverage within 60 days of giving birth, leading to difficulties in obtaining primary care follow-up [11].

While the federal government is responsible for allocating funds and establishing national guidelines that states and local actors can follow, the actual implementation of policies to reduce the maternal mortality rate will largely occur at the local level. Despite a renewed federal effort to address this crisis, the success of these initiatives will depend on how effectively they are applied and adapted to the specific needs of communities across the country.

5.2.1 Federal Initiatives: Driving Change in Maternal Health

The federal government has been the primary driving force behind state adoption of high-value maternity services through various means, including educating states, instituting requirements for payers through the Affordable Care Act (ACA), Medicare, and Medicaid expansion, and creating funding blocks for initiatives aimed at reducing maternal mortality. The Biden administration has made addressing the maternal mortality crisis a priority, allocating a $470 million budget in December 2022 for a range of measures, including rural maternal health, addressing implicit bias among healthcare providers, and supporting the Centers for Medicare and Medicaid Services' (CMS's) Maternal Care Action Plan [12].

CMS has implemented a significant number of data collection, quality, and social support-related interventions to lower maternal mortality, in addition to expanding Medicaid coverage for postpartum women up to a year [13]. For instance, CMS created a health screening tool that assesses "health-related social needs," gathering information on food insecurity, housing instability, transportation needs, difficulty with utilities, and interpersonal safety. Starting in 2024, hospitals participating in the Medicare

---

2 Toxic stress, the result of race-related aggressions and insults that impact an individual, is proven to have a physical effect on the body, having an impact and causing it to age prematurely.

Hospital Inpatient Quality Reporting Program are required to send this data. Furthermore, CMS is conducting an equity assessment to analyze the quality of postpartum care in Medicaid and Children's Health Insurance Program (CHIP) and is developing a data system capable of identifying individuals losing Medicaid coverage and providing targeted outreach to transition them onto marketplace plans. CMS has also proposed creating a "birthing-friendly hospital" designation to help consumers identify hospitals committed to providing high-quality maternal care. However, rural women often lack the ability to "shop around" when choosing where to give birth, and underfunded areas may not have the resources to improve outcomes without additional interventions.

The Maternal, Infant, and Early Childhood Home Visiting Program, administered by Health Resources and Services Administration (HRSA) and the Administration for Children and Families (ACF), provides funding to states and territories to develop evidence-based home-visiting programs led by various professionals [14]. These programs educate parents about safe sleep practices, the importance of postpartum care, and screen for maternal depression. During the COVID-19 pandemic, HRSA awarded $121 million in American Rescue Plan Act funding to support this program [15]. In 2019, the program conducted over 1 million home visits, serving more than 154 000 families across all states and DC [16]. The majority of enrollees were young, low income, and racially and ethnically diverse, with approximately 70% being women of color. While ACF found that home visiting may improve maternal health through better general health, increased rates of health insurance coverage, reduced symptoms of depression, and the effects on family outcomes were mixed.

5.2.2 State-Level Initiatives: Medicaid Expansion and Targeted Interventions

Medicaid plays a crucial role in maternal health, covering 45% of all births in the United States and 66% of births to Black mothers [17]. States that expanded Medicaid under the ACA experienced a significant reduction in maternal mortality, with 7.01 fewer maternal deaths per 100,000 live births compared to non-expansion states [18]. Medicaid covers pregnancy-related services, prenatal care, delivery, postpartum care, family planning services, and conditions that may complicate pregnancy. Notably, four out of the 12 states that have not expanded Medicaid under the ACA have adopted 15 or more policies to improve maternal health outcomes, including legislation supporting postpartum coverage [19].

The American Rescue Plan Act provided states with a new five-year option to extend postpartum coverage to a full year. As of December 2022, 36 states and Washington, DC had implemented this extension, with an additional 7 states planning to follow suit [20]. Some non-expansion states also decided to extend Medicaid coverage beyond the initial 60-day window. For instance, on March 7, 2023, Mississippi's legislature agreed to expand their Medicaid coverage window in response to the end of the federal emergency Medicaid coverage mandate.

Despite these developments, states have further options to expand Medicaid and address maternal mortality. Some states allow for presumptive eligibility, which automatically enrolls low-income pregnant women in Medicaid, making them eligible for prenatal services [21]. This increases access to care, provided that states also offer education about available interventions for targeted groups.

Furthermore, CMS is encouraging states to expand Medicaid access to doula care through community-based maternity services and freestanding birth centers [22]. However, few states currently have robust networks of birth centers, midwives, doulas, or community health workers.

Maternal Mortality Review Committees (MMRCs) are multidisciplinary committees that operate at the state or local level, reviewing pregnancy-associated deaths using clinical and nonclinical information [23]. As the primary data source for pregnancy-associated and pregnancy-related deaths, MMRCs conduct more detailed investigations than death certificates, allowing them to gather additional information on racial, income-related, and geographic disparities in maternal mortality rates. These committees also provide recommendations for changes in clinical protocols and provider training, which can help state legislatures and public health departments create targeted interventions. Currently, 49 states, the District of Columbia, New York City, Philadelphia, and Puerto Rico, have MMRCs or a legal requirement to review pregnancy-related deaths. Most of these states (36) are required to review deaths occurring up to 1-year postpartum, and 14 states must determine whether the investigated pregnancy-related death was preventable. Nine states, DC, and New York City require the investigation or consideration of racial disparities and equity when conducting MMRC reviews.

In 2018, Congress passed the Preventing Maternal Deaths Act, aiming to assist states in addressing mothers' needs during pregnancy, childbirth, and postpartum, eliminating disparities in maternal health outcomes for pregnancy-related and pregnancy-associated deaths, and identifying solutions to improve healthcare quality and maternal health outcomes [24]. This legislation encourages the establishment of MMRC committees and authorizes the CDC to support states in funding these programs.

The California Maternal Quality Care Collaborative serves as an example of how targeted MMRC data can be used effectively [25]. The Collaborative analyzed the data to identify the most common clinical problems and complications related to maternal mortality. Based on these findings, they developed evidence-based toolkits to help healthcare providers better prepare for and manage complications such as maternal hemorrhage (one of the most common and preventable causes of death in California) and preeclampsia. California also provides a database that allows providers to compare their progress against other providers in the state.

Complementing the HRSA funding described in the federal program section, which is available in every state, some states have enacted legislation to standardize home visiting measures, emphasizing screening for mental health conditions and intimate partner visits [26]. These state-level initiatives aim to improve maternal and infant health outcomes by providing targeted support to expectant and new mothers. In Michigan, for example, five years after implementing a home visiting program, 87% of enrolled mothers delivered their babies at full term, demonstrating the effectiveness of such interventions. Similarly, New Jersey recently passed legislation establishing a three-year Medicaid home visitation demonstration project, building upon the success of these programs and expanding access to essential services for low-income families. By investing in home visiting programs and standardizing their focus on critical issues like mental health and intimate partner violence, states are taking proactive steps to address the complex factors contributing to maternal mortality and morbidity.

In an effort to provide comprehensive and coordinated care for expectant mothers, some states have implemented patient-centered medical home models that focus on developing care pathways for specific conditions, such as hypertension and substance abuse disorders. These medical home models aim to improve maternal health outcomes by ensuring that women receive timely, appropriate, and evidence-based care throughout their pregnancy and postpartum period. By establishing clear protocols and guidelines for managing common pregnancy-related conditions, these initiatives help healthcare providers deliver consistent, high-quality care tailored to each patient's individual needs. Furthermore, by addressing the unique challenges posed by hypertension and substance abuse disorders, these medical home models recognize the complex interplay between physical and mental health factors in shaping maternal health outcomes. Through the adoption of these innovative care delivery models, states are taking important steps to reduce maternal morbidity and mortality rates and promote the well-being of mothers and their families.

Policy Recommendations and Equity Considerations for Improving Maternal Health

Area of Policy	Key Recommendations	Equity Considerations
Social Determinants of Health (SDOH)	Focus on maternal mental health, expand telehealth, extend health coverage, and tackle structural racism	Improve environmental conditions affecting health outcomes, prioritizing communities of color
Legislative and Federal Actions	Support legislation to lower maternal morbidity and mortality rates, and enhance the healthcare coverage throughout pregnancy and postpartum	Aim policies to specifically reduce racial and geographic disparities in maternal health
Healthcare Access and Quality	Enhance access to quality maternity care and support Medicaid coverage for a full-year postpartum	Increase care accessibility for people of color and those in rural areas
Community-Based Solutions	Fund community-based organizations and expand successful local initiatives improving maternal health in communities of color	Ensure equitable support and funding for Black-led Community Based Organizations (CBOs)
Workforce Diversity and Training	Diversify the perinatal workforce and integrate cultural competency in healthcare training	Encourage policies that foster racial and ethnic diversity in healthcare professions
Data Collection and Quality Improvement	Improve data collection on maternal health to inform better clinical practices and policymaking	Use data to enhance understanding and care for marginalized groups, focusing on patient experiences

5.3 Overcoming Fragmentation: Collaboration and Bias Training

The fragmented and inconsistent implementation of federal guidelines and maternal mortality initiatives across states poses a significant challenge to achieving long-term, meaningful change in addressing the maternal health crisis [27]. To ensure that the federal government has accurate information about the most common complications leading to maternal mortality, the Department of Health and Human Services (HHS) and the CMS should continue collaborating with state MMRCs.

However, gathering more information and gaining deeper insights into the clinical causes of maternal mortality is only one aspect of the solution. Healthcare providers must also develop a greater understanding of the social determinants of health and recognize their own internal biases. To address this, medical schools and employers should implement policies and training programs, starting from the licensure phase, that aim to identify and combat unconscious bias among healthcare professionals.

5.4 Conclusion: Strengthening Legislation: Equity-Focused Interventions

To effectively address the maternal health crisis, future legislation should place stronger requirements on HHS, CMS, and the CDC to actively reduce disparities, rather than simply permitting the Secretary to conduct research, as is the case with the 2018 Preventing Maternal Deaths Act [28]. At the federal level, more efforts are needed to fund educational programs focused on anti-racism and anti-discrimination initiatives, develop techniques for providing culturally sensitive support, and promote equity within existing health programs.

Lawmakers must also consider how interventions implemented prior to pregnancy can contribute to better health outcomes during and after pregnancy. This includes addressing both access to healthcare and social determinants of health, such as income, education, and living conditions. By taking a comprehensive approach that tackles the root causes of maternal health disparities, policymakers can create a more equitable and effective system that supports the well-being of all mothers and families.

References

1 Xu, J., Murphy, S.L., Kochanek, K.D., and Arias, E. (2021). *Deaths: Final Data for 2019*. https://www.cdc.gov/nchs/data/nvsr/nvsr70/nvsr70-08-508.pdf.

2 Hoyert, D.L. and Miniño, A.M. (2020). Maternal mortality in the United States: changes in coding, publication, and data release, 2018. National vital statistics reports: from the Centers for Disease Control and Prevention, National Center for Health Statistics. *National Vital Statistics System* 69 (2): 1–18.

3 Abbasi, J. (2023). US maternal mortality is unacceptably high, unequal, and getting worse—what can be done about it? *JAMA* 330 (4): 302–305.

4 Jang, C.J. and Lee, H.C. (2022). A review of racial disparities in infant mortality in the US. *Children* 9 (2): 257.

5 Njoku, A., Evans, M., Nimo-Sefah, L., and Bailey, J. (2023). Listen to the whispers before they become screams: addressing black maternal morbidity and mortality in the United States. *Healthcare (Basel, Switzerland)* 11 (3): 438. https://doi.org/10.3390/healthcare11030438.

6 Kennedy-Moulton, K., Miller, S., Persson, P. et al. (2022). *Maternal and Infant Health Inequality: New Evidence from Linked Administrative Data (No. w30693)*. National Bureau of Economic Research.

7 Lin, B. and Appleton, A.A. (2022). Developmental origins of pregnancy-related morbidity and mortality in Black US women. *Frontiers in Public Health* 10: 853018.

8 Howell, E.A., Egorova, N., Balbierz, A. et al. (2016). Black-white differences in severe maternal morbidity and site of care. *American Journal of Obstetrics and Gynecology* 214 (1): 122–e1.

9 Morello-Frosch, R. and Shenassa, E.D. (2006). The environmental "riskscape" and social inequality: implications for explaining maternal and child health disparities. *Environmental Health Perspectives* 114 (8): 1150–1153.

10 Nelson, D. and Fomina, Y. (2023). How can we prevent pregnancy-related deaths? *Contemporary OB/GYN Journal* 68 (03): 10–14.

11 Rosenbaum, S., Handley, M., Casoni, M., and Morris, R. (2021). *Medicaid and the American Rescue Plan: How It All Fits Together*. Health Affairs Forefront.

12 Knocke, K., Chappel, A., Sugar, S. et al. (2022). *Doula Care and Maternal Health: An Evidence Review*. Department of Health and Human Services, Office of Health Policy.

13 Abboud, K. (2020). Why the United States is failing new mothers and how it can counteract its rapidly climbing maternal mortality rate. *Health Matrix* 30: 407.

14 Fernandes-Alcantara, A.L. (2018). Maternal, infant, and early childhood home visiting (MIECHV) program: background and funding. *Congressional Research Service* 18: 1–51.

15 Napili, A. and Colello, K.J. (2013). *Funding for the Older Americans Act and Other Aging Services Programs*, 196. Washington, DC: Congressional Research Service.

16 Platt, T. and VanLandgehem, K. *Public Insurance Financing of Home Visiting Services: Insights from a Federal/State Discussion*. National Academy for State Health Policy.

17 Markus, A.R. and Rosenbaum, S. (2010). The role of Medicaid in promoting access to high-quality, high-value maternity care. *Women's Health Issues* 20 (1): S67–S78.

18 Eliason, E.L. (2020). Adoption of Medicaid expansion is associated with lower maternal mortality. *Women's Health Issues* 30 (3): 147–152.

19 Searing, A. and Ross, D.C. (2019). *Medicaid Expansion Fills Gaps in Maternal Health Coverage Leading to Healthier Mothers and Babies*. Washington, DC: Georgetown University Health Policy Institute Center for Children and Families.

20 Johnston, E.M., Haley, J.M., Long, J., and Kenney, G.M. (2023). *New Mothers' Coverage Improved During the Public Health Emergency*. Urban Institute.

21 Hill, I., Hogan, S., Palmer, L. et al. (2009). *Medicaid Outreach and Enrollment for Pregnant Women: What Is the State of the Art?* Washington, DC: The Urban Institute and The National Academy for State Health Policy http://www.urban.org/publications/411898.html.

22 Backes, E.P., Scrimshaw, S.C., and National Academies of Sciences, Engineering, and Medicine (2020). Maternal and newborn care in the United States. In: *Birth Settings in America: Outcomes, Quality, Access, and Choice*. National Academies Press (US).

23 Zaharatos, J., St. Pierre, A., Cornell, A. et al. (2018). Building US capacity to review and prevent maternal deaths. *Journal of Women's Health* 27 (1): 1–5.

24 Kronemyer, B. (2018). Preventing maternal deaths gains support in congress. *Contemporary OB/GYN* 63 (2): 14–15.

25 Markow, C. and Main, E.K. (2019). Creating change at scale: quality improvement strategies used by the California maternal quality care collaborative. *Obstetrics and Gynecology Clinics* 46 (2): 317–328.

26 Johnson, K.A. (2001). *No Place like Home: State Home Visiting Policies and Programs (vol. 452)*. Commonwealth Fund.

27 Barnea, E.R., Nicholson, W., Theron, G. et al. (2021). From fragmented levels of care to integrated health care: framework toward improved maternal and newborn health. *International Journal of Gynecology & Obstetrics* 152 (2): 155–164.

28 Mehta, L.S., Sharma, G., Creanga, A.A. et al. (2021). Call to action: maternal health and saving mothers: a policy statement from the American Heart Association. *Circulation* 144 (15): e251–e269.

6

Mitigating Algorithmic Bias in Healthcare AI for Equitable Care

Abstract

The healthcare industry is exploring the use of artificial intelligence (AI) to improve patient outcomes, but the datasets used to train these systems raise concerns about algorithmic bias and its potential to exacerbate racial disparities in care. This chapter explores the issue of algorithmic bias in healthcare AI and its potential to exacerbate racial disparities in patient care. The chapter begins by explaining how AI systems, particularly those using machine learning (ML), rely on datasets that may be incomplete or under-representative, leading to systematic errors and racial bias. It then discusses the current legal landscape and challenges in regulating algorithmic bias, emphasizing the need for collaboration among stakeholders to identify, prevent, and mitigate bias. The chapter also explores strategies for enhancing data quality and diversity, the role of regulatory oversight and transparency, and the importance of diverse teams and inclusive datasets in addressing algorithmic bias. Finally, the chapter concludes by discussing the challenges faced by developers in gathering representative datasets, the need for legal frameworks to keep pace with technological advancements, and the importance of funding and accountability in creating a more equitable healthcare AI landscape.

Keywords   *algorithmic bias; healthcare AI; racial disparities; data quality; legal frameworks; regulatory oversight; diversity in development; equity in healthcare*

> *James, an African American patient, was inaccurately classified by a healthcare artificial intelligence (AI) system during a routine screening. The AI, trained primarily on data from non-African American populations, failed to recognize the specific risk factors associated with his demographics, leading to delayed diagnosis and treatment.*
>
> *Dr. Lee, a physician in an urban clinic, noticed a pattern of AI misdiagnoses among her Hispanic patients. The AI tool, designed to predict cardiovascular risk, systematically underestimated the risk for her patients, contributing to a cycle of undertreatment.*
>
> *A rural hospital adopted an AI system for patient management but soon discovered that the system was not optimized for the local demographic, which had a higher prevalence of chronic conditions not well-represented in the training data.*

Achieving Health Equity: The Role of Law and Policy, First Edition. Y. Tony Yang.

6.1 Addressing Algorithmic Bias in AI to Ensure Fair Healthcare

AI systems, particularly those utilizing ML, rely on datasets to function effectively. ML algorithms are trained to learn from and act upon data, with the potential to enhance patient care by deriving valuable insights from vast amounts of individual and collective patient data. However, incomplete or under-representative datasets can lead to systematic errors in AI's ability to classify patients, estimate risk levels, or make predictions, resulting in racial bias and negative outcomes for minority patients when their health needs are not accurately assessed [1, 2].

Algorithmic bias occurs when algorithms identify disease causes and recommend treatments based on input factors such as weight, height, and blood pressure, but generate less accurate predictions for certain groups, negatively impacting their health outcomes. Even if race is not explicitly considered in the algorithm's decision-making process, it may correlate with other factors affecting outcomes. For instance, Black patients may have a higher prevalence of comorbidities, which can influence overall health outcomes. The perceived "race neutrality" of algorithms can affect how ML adjusts for the relationship between race and health conditions, with studies showing that some AI devices fail to accurately detect racial differences before adjusting for clinical comorbidities and health status, thereby widening existing healthcare disparities [1].

Healthcare providers may unknowingly rely on outputs generated by systems with algorithmic bias when recommending medical care, potentially harming minority patients. Algorithmic bias is challenging to control as it can be introduced at any stage of the development process, from study design and data collection to implementation and dissemination of results, creating a compounding effect that necessitates early prevention or mitigation.

Selection bias may also contribute to the development of biased medical AI datasets. If racial groups, such as Black patients, have limited access to treatments or are ineligible for certain therapies due to baseline health status or comorbidities, there will be less data available on those groups, affecting the algorithm's ability to make accurate predictions and recommend appropriate treatments for patients with different health risks [3].

Experts caution that there is a tradeoff between algorithmic performance and bias, as efforts to decrease bias may impact the overall effectiveness of the AI. Addressing algorithmic bias to protect one racial group may reduce overall accuracy, but it is essential to ensure disadvantaged groups receive equitable care. Protecting these groups is crucial to promote better healthcare for all.

> *"As a society, we must be clear-eyed about both the promise and the perils of generative AI and work together to ensure that AI is always in service of humanity."*
>
> Brad Smith, Vice Chair and President, Microsoft

6.2 Legal Landscape and Challenges in Regulating Algorithmic Bias in Healthcare AI

The adoption of AI in healthcare is becoming increasingly prevalent, but the potential impacts of algorithmic bias are still being studied. As this is a relatively new and evolving area of law, there are limited regulations specifically addressing racial bias in algorithms used for medical care, and few avenues for legal challenges to algorithmic bias [4]. Despite emerging laws tackling bias in AI, only a small number explicitly cover racial bias in healthcare AI [5]. Moreover, regulatory tools for identifying and mitigating algorithmic biases often lack provisions for developers to self-regulate and audit their systems [6]. This section provides an overview of existing laws and their potential interaction with the regulation of algorithmic bias in healthcare.

The US Affordable Care Act prohibits discrimination against patients based on race, ethnicity, national origin, sex, age, or disability. However, it remains unclear whether racial bias in algorithms could be challenged under this law, as some courts have interpreted it to apply only when there is evidence of intent or motivation to discriminate. Algorithmic bias is often unintentional or caused by other difficult-to-trace systemic factors, making it unlikely that the current interpretation of the Affordable Care Act would cover algorithmic bias without evidence of intentional discrimination.

Scholars have explored the possibility of US Food and Drug Administration (FDA) regulation of AI algorithms, but changes to the law would be necessary to ensure these devices fall under FDA jurisdiction, as many currently do not. In 2021, the FDA released an action plan emphasizing the importance of identifying and mitigating bias in medical AI devices, but no concrete laws regulating this area exist yet. As the technology becomes more common, making the FDA a regulator of algorithmic bias should be a priority.

The Federal Trade Commission (FTC) has indicated its intent to consider the "sale or use of ... racially based algorithms" as potentially violating Section 5 of the FTC Act, which prohibits "unfair or deceptive practices" [7]. If the FTC proceeds with this type of regulation and includes medical AI devices within its scope, it could create a new avenue for legal liability. As this regulatory scheme develops, it will be crucial to determine if it applies to AI in healthcare and if there are requirements to demonstrate intent to discriminate.

Some scholars have considered challenging racial bias using a tort law theory of negligence but are skeptical about the likelihood of success because algorithmic errors may not be foreseeable. However, if AI errors become more foreseeable as technology and data improve, negligence claims could potentially prevail in this context.

State insurance regulators may also be able to exert pressure on the medical AI industry. For example, New York state insurance regulators announced an investigation into users of an algorithm that helped payers and health systems target patients for high-risk care management but was found to treat Black patients worse than white patients with the same health status [8]. This may signal a new trend for insurance regulators to investigate and police bias in medical device AI.

6.3 Collaborative Efforts to Address Algorithmic Bias in Healthcare AI

Addressing systemic bias in healthcare AI requires context-dependent and system-level solutions, as bias is often unconsciously infused into datasets, and there are limited practical solutions to eliminate unintended bias from an algorithm without compromising its overall accuracy. Consequently, there is no simple solution to the problem, and properly addressing algorithmic bias in healthcare AI necessitates collaboration among regulators, developers, and other stakeholders to identify, prevent, and mitigate bias. Policymakers must take action to implement a uniform approach to prevent health biases in AI, which includes improving algorithm evaluation. Evaluating algorithms for bias and disparate impacts should be an ongoing process to ensure that new biases and developments are addressed in a timely manner. Failure to recognize and address these flaws has the potential to exacerbate existing health injustices and create new ones. By working together and maintaining vigilance, stakeholders can strive to create a more equitable and unbiased healthcare AI landscape that benefits all patients, regardless of their racial or ethnic background [9].

6.3.1 Enhancing Data Quality and Diversity to Address Algorithmic Bias

Improving data collection and preparation is the first step in addressing racial bias in healthcare AI. The core of the issue lies in the quality of the datasets, and enhancing data diversity can lead to better health outcomes and promote equity [10]. Experts recommend compiling large and diverse datasets that better represent all patient groups, including expanding the dataset to encompass the full range of patients who may be referred and evaluated for treatment, rather than limiting it to those who received the treatment.

More representative datasets would have the appropriate statistical properties concerning the persons or groups of persons on which the high-risk AI system is intended to be used. Datasets should be examined to determine whether they contain any potential for racial bias due to statistical disproportions by race in the data, as disproportionate data creates potential for racial bias in the relevance and accuracy of predictions for minorities [11].

Experts recommend that algorithm development should prioritize addressing four crucial questions to ensure fairness and accuracy [12]. First, developers must assess the representativeness of the dataset, determining whether it adequately captures the diversity of the target population. Second, they should examine if the data model actively accounts for and mitigates potential biases that may be present in the dataset. Third, the accuracy of predictions based on large datasets must be rigorously evaluated to ensure their reliability and validity [13]. Finally, developers must consider the ethical and fairness implications of relying heavily on big data, as this reliance may perpetuate or amplify existing societal biases and disparities. While these guiding questions provide a strong foundation for developing policies and strategies to mitigate algorithmic bias, improving data sets may be more complex than it appears [14]. Barriers to generating or synthesizing relevant data may exist, and some experts propose addressing the larger societal and systemic sources of bias, calling on developers to collect data beyond their current regulatory gaze and legal mandate. However, this instruction lacks clarity, and there are no established best practices for developers to self-regulate and audit their systems. Moreover, this approach implies that developers should allocate limited time, funding, and other resources to information gathering that may or may not improve context-dependent outcomes and the existence of racial bias in data sets.

6.3.2 Regulatory Oversight and Transparency in Medical AI Development and Implementation

Policymakers should regulate medical device AI throughout all stages, from design to execution, to ensure diversity, nondiscrimination, fairness, and equity. Proposed regulatory schemes suggest high standards in development and evaluation to improve algorithmic fairness and accuracy. To achieve this, developers should be required to monitor error rates for patient groups of different demographics and evaluate models to assess the quality of predictions and validate the model's decision-making process. Evaluating the models can help developers identify bias and pinpoint potentially biased predictors [15].

Experts recommend that developers assess the risks of bias and use reporting checklists that could be referenced by regulating agencies during authorization [16]. Disclosing data about the datasets, errors, and performance levels can also be used by end users, such as physicians, to better understand whether the system is appropriate for specific groups of patients [17]. Once a medical device using AI is implemented in clinical practice, the system should be continuously monitored to ensure the performance does not degrade and to identify potential sources of error [18].

A transparent review and disclosure process are essential to reduce the risk of racial bias in AI. Developers must use the highest possible quality data to minimize risks and discriminatory outcomes. Additionally, human oversight measures must be implemented to reduce risk, including oversight during development and monitoring when the systems are used in practice to account for changes or new biases as the machines learn [19]. By implementing these measures, policymakers and developers can work together to create a more equitable and trustworthy AI ecosystem in healthcare, ensuring that all patients receive fair and accurate treatment regardless of their racial or ethnic background [20, 21].

6.3.3 Diverse Teams and Inclusive Datasets: Strategies for Mitigating Algorithmic Bias

Unconscious bias is often infused in datasets, and there are limited practical solutions to eliminate unintended bias from an algorithm without impairing its efficacy. Addressing this cross-cutting issue requires diverse disciplinary teams to develop and review the algorithms. Diverse teams of experts can provide a deep understanding of the clinical context, improving the modeling process. While data scientists may have a technical understanding of the AI, other professionals may have a better sense of how the machine will be used in practice and can better predict where bias may be implicated. Involving diverse groups of stakeholders should also raise awareness of the effects of datasets and bias in algorithms [22].

As this area of healthcare continues to develop, experts are still learning about the effects of algorithmic bias and exploring ways to prevent and mitigate the disparate effects on racial groups. As technology advances, AI systems should be designed to account for bias in the data to mitigate the chances that underrepresented groups are affected by inaccurate predictions. New technology is becoming available to "de-bias" the data while simultaneously achieving better performance and greater accuracy [23]. However, these techniques are still in their early stages, and more research is needed to confirm their reliability.

While experts work to expand datasets to encompass the full range of potential patients, some scholars suggest labeling medical devices to better describe for whom they work (e.g. "not cleared for Black women under the age of 40") [24]. Although labeling practices may clarify who is best suited for certain treatments, they do not actually mitigate racial bias or address the core problem. In fact, this approach may exacerbate the justice-based concern of racial bias by making treatments available only to certain racial or demographic groups. This strategy should be used sparingly and only while improving data to make the algorithm better suited for widespread use, regardless of demographics.

Overview of Key Policy Areas and Actions for Addressing Algorithmic Bias in Healthcare AI

Category	Policy Area	Key Actions and Considerations
Algorithmic Bias and Data Management	Algorithmic Bias and Data Quality and Diversity	• Address systematic errors and racial bias with more representative datasets • Enhance data collection and ensure broad demographic representation
Legal and Regulatory Frameworks	Legal Landscape and Regulatory Oversight and Transparency	• Amend existing laws to incorporate AI-specific regulations • Implement comprehensive oversight throughout AI development and deployment stages
Collaboration and Diversity	Collaborative Efforts and Diverse Teams and Inclusive Datasets	• Foster collaboration among stakeholders to identify and mitigate biases • Involve diverse teams in AI development to predict and address biases
Funding and Resource Allocation	Addressing Racial Bias	• Secure funding for research on racial biases in datasets • Develop legal and regulatory strategies to ensure equitable AI application

6.4   Conclusion: Overcoming Challenges in Addressing Racial Bias in Medical AI

Developers working on medical AI may face challenges in gathering representative datasets that mitigate concerns of racial bias in algorithms due to limited funding or resources. Simultaneously, the law has not kept pace with the rapid advancements in technology, leaving developers with potentially no legal obligation to control for racial bias and, consequently, limited incentives to do so. However, as AI becomes increasingly prevalent in healthcare, it is crucial that the algorithm development process and the legal framework evolve to effectively regulate racial bias in medical devices using AI, as this pressing issue directly impacts health outcomes [25].

Refining the algorithm development process to minimize bias is an important ethical consideration that demands attention from researchers. Incorporating checks and balances, such as regulatory accountability and dataset improvements, will contribute to greater health equity over time and help avoid exacerbating inequalities and bias. To better understand the problem and identify solutions, stakeholders must make concerted efforts to document race and associated variables, enabling systemic inquiries into potential sources of racial bias. Additionally, funding should be made available to developers to examine underlying datasets for racial gaps and develop mitigation strategies. Furthermore, exploring policy and regulatory solutions is essential to improve accountability in this context. By addressing these challenges head-on, the medical AI community can work toward creating a more equitable and unbiased healthcare landscape that benefits all patients, regardless of their racial or ethnic background [26].

References

1 Obermeyer, Z., Powers, B., Vogeli, C., and Mullainathan, S. (2019). Dissecting racial bias in an algorithm used to manage the health of populations. *Science (New York, N.Y.)* 366 (6464): 447–453. https://doi.org/10.1126/science.aax2342.

2 Benjamin, R. (2019). Assessing risk, automating racism. *Science* 366 (6464): 421–422.

3 Gianfrancesco, M.A., Tamang, S., Yazdany, J., and Schmajuk, G. (2018). Potential biases in machine learning algorithms using electronic health record data. *JAMA Internal Medicine* 178 (11): 1544–1547. https://doi.org/10.1001/jamainternmed.2018.3763.

4 Hoffman, S. and Podgurski, A. (2019). Artificial intelligence and discrimination in health care. *The Yale Journal of Health Policy, Law, and Ethics* 19: 1.

5 Price, W. and Nicholson, I.I. (2019). Medical AI and contextual bias. *The Harvard Journal of Law & Technology* 33: 65.

6 Wiens, J., Price, W.N., and Sjoding, M.W. (2020). Diagnosing bias in data-driven algorithms for healthcare. *Nature Medicine* 26 (1): 25–26.

7 Selbst, A.D. and Barocas, S. (2022). Unfair artificial intelligence: how FTC intervention can overcome the limitations of discrimination law. *The University of Pennsylvania Law Review* 171: 1023.

8 Kostick-Quenet, K.M., Cohen, I.G., Gerke, S. et al. (2022). Mitigating racial bias in machine learning. *The Journal of Law, Medicine & Ethics* 50 (1): 92–100.

9 Chen, I.Y., Szolovits, P., and Ghassemi, M. (2019). Can AI help reduce disparities in general medical and mental health care? *AMA Journal of Ethics* 21 (2): 167–179.

10 Ferryman, K., & Pitcan, M. (2018). Fairness in Precision Medicine. https://datasociety.net/wp-content/uploads/2018/02/DataSociety_Fairness_In_Precision_Medicine_Feb2018.pdf

11 Goodman, S.N., Goel, S., and Cullen, M.R. (2018). Machine learning, health disparities, and causal reasoning. *Annals of Internal Medicine* 169 (12): 883–884.

12 Rajkomar, A., Hardt, M., Howell, M.D. et al. (2018). Ensuring fairness in machine learning to advance health equity. *Annals of Internal Medicine* 169 (12): 866–872. https://doi.org/10.7326/M18-1990.

13 Chen, M., Hao, Y., Hwang, K. et al. (2017). Disease prediction by machine learning over big data from healthcare communities. *IEEE Access* 5: 8869–8879.

14 Panch, T., Mattie, H., and Celi, L.A. (2019). The "inconvenient truth" about AI in healthcare. *npj Digital Medicine* 2 (1): 1–3.

15 Parikh, R.B., Teeple, S., and Navathe, A.S. (2019). Addressing bias in artificial intelligence in health care. *JAMA* 322 (24): 2377–2378.

16 Page, M.J., McKenzie, J.E., and Higgins, J.P. (2018). Tools for assessing risk of reporting biases in studies and syntheses of studies: a systematic review. *BMJ Open* 8 (3): e019703.

17 Nordling, L. (2019). A fairer way forward for AI in health care. *Nature* 573 (7775): S103–S103.

18 Rajkomar, A., Dean, J., and Kohane, I. (2019). Machine learning in medicine. *New England Journal of Medicine* 380 (14): 1347–1358.

19 Gerke, S., Minssen, T., and Cohen, G. (2020). Ethical and legal challenges of artificial intelligence-driven healthcare. In: *Artificial Intelligence in Healthcare*, 295–336. Academic Press.

20 Char, D.S., Shah, N.H., and Magnus, D. (2018). Implementing machine learning in health care – addressing ethical challenges. *The New England Journal of Medicine* 378 (11): 981–983. https://doi.org/10.1056/NEJMp1714229.

21 Vayena, E., Blasimme, A., and Cohen, I.G. (2018). Machine learning in medicine: addressing ethical challenges. *PLoS Medicine* 15 (11): e1002689.

22 Sendak, M., Gao, M., Nichols, M. et al. (2019). Machine learning in health care: a critical appraisal of challenges and opportunities. *EGEMs* 7 (1).

23 Zhang, B.H., Lemoine, B., and Mitchell, M. (2018). Mitigating unwanted biases with adversarial learning. *Proceedings of the 2018 AAAI/ACM Conference on AI, Ethics, and Society*, pp. 335–340.

24 Benjamens, S., Dhunnoo, P., and Meskó, B. (2020). The state of artificial intelligence-based FDA-approved medical devices and algorithms: an online database. *npj Digital Medicine* 3 (1): 118.

25 Matheny, M.E., Whicher, D., and Israni, S.T. (2020). Artificial intelligence in health care: a report from the National Academy of Medicine. *JAMA* 323 (6): 509–510.

26 Cohen, I.G., Amarasingham, R., Shah, A. et al. (2014). The legal and ethical concerns that arise from using complex predictive analytics in health care. *Health Affairs* 33 (7): 1139–1147.

7

Confronting Inequities in the US Organ Transplant System

Abstract

This chapter explores the pervasive inequities in the US organ transplant system, which disproportionately affect communities of color. Despite higher rates of conditions that lead to organ failure, Black and Latino patients face lower probabilities of being placed on transplant waitlists and receiving transplants. The chapter delves into the various stages of the transplant process, identifying barriers and biases that perpetuate these disparities, such as limited access to specialist referrals, race-based clinical policies, and socioeconomically advantageous waitlist policies. It also examines the challenges faced by organ procurement organizations (OPOs) in effectively communicating with and supporting diverse communities, as well as the impact of provider bias and insurance disparities on Black patients' transplant access. The chapter highlights recent efforts to address these inequities, such as the Organ Procurement and Transplant Network's (OPTNs) mandate for race-neutral transplant eligibility calculations. It presents recommendations for improving equity at each stage of the transplant process, drawing from a 2022 report by the National Academies. These recommendations include increasing data collection, standardizing referral pathways and waitlist placement criteria, and implementing policies that promote equal access to transplantation services. Additionally, the chapter addresses discrimination based on disability in organ transplantation, which persists despite legal protections under the Americans with Disabilities Act (ADA). It concludes by emphasizing the need for a comprehensive, multi-stage approach to ensure equitable organ allocation in the highly complex US organ transplant system, calling for a concerted effort to address systemic issues that perpetuate inequities and work toward a more just and equitable system for all patients in need.

Keywords *organ transplantation; racial disparities; access to care; waitlist inequities; organ procurement organizations (OPOs); implicit bias; disability discrimination*

> *Denzel, a 35-year-old Black man, had been battling kidney disease for years. Despite his deteriorating condition, his primary care doctor never referred him to a transplant specialist. By the time he was evaluated, his chances of being placed on the transplant waitlist were slim. The lack of early specialist referrals severely impacted Denzel's health, prolonging his suffering and reducing his chances of receiving a life-saving transplant.*

Achieving Health Equity: The Role of Law and Policy, First Edition. Y. Tony Yang.
© 2025 John Wiley & Sons Ltd. Published 2025 by John Wiley & Sons Ltd.

> *Ana, a 28-year-old Latina, struggled with the organ transplant system's complexities. Her family's limited English proficiency made communication with organ procurement organizations (OPOs) difficult. When her younger brother, who was a match, passed away unexpectedly, Ana felt overwhelmed and unsupported. The OPO's lack of resources to effectively engage with diverse communities meant Ana missed out on crucial guidance and support during a critical time.*
>
> *Mark, a middle-aged man with Down Syndrome, faced an uphill battle when he needed a liver transplant. Despite legal protections under the Americans with Disabilities Act (ADA), Mark encountered discrimination and delays. Transplant centers were hesitant to place him on the waitlist, citing unfounded concerns about his ability to comply with post-transplant care. Mark's experience highlights the persistent biases and inequities that individuals with disabilities face within the organ transplant system.*

7.1 Inequities in Organ Transplantation Disproportionately Affect Communities of Color

Communities of color face higher rates of diabetes and high blood pressure, conditions that increase the risk of organ failure and the need for transplantation [1]. However, the US organ transplant system is plagued by inequities [2]. Despite being three to four times more likely to experience kidney failure compared to white Americans, Black and Latino patients on dialysis have a lower probability of being placed on the transplant waitlist and receiving a transplant [3].

Efforts to address these disparities over the past two decades have been insufficient, with the gap in live donor kidney transplantation widening between 1995–1999 and 2010–2014 [4]. The scarcity of available organs exacerbates the issue, with the Health Resources and Services Administration reporting 105,800 individuals on the national transplant waiting list as of March 2022, and average wait times spanning three to five years [5]. In 2020, white patients received 48% of available organs, while Black patients received only 28% [6].

The organ transplant process begins with a patient's evaluation at a transplant hospital, which determines their suitability for transplantation based on a combination of standardized and hospital-specific criteria. Inequities arise throughout the process due to a lack of organ matches for people of color, fewer specialist referrals, biases in waitlist placement, and provider prejudices. These factors contribute to downstream health disparities. Black patients, who are disproportionately affected by kidney failure and face structural barriers to care and transplantation [7], experience longer waiting times from the start of dialysis to waitlist placement, are more frequently deemed psychologically unfit for transplantation [8], and are less likely to be waitlisted compared to white patients [9].

> *"In the U.S., Black people are four times as likely to develop kidney failure as White people, but they are much less likely to receive a lifesaving kidney transplant. Black people also experience the highest rates of heart failure, but receive heart transplants at lower rates than their White counterparts."*
>
> Jewel Mullen, M.D., Dell Medical School

7.2 Barriers to Specialist Referrals and Data Gaps Perpetuate Inequities

Communities of color often face barriers in accessing consistent preventative care and regular visits to primary care providers, which can hinder their referral to transplant hospitals or specialists for further evaluation. Black patients, in particular, are less likely than white patients to receive timely referrals for transplant evaluation or complete the necessary pretransplant medical assessments [10]. This delay in referral can lead to worsening health conditions, increased morbidity, mortality, and resource utilization, and missed opportunities for preemptive transplantation [11].

The lack of necessary specialist referrals not only affects individual patients but also hinders the transplant system's ability to accurately assess patient population and demand. The absence of a national database that facilitates studies on equitable referral and evaluation practices in organ transplantation creates a data gap in referral and admissions information. Without comprehensive data on socioeconomic status and social determinants of health, patients may be incorrectly labeled as noncompliant, further limiting their access to transplantation and contributing to poorer outcomes.

7.3 Race-Based Clinical Policies Hinder Equitable Waitlist Placement

Disparities persist even when patients receive a referral, as transplant hospitals may not determine that the patient should be added to the national waitlist. Black and Hispanic candidates face a more than 50% lower likelihood of being preemptively listed for a kidney transplant compared to white candidates [12]. While national standards serve as a baseline for hospitals when deciding if a patient is a suitable candidate, most transplant centers also consider their own factors. Clinical policies that incorporate race as a factor in determining disease severity can delay the timely placement of Black patients on transplant waitlists [13]. For instance, estimated Glomerular Filtration Rate (eGFR), a measurement of the kidneys' efficiency in removing creatinine from blood, was previously used as a qualifier for initiating time on the kidney transplantation waitlist [14]. However, as Black patients generally have higher creatinine levels, some providers historically incorporated a Black race variable that automatically increased eGFR values for all Black patients [15]. This variable overestimated the kidney function of Black patients, disadvantaging them by prolonging their wait time.

7.4 Waitlist Policies Favor Socioeconomically Advantaged Patients

Even if a patient successfully navigates the initial referral and waitlist placement, the transplant waitlist itself may contribute to inequitable outcomes. Black patients have a nearly 50% lower likelihood of receiving a living donor kidney compared to white patients [16], while Hispanic patients face a higher risk of being removed from the waiting list due to death or deterioration [17]. Moreover, Black patients experience a longer median wait time from waitlist placement to kidney transplantation than white patients [18]. While these outcomes cannot be attributed to a single source, some may be linked to United Network for Organ Sharing (UNOS) and OPTN rules that favor patients from higher socioeconomic backgrounds.

One such rule, implemented by UNOS in 1987, allows organ transplant candidates to pursue "multiple listing," which involves registering for transplants at multiple hospitals [19]. This approach often requires additional temporary housing and transportation costs not covered by insurance, as well as out-of-state care that may not be covered by Medicaid. A 2015 study reveals that patients added to the national waitlist through multiple listings tend to have higher income and private insurance, yet appear to have less medical need than single-list patients for most of their waiting time [15]. Despite the controversy surrounding the multiple listing rule, with some states like New York banning it for certain transplant types, a ban based on inequality failed in 1988 due to strong opposition from patient advocacy groups [20]. This policy conflicts with the principle of allocating organs based on "sound medical judgment" and "objective and measurable medical criteria."

7.5 Communication Barriers and Resource Limitations Hinder Diverse Organ Donation

OPOs often struggle to effectively communicate with potential donors and provide adequate support to communities of color. Given that same-ethnicity donors and recipients are more likely to be clinical matches for transplants, ensuring diverse organ sources is crucial. However, Black patients are less likely to be referred to OPOs, and self-reported donor registration rates are lower among Black and Asian Americans compared to other racial and ethnic groups [21]. This disparity can be attributed to OPOs' limited resources and the pressure to prioritize opportunities with a higher likelihood of success. Black families often experience less comprehensive discussions about the possibility of donation and are more likely to report insufficient time to make the decision to donate [22]. Cultural differences and language barriers may hinder OPO representatives' ability to communicate effectively and empathetically with a family that has recently lost a loved one [23].

7.6 Provider Bias and Insurance Disparities Impede Black Patients' Transplant Access

Black individuals face persistent access barriers related to higher rates of un- and underinsurance, which are further exacerbated by implicit bias from healthcare providers [24]. This bias permeates every stage of the transplant process, from providers failing to trust patients who request referrals to harboring ingrained beliefs about a cultural group's tendency toward altruism. These factors interact with and compound the challenges Black patients encounter throughout their transplant journey.

7.7 OPTN Mandates Race-Neutral Transplant Eligibility Calculations

The OPTN, a Board established by the Department of Health and Human Services, is responsible for developing policies that ensure "equitable allocation of cadaveric organs" among its member transplant hospitals, OPOs, and histocompatibility labs. On June 27, 2022, the OPTN approved a policy mandating that all transplant hospitals use race-neutral calculations when determining a patient's eligibility for the transplant waitlist [25]. This policy is retroactive, allowing transplant programs the discretion to update the date a patient qualified for transplant waitlist time if the hospital determines that the wait time was based on a race-based policy. This policy represents a crucial step in ensuring equity in transplant allocation by requiring transplant hospitals to ensure that their calculations are race-neutral and do not include adjustments for Black or other minority patients. However, hospitals still retain the discretion to determine their "scoring" system, provided it does not include race as a factor.

7.8 Recommendations for Improving Equity at Each Stage of the Transplant Process

A 2022 report highlighted the importance of increasing data collection and disaggregating existing data categories to enable OPTN to explicitly include and measure equity initiatives and their impact on the transplant process [26]. This approach would provide more comprehensive information about the types of patients placed on the waitlist and their outcomes. The report also outlined several interventions that OPTN could implement to enhance equity at each stage of the organ transplant process. This section categorizes potential recommendations based on the specific "area" of the transplant process they would impact, recognizing that addressing implicit bias, inadequate data collection, and unequal access remain consistent themes throughout the cycle.

To promote equality in the referral process, the government should prioritize access to primary care and preventative screening services [27]. Dialysis clinics and similar interventions should have patient navigators trained to discuss options and connect patients with transplant hospitals and specialists [28]. Dialysis providers and others caring for patients with end-stage organ failure can establish systematic referral and screening pathways to transplant centers.

While OPTN's policy requiring transplant hospitals to use race-neutral calculations for waitlist qualification is a significant step, further standardization of waitlist placement requirements is needed. Given the national transplant waiting list's purpose of ensuring equal organ access without significant geographical bias, it is counterproductive for hospitals to have varying standards. The Board should set national standards for waitlist placement, allowing discretion within those ranges.

OPTN currently grants allocation credits to patients who accrue waiting list time before beginning dialysis, despite many patients requiring dialysis until a kidney becomes available. The National Academies of Sciences, Engineering, and Medicine recommends discontinuing this practice, as it favors patients with better insurance and socioeconomic status who can access early referral and listing [20]. Instead, waiting time points should be based on the date the patient began dialysis. The Board should also disincentivize "Double Listing," which favors those who can afford access to multiple transplant hospitals.

Transitioning from an opt-in to an opt-out organ donation system could address organ shortages and lessen pressure on the allocation system, but this change may face political challenges. On a smaller scale, HHS should scrutinize the work of OPOs in communities of color and require these organizations to increase staff with backgrounds that reflect the communities they engage with [29]. This change should lead to more empathetic and productive conversations, resulting in higher donation levels and better clinical matches for patients of color.

To address implicit bias, hospitals and the government must work to increase diversity in the biomedical services workforce and among transplant surgeons [30]. One policy initiative is to increase funding for students of color to attend biomedical conferences and learn about the field. Additionally, hospitals should increase continuing legal education (CLE) focused on disparities in transplantation.

7.9 Discrimination Based on Disability in Organ Transplantation Persists

Denying access to organ transplants based on disabilities, such as Down Syndrome or Autism, is a common practice despite being illegal under the ADA [31]. Some states have enacted laws prohibiting physicians from denying an organ transplant solely on the basis of a patient's disability. In 2020, the Department of Justice (DOJ) reached a settlement agreement with a Massachusetts hospital's transplant center to resolve allegations of discrimination against patients with opioid use disorders [32]. The hospital allegedly refused to treat a patient who was taking a legal, prescription medication while actively participating in a supervised rehabilitation treatment program. The settlement agreement required the hospital to develop and enforce nondiscrimination transplant policies, provide employee training on ADA requirements, and comply with specific reporting obligations set by the DOJ.

7.10 A Comprehensive, Multistage Approach for Equitable Organ Allocation

The US organ transplant system is highly complex, and interventions to address equity issues must target each stage of the process, from initial referral to waitlist designations and transplant assignment. While the OPTN recently took a crucial step by banning the use of race in calculating a patient's eligibility for the transplant waitlist, further measures can be implemented to ensure equitable allocation of organ donations [33]. To achieve this goal, a comprehensive approach that addresses disparities at every point in the transplantation process is necessary. This may include standardizing referral pathways, establishing consistent waitlist placement criteria, and implementing policies that promote equal access to transplantation services [34]. By addressing the systemic issues that perpetuate inequities, the United States can work toward a more just and equitable organ transplant system for all patients in need.

Key Policy and Equity Issues in Organ Transplantation and Recommended Actions

Policy/Aspect	Issue/Disparity	Recommendation/Action
Referral Process	Limited referrals for Black and Hispanic patients; delays in specialist referrals.	Increase primary-care access and systematic referral pathways. Implement patient navigators at dialysis clinics to discuss options and connect patients with transplant hospitals and specialists.
Implicit Bias	Bias in provider attitudes affects referral and evaluation processes.	Increase diversity in the biomedical services workforce and among transplant surgeons. Provide continuing education on disparities and implicit bias in transplantation.

Policy/Aspect	Issue/Disparity	Recommendation/Action
Waitlist Placement	Black and Hispanic patients are less likely to be preemptively listed for kidney transplants.	Standardize waitlist placement criteria across hospitals. Mandate national standards for transplant waitlist placement, removing geographical biases, and ensuring equity.
Race-Based Clinical Policies	Use of race-based factors like eGFR leads to delayed waitlist placement for Black patients.	Implement race-neutral eligibility calculations. Require transplant hospitals to update waitlist times retroactively for patients affected by race-based policies.
Insurance and Socioeconomic Barriers	Black patients face higher rates of un- and underinsurance, impacting their transplant access.	CMS should adopt payment policies that incentivize equity in care from primary care to posttransplant care. Expand insurance coverage and support for all patients to ensure equal access to transplant services.
Organ Procurement Organizations (OPOs)	Communication barriers and limited resources hinder effective engagement with diverse communities.	Increase OPO staff diversity to reflect communities served. Enhance training in cultural sensitivity and empathy for OPO representatives.
Living donor Transplants	Lower rates of living donor transplants among Black patients due to socioeconomic factors.	Implement targeted educational interventions and patient navigator programs to increase living donor kidney transplantation among minority communities.
Data collection and transparency	Gaps in data on socioeconomic status and social determinants of health hinder equitable policymaking.	Improve data collection to include socioeconomic factors and social determinants of health. Implement a national database for referral and evaluation practices. Develop an equity dashboard to track disparities and progress in real time.
Legal protections and disabilities	Discrimination based on disability persists despite ADA protections.	Ensure compliance with ADA and enact specific laws prohibiting discrimination in organ transplantation based on disabilities. Provide training for transplant centers on nondiscrimination policies.
Public education and engagement	Lack of awareness and engagement among minority communities regarding organ donation.	Conduct ongoing, culturally targeted public education campaigns about the benefits and process of organ donation and transplantation.

References

1 Vanholder, R., Domínguez-Gil, B., Busic, M. et al. (2021). Organ donation and transplantation: a multi-stakeholder call to action. *Nature Reviews Nephrology* 17 (8): 554–568.

2 Bratton, C., Chavin, K., and Baliga, P. (2011). Racial disparities in organ donation and why. *Current Opinion in Organ Transplantation* 16 (2): 243–249.

3 El-Khoury, B. and Yang, T.C. (2024). Reviewing racial disparities in living donor kidney transplantation: a socioecological approach. *Journal of Racial and Ethnic Health Disparities* 11 (2): 928–937. https://doi.org/10.1007/s40615-023-01573-x.

4 Chopra, B. and Sureshkumar, K.K. (2015). Changing organ allocation policy for kidney transplantation in the United States. *World Journal of Transplantation* 5 (2): 38.

5 Morrison, L.J., Sandroni, C., Grunau, B. et al. (2023). Organ donation after out-of-hospital cardiac arrest: a scientific statement from the International Liaison Committee on Resuscitation. *Circulation* 148 (10): e120–e146.

6 HRSA (2022). U.S. organ procurement and transplantation network (OPTN). Based on OPTN data as of October 31, 2022. https://optn.transplant.hrsa.gov/data/view-data-reports/national-data/ (accessed 30 August 2024).

7 Kulkarni, S., Ladin, K., Haakinson, D. et al. (2019). Association of racial disparities with access to kidney transplant after the implementation of the new kidney allocation system. *JAMA Surgery* 154 (7): 618–625.

8 Joshi, S., Gaynor, J.J., Bayers, S. et al. (2013). Disparities among Blacks, Hispanics, and Whites in time from starting dialysis to kidney transplant waitlisting. *Transplantation* 95 (2): 309–318.

9 Gosto, M. (2015). Current allocation policies and disparities within liver and kidney transplantation. Doctoral Dissertation. University of Pittsburgh.

10 Gander, J.C., Zhang, X., Plantinga, L. et al. (2018). Racial disparities in preemptive referral for kidney transplantation in Georgia. *Clinical Transplantation* 32 (9): e13380.

11 Steinman, T.I., Becker, B.N., Frost, A.E. et al. (2001). Guidelines for the referral and management of patients eligible for solid organ transplantation. *Transplantation* 71 (9): 1189–1204.

12 Reese, P.P., Mohan, S., King, K.L. et al. (2021). Racial disparities in preemptive waitlisting and deceased donor kidney transplantation: ethics and solutions. *American Journal of Transplantation* 21 (3): 958–967.

13 Patzer, R.E. and Pastan, S.O. (2020). Policies to promote timely referral for kidney transplantation. *Seminars in Dialysis* 33 (1): 58–67.

14 Ku, E., McCulloch, C.E., Adey, D.B. et al. (2021). Racial disparities in eligibility for preemptive waitlisting for kidney transplantation and modification of eGFR thresholds to equalize waitlist time. *Journal of the American Society of Nephrology* 32 (3): 677–685.

15 Gillespie, N. and Mohandas, R. (2023). New eGFR equations: implications for cardiologists and racial inequities. *American Heart Journal Plus: Cardiology Research and Practice* 27: 100269.

16 Wesselman, H., Ford, C.G., Leyva, Y. et al. (2021). Social determinants of health and race disparities in kidney transplant. *Clinical Journal of the American Society of Nephrology: CJASN* 16 (2): 262–274. https://doi.org/10.2215/CJN.04860420.

17 Thuluvath, P.J., Amjad, W., and Zhang, T. (2020). Liver transplant waitlist removal, transplantation rates and post-transplant survival in Hispanics. *PLoS One* 15 (12): e0244744. https://doi.org/10.1371/journal.pone.0244744.

18 Kasiske, B.L., London, W., and Ellison, M.D. (1998). Race and socioeconomic factors influencing early placement on the kidney transplant waiting list. *Journal of the American Society of Nephrology* 9 (11): 2142–2147.

19 Givens, R.C., Dardas, T., Clerkin, K.J. et al. (2015). Outcomes of multiple listing for adult heart transplantation in the United States: analysis of OPTN data from 2000 to 2013. *JACC Heart Failure* 3 (12): 933–941. https://doi.org/10.1016/j.jchf.2015.07.012.

20 White, A.J., Ozminkowski, R.J., Hassol, A. et al. (1998). The effects of New York state's ban on multiple listing for cadaveric kidney transplantation. *Health Services Research* 33 (2 Pt 1): 205–222.

21 Bodenheimer, H.C. Jr., Okun, J.M., Tajik, W. et al. (2012). The impact of race on organ donation authorization discussed in the context of liver transplantation. *Transactions of the American Clinical and Climatological Association* 123: 64–78.

22 Siminoff, L.A., Lawrence, R.H., and Arnold, R.M. (2003). Comparison of black and white families' experiences and perceptions regarding organ donation requests. *Critical Care Medicine* 31 (1): 146–151. https://doi.org/10.1097/00003246-200301000-00023.

23 Siminoff, L.A., Traino, H.M., and Genderson, M.W. (2015). Communicating effectively about organ donation: a randomized trial of a behavioral communication intervention to improve discussions about donation. *Transplantation Direct* 1 (2): e5. https://doi.org/10.1097/TXD.0000000000000513.

24 Hall, W.J., Chapman, M.V., Lee, K.M. et al. (2015). Implicit racial/ethnic bias among health care professionals and its influence on health care outcomes: a systematic review. *American Journal of Public Health* 105 (12): e60–e76. https://doi.org/10.2105/AJPH.2015.302903.

25 OPTN (2022). OPTN board approves elimination of race-based calculation for transplant candidate listing. https://optn.transplant.hrsa.gov/news/optn-board-approves-elimination-of-race-based-calculation-for-transplant-candidate-listing/ (accessed 30 August 2024).

26 National Academies of Sciences, Engineering, and Medicine, Health and Medicine Division, Board on Health Care Services et al. (2022). Confronting and eliminating inequities in the organ transplantation system. Chapter 4. In: *Realizing the Promise of Equity in the Organ Transplantation System* (ed. M. Hackmann, R.A. English, and K.W. Kizer). Washington, DC: National Academies Press (US) https://www.ncbi.nlm.nih.gov/books/NBK580030/.

27 Persaud, N., Sabir, A., Woods, H. et al. (2023). Preventive care recommendations to promote health equity. *CMAJ: Canadian Medical Association Journal* 195 (37): E1250–E1273. https://doi.org/10.1503/cmaj.230237.

28 Cervantes, L., Hasnain-Wynia, R., Steiner, J.F. et al. (2020). Patient navigation: addressing social challenges in dialysis patients. *American Journal of Kidney Diseases: The Official Journal of the National Kidney Foundation* 76 (1): 121–129. https://doi.org/10.1053/j.ajkd.2019.06.007.

29 Rosenberg, P., Ciccarone, M., Seeman, B. et al. (2020). *Transforming Organ Donation in America.* The Bridgespan Group Bridgespan.org.

30 Vela, M.B., Erondu, A.I., Smith, N.A. et al. (2022). Eliminating explicit and implicit biases in health care: evidence and research needs. *Annual Review of Public Health* 43: 477–501.

31 Peña, A. (2022). Recalibrating transplant eligibility criteria: ensuring equitable access to organ transplantation for intellectually disabled persons. *American Journal of Law & Medicine* 48 (4): 380–411.

32 U.S. Attorney's Office, District of Massachusetts (2020). Massachusetts general hospital enters agreement with U.S. Attorney's office to better ensure equal access for individuals with disabilities. https://www.justice.gov/usao-ma/pr/massachusetts-general-hospital-enters-agreement-us-attorney-s-office-better-ensure-equal (accessed 30 August 2024).

33 Nishio Lucar, A.G., Patel, A., Mehta, S. et al. (2024). Expanding the access to kidney transplantation: strategies for kidney transplant programs. *Clinical Transplantation* 38 (5): e15315.

34 Bergeron, M. (2020). Transplant Center Criteria and Inequalities Within Transplant Wait Listing Process. https://stars.library.ucf.edu/cgi/viewcontent.cgi?article=1174&context=etd2020.

8

Transforming Blood Donation: Path to Inclusivity and Science-Based Guidelines

Abstract

The chapter discusses the evolution of the Food and Drug Administration's (FDA) blood donation guidelines for men who have sex with men (MSM) and the implications of these policies. It begins by introducing the FDA's proposal in January 2023 to revise its guidelines and eliminate categorical deferrals based on sexual orientation, replacing them with individualized risk assessments for all potential donors. The chapter then provides an overview of the finalized guidelines, which were announced on May 11, 2023, and how they aim to reduce stigma and increase the safety and availability of the US blood supply. Next, the chapter delves into the history of the FDA's restrictions on blood donation by MSM, starting from the initial nonmandatory guidance in 1983 to the evolution of the policy over time, including the one-year deferral period implemented in 2015 and the subsequent reduction to a three-month deferral during the COVID-19 pandemic. The chapter then examines the constitutionality of the FDA's previous MSM blood donation policies, arguing that they were both underinclusive and overinclusive, lacking a rational connection to the legitimate governmental interest of preventing the transmission of infectious diseases through blood transfusions. It highlights how advancements in testing technology have rendered the previous policies outdated and unnecessary. The chapter goes on to discuss how the FDA's prior guidance perpetuated harmful stereotypes and homophobia, contributing to negative mental health outcomes and higher substance abuse rates among affected individuals. It emphasizes the importance of the new guidelines in combating stigma and promoting inclusivity. Finally, the chapter addresses the need to rebuild trust and encourage inclusive blood donation among gay and bisexual men who may remain hesitant due to previous discriminatory policies. It suggests strategies for federal, state, and local governments, as well as blood collection organizations, to communicate the scientific basis for the policy change and engage in intentional outreach to LGBT communities to promote understanding and inclusivity.

Keywords   *blood donation; FDA guidelines; men who have sex with men (MSM); individual risk assessment; inclusivity; stigma reduction; HIV testing; public health policy*

> *John, a gay man in a monogamous relationship, has always wanted to donate blood to help others in need. However, due to the Food and Drug Administration's (FDA) previous lifetime deferral policy for men who have sex with men (MSM), he was barred from doing so, despite being HIV-negative and practicing safe sex. The new guidelines, which focus on individual risk assessments rather than sexual orientation, finally allow John to fulfill his desire to contribute to the blood supply.*
>
> *Sarah, a medical student, learns about the history of the FDA's blood donation policies for MSM during a lecture on public health. She is surprised to discover that the previous policies were not based on the latest scientific evidence and testing capabilities, but rather on outdated assumptions and stereotypes. Sarah realizes the importance of regularly reviewing and updating health policies to ensure they align with current medical knowledge and promote equity.*
>
> *Michael, a gay rights activist, has long advocated for the removal of the discriminatory blood donation ban on MSM. He has witnessed firsthand how the stigma perpetuated by these policies has negatively impacted the mental health and well-being of the Lesbian, Gay, Bisexual, and Transgender (LGBT) community. With the implementation of the new guidelines, Michael sees an opportunity to rebuild trust between the LGBT community and the healthcare system, and he works to encourage inclusive blood donation through targeted outreach and education efforts.*

8.1 Updated FDA Blood Donation Guidelines Promote Inclusivity and Safety

In January 2023, the FDA sought public input on a proposal to revise its guidelines regarding blood donations from MSM [1]. This proposal followed decades of restrictive policies that either banned MSM from donating blood or imposed deferral periods based on sexual activity. The outdated policies were both underinclusive and overinclusive, as they were based solely on whether a man had ever had sex with another man, without considering the actual risk of HIV infection. With advanced testing options now available, these restrictions are no longer justified. The ban has resulted in a 2–4% reduction in the total annual blood supply, equivalent to 345,400–615,300 pints of blood each year [2].

The FDA, responsible for licensing blood banks and ensuring the safety of the blood supply, has regulations that require blood collection establishments to screen donors for risk factors related to infectious diseases like HIV. Although these regulations do not specifically identify MSM as a high-risk group, the FDA has historically categorized them as such, preventing them from donating blood.

On May 11, 2023, the FDA finalized its updates to the blood donation guidelines for MSM [3]. The new guidelines eliminate categorical deferrals based on sexual orientation and implement individualized risk assessments for all potential donors. This shift aims to reduce stigma against gay and bisexual men and increase the safety and availability of the US blood supply. The updated policy aligns with practices in many other countries and focuses on recent sexual behavior rather than sexual orientation, promoting a more inclusive approach to blood donation.

Under the new guidelines, all potential donors, regardless of gender or sexual orientation, must disclose new or multiple sexual partners within the past three months and any history of anal sex within the same period. Those who have engaged in anal sex with new or multiple partners within the past three months will be deferred. Additionally, individuals taking oral pre-exposure prophylaxis (PrEP) for HIV prevention will be deferred for three months after their last dose, and those on injectable PrEP will be deferred for two years. This is to mitigate the risk of delayed HIV detection due to PrEP's impact on viral load.

The updated policy represents significant progress toward a more inclusive and safe blood donation system. It allows HIV-negative MSM with low transmission risk, such as those in monogamous relationships, to donate blood. By focusing on behaviors rather than sexual orientation, the new guidelines aim to enhance blood safety and remove previous discriminatory barriers. The FDA's changes are a crucial step forward in ensuring a sufficient and safe blood supply while fostering trust within the LGBTQ+ community.

> *"FDA's outdated ban was not supported by the science and further, it served to stigmatize gay men, bisexual men, and other men who have sex with men as a group that were considered 'unclean' or who are not worthy of being full participants in society."*
>
> Gretchen Newman, MD, Detroit Receiving Hospital

8.2 The Evolution of FDA Blood Donation Policies for Men Who Have Sex with Men

The FDA's restrictions on blood donation by MSM began in 1983 with nonmandatory guidance recommending that at-risk groups refrain from donating plasma or blood [4]. This guidance evolved over time, and by 1992, it had become a policy that excluded men who had sex with another man one or more times since 1977, with language recommending a "lifetime deferral" for MSM.

In December 2015, the FDA revised the ban, replacing it with a one-year deferral period [5]. Gay and bisexual men were allowed to donate blood if they had not engaged in any sexual activity with other men in the year prior to the donation. During the COVID-19 pandemic, the deferral period was further shortened to three months [6]. However, these restrictions applied even to gay men who were monogamous, tested HIV negative, and practiced safe sex.

Both of these policies were based on the premise that, at the time, existing blood donor testing would fail to detect all infected donors, leading to undetected infected donations slipping through the cracks if the ban were lifted. However, as will be explained later, this is no longer the case and has not been since 2002. There are many situations where MSM can safely give blood with minimal to no risk of it carrying HIV.

In January 2023, the FDA announced draft guidance to receive comments on revised recommendations for evaluating donor eligibility based on individual risk, rather than sexual orientation [1]. The guidance aimed to eliminate time-based deferrals for MSM and women who have sex with MSM. Instead, it recommends assessing donor eligibility using gender-inclusive individual risk-based questions relevant to HIV risk. These questions would ask all potential donors about new or multiple sex partners they have had in the past three months. Those who report having more than one new sexual partner during that time frame would be deferred if they reported having anal sex.

On May 11, 2023, the FDA finalized the guidelines proposed in January 2023 [3]. The new policy eliminates the categorical deferral for MSM and instead uses individualized risk assessments to screen potential donors for eligibility. All prospective donors, regardless of sex, sexual orientation, or gender identity, must disclose new or multiple sexual partners within the past three months, followed by a question on a history of anal sex in the same time frame. Individuals who have engaged in anal sex with either new or multiple partners in the past three months would be deferred. The three-month deferrals for individuals with a history of exchanging sex for money or nonprescription injection drug use, as well as the lifetime deferral for individuals with a history of a positive HIV test, remain unchanged. Additionally, the guidance recommends that individuals who take oral medications to prevent HIV (PrEP) would be subject to a three-month deferral period starting from their last dose, while those receiving injectable PrEP would be subject to a two-year deferral period.

8.3 Challenging the Constitutionality of FDA's MSM Blood Donation Policies

Advocates argue that the FDA's previous "lifetime deferral policy" and time-bound deferral policies for gay men donating blood were unconstitutional because they treated gay men differently than similarly situated straight donors without a rational connection to a permissible state end. When determining the constitutionality of laws that do not affect an individual's fundamental rights, judges apply rational basis review. In her concurrence in Lawrence v. Texas, Justice O'Connor stated that rational basis scrutiny applied, but her reasoning suggested that a higher level of scrutiny could be appropriate when laws disparately impact LGBT communities [7]. Although lower courts have applied this unevenly since then, it indicates that laws based solely on moral disapproval of a group, like a bare desire to harm the group, are an interest that is insufficient to satisfy rational basis review under the Equal Protection Clause [8]. Without further clarification, the FDA's previous "lifelong deferral" and time-bound deferral policies would likely have been subject to rational basis review [9].

To satisfy rational basis review, a government policy or law must (i) serve a legitimate governmental interest and (ii) have a rational connection to that permissible state end. The FDA has a legitimate interest in regulating blood donations to prevent the transmission of infectious diseases [10]. However, if the government interest is framed differently, there is a narrow chance that the previous policies could have failed this prong. In her Lawrence concurrence, Justice O'Connor explained that the only governmental interest furthered by the Texas sodomy law was moral disapproval of homosexuality – an illegitimate government interest because legal classifications must not be "drawn for the purpose of disadvantaging the group burdened by the law." Although Justice O'Connor was not in the majority on this issue and it's unclear how the current Court would rule, some advocates argue that the FDA's previous deferral guidance operated separately, drawn merely for the purpose of targeting MSMs, even though HIV transmission can occur among other populations [11].

The stronger argument against the constitutionality of the FDA's previous rules on MSM blood donations under rational basis review is that the FDA's chosen method lacked a "rational connection to the legitimate governmental interest." If the FDA's purpose of avoiding infectious disease transmission through blood transfusions is valid, the government must demonstrate that its chosen solution was reasonably related to addressing that policy goal. There is a strong argument that the second prong was not satisfied by either the time or lifetime deferral policies because a bright-line rule that only considered sexual orientation was both under- and over-inclusive [12].

The previous policies were underinclusive because they failed to identify other high-risk populations for contracting HIV and AIDS. While gay, bisexual, and other MSM are most likely to be affected by AIDS, women can still contract it, and the policy did not require blood collection centers to inquire further if a man stated he did not have sex with other men. In 2019, heterosexual people accounted for 22%

of new HIV infections [13]. Men who do not identify as having sexual contact with other men were not asked about sexual activity and did not have to undergo any waiting period before donating blood. Moreover, under the more recent time deferral policies, the FDA allowed for self-identification and self-reporting of gender, making no distinction in the policy between cisgender MSM and transgender MSM [14]. If the FDA's true goal was to eliminate the potential for undetected infected donations to enter the "blood pool," these populations could still have posed a threat [15].

Simultaneously, the previous policies were also overinclusive. The lifetime deferral applied to MSM at any point since 1977, regardless of whether it was only one partner or one time. This meant that men in monogamous relationships or men who no longer had sex with men would have been excluded from the donor population, even if there was no chance of them carrying HIV. Additionally, MSM's risk of contracting HIV has decreased. Medical interventions, such as PrEP, have been shown to be highly effective, reducing the risk of HIV infection from sex by about 99% [16]. Thus, the FDA's previous policies no longer served their intended goal because they prevented MSM from giving blood solely based on prior sexual encounters without considering medical realities [17].

Finally, the lifetime deferral and time-bound deferrals were not reasonably connected to the FDA's goal of avoiding infectious disease transmission through blood transfusions because the technological reality has changed since 1983 [18]. During the initial AIDS epidemic, there was no way to identify and test for AIDS and HIV, so the expansive policy made sense as there was no other way for the FDA and blood collection centers to detect the virus. However, as testing developed and became more reliable in identifying the virus, the lifetime deferral policy became outdated. Now, there is universal testing of blood donations that can detect human antibodies produced in response to HIV exposure, and the initial risk of a false positive has decreased with a confirmatory test that is 100% effective for detecting HIV antibodies [19]. Furthermore, since 2002, the routine use of nucleic acid testing for HIV has further reduced the risk of transmission to about one unit per two million donations [20].

In May 2023, the FDA finalized its updated guidance, which eliminates the categorical deferral for MSM and instead uses individualized risk assessments to screen potential donors for eligibility. This new policy addresses many of the constitutional concerns raised by advocates regarding the previous deferral policies. The FDA's original rationale for the previous guidance no longer holds and should not be considered to have a rational connection to its purpose [21].

Policy and Equity in FDA's MSM Blood Donation Guidelines

Aspect	Previous Policy	New Policy (May 2023 Update)	Equity Implications
Deferral Basis	Categorical exclusion based on sexual orientation	Individual risk assessment based on recent sexual behavior	Reduces discrimination by eliminating categorical exclusions; focuses on actual risk behavior rather than sexual orientation
Deferral Period for MSM	Lifetime deferral (pre-2015), one-year deferral (2015), three-month deferral (COVID-19 pandemic adjustment)	No categorical deferral; deferrals based on reporting new or multiple sexual partners and anal sex within three months	More inclusive, allowing MSM in monogamous relationships or those who practice safe sex to donate, thus reducing stigma and promoting equality

(Continued)

Aspect	Previous Policy	New Policy (May 2023 Update)	Equity Implications
PrEP Users	Not specifically addressed	Three-month deferral after last dose for oral PrEP users; two-year deferral for injectable PrEP users	Acknowledges advancements in HIV prevention but still imposes some deferral to ensure safety due to potential impacts on HIV detection
Screening Questions	Focused on whether a man has ever had sex with another man	Focused on recent sexual behavior (new or multiple partners, history of anal sex)	Shifts from broad exclusion based on sexual orientation to specific risk-related questions applicable to all donors, promoting fairness, and reducing unnecessary exclusions
Communication and Outreach	Minimal targeted outreach	Emphasis on communicating scientific advancements and engaging LGBT communities	Essential for rebuilding trust and encouraging participation from previously excluded groups, ensuring equitable access to donation opportunities
Impact on Blood Supply	Estimated reduction of 2–4% in total annual blood supply due to MSM deferral	Potential increase in blood supply by including low-risk MSM donors	Addresses blood shortages by allowing more individuals to donate, improving overall supply while maintaining safety

8.4   FDA's New Guidelines Combat Stigma and Promote Inclusivity

The FDA's prior guidance on blood donations not only lacked scientific grounding but also perpetuated harmful stereotypes and homophobia [22]. By basing deferral decisions solely on whether a potential donor was a man who had ever had sex with another man, the policy reinforced the false perception that being gay or bisexual is inherently unsafe or unhealthy. This stereotype, exacerbated during the AIDS epidemic and pervasive in pop culture and American discourse, fails to recognize the diversity and actual risks within these communities. Such stigmatization contributes to negative mental health outcomes and higher substance abuse rates among affected individuals [23].

Additionally, when healthcare regulations are not grounded in medical science, they can foster a perception that the healthcare system is unwelcoming and unsupportive. This can lead individuals from targeted groups to delay or avoid seeking preventive care. The shift to gender-neutral, risk-based guidelines, as finalized in May 2023, aims to combat this stigma [24]. By evaluating individual risk rather than applying broad, population-based exclusions, the new approach promotes inclusivity and reduces the negative impacts of previous discriminatory policies.

8.5   Conclusion: Rebuilding Trust and Encouraging Inclusive Blood Donation

Even as the FDA accepts comments on its proposed guidance, gay and bisexual men may remain hesitant to donate blood due to previous discriminatory policies and lingering stigma around HIV transmission. Once the new guidelines are finalized, it will be crucial for federal, state, and local governments, as well as blood collection organizations, to clearly communicate that improved science around HIV transmission and increased availability of treatments support this shift in donor requirements [25]. Intentional outreach to LGBT communities will be essential [26].

These institutions should provide resources to help men determine their eligibility for blood donation [27]. This can include local discussions, community-driven social marketing, and other outreach efforts tailored to the specific needs and concerns of LGBT individuals [28]. By promoting understanding and inclusivity, these efforts can help rebuild trust and encourage more people to participate in blood donation [29].

References

1 FDA (2023). *FDA Proposes Individual Risk Assessment for Blood Donations, While Continuing to Safeguard U.S. Blood Supply*. U.S. Food and Drug Administration https://www.fda.gov/news-events/press-announcements/fda-proposes-individual-risk-assessment-blood-donations-while-continuing-safeguard-us-blood-supply.

2 Williams Institute (2014). *Update: Effects of Lifting Blood Donation Bans on Men Who Have Sex with Men*. UCLA School of Law.

3 FDA (2023). *FDA Finalizes Move to Recommend Individual Risk Assessment to Determine Eligibility for Blood Donations*. U.S. Food and Drug Administration https://www.fda.gov/news-events/press-announcements/fda-finalizes-move-recommend-individual-risk-assessment-determine-eligibility-blood-donations.

4 Bensing, D.J. (2011). Science or stigma: Potential challenges to the FDA's ban on gay blood. *University of Pennsylvania Journal of Constitutional Law* 14: 485.

5 FDA (2015). Revised recommendations for reducing the risk of human immunodeficiency virus transmission by blood and blood products. https://www.fda.gov/media/92490/download (accessed 29 August 2024).

6 FDA (2020). Coronavirus (COVID-19) update: FDA provides updated guidance to address the urgent need for blood during the pandemic. https://www.fda.gov/news-events/press-announcements/coronavirus-covid-19-update-fda-provides-updated-guidance-address-urgent-need-blood-during-pandemic (accessed 29 August 2024).

7 Leslie, C.R. (2004). Lawrence v. Texas as the perfect storm. *UCD Law Review* 38: 509.

8 Lund, N. and McGinnis, J.O. (2003). Lawrence v. Texas and judicial hubris. *Michigan Law Review* 102: 1555.

9 Gallagher, B. (2018). A decade of progress, but continued disparities: a look at the FDA's blood donor deferral policy for men who have sex with men. *Quinnipiac Health Law Journal* 21: 215.

10 Galarneau, C. (2010). Blood donation, deferral, and discrimination: FDA donor deferral policy for men who have sex with men. *The American Journal of Bioethics* 10 (2): 29–39.

11 Casey, B. (2007). Illicit regulation: a framework for challenging the procedural validity of the gay blood ban. *Food and Drug Law Journal* 62: 551.

12 Larkin, E. (2009). *The Exclusion of Gay Men from Blood Donation: A Constitutional Analysis*, 1–33. American University Washington College of Law.

13 Crepaz, N., Hess, K.L., Purcell, D.W., and Hall, H.I. (2019). Estimating national rates of HIV infection among MSM, persons who inject drugs, and heterosexuals in the United States. *AIDS* 33 (4): 701–708.

14 Morrison, M.A., Hoehn, D., and Cawston, A. (2021). Cisgender and transgender men who have sex with men and blood donation policy in the United States and Canada. *Transfusion* 61 (5): 1492–1502.

15 Piliavin, J.A. and Callero, P.L. (1991). *Giving Blood: The Development of an Altruistic Identity*. Johns Hopkins University Press.

16 Spinner, C.D., Boesecke, C., Zink, A. et al. (2016). HIV pre-exposure prophylaxis (PrEP): a review of current knowledge of oral systemic HIV PrEP in humans. *Infection* 44: 151–158.

17 Goldberg, N.G. (2010). The impact of blood donor policy on the health and well-being of gay and bisexual men. *Dissertation Abstracts International* 71 (03).

18 Adkins, R. (2016). Blood donations and the lifetime ban: an examination of the policy and constitutional concerns surrounding the prohibition on blood donations from men who have sex with men. *University of Louisville Law Review* 55 (1): 1–29.

19 Custer, B., Kessler, D., Vahidnia, F. et al. (2015). Risk factors for retrovirus and hepatitis virus infections in accepted blood donors. *Transfusion* 55 (5): 1098–1107.

20 Stramer, S.L. (2007). Current risks of transfusion-transmitted agents: a review. *Archives of Pathology & Laboratory Medicine* 131 (5): 702–707.

21 Miyashita, A. and Gates, G.J. (2014). *An Analysis of the FDA's Rationale for Excluding Men Who Have Sex with Men From Donating Blood*. Williams Institute, UCLA School of Law.

22 Caplan, A.L. (2010). Blood stains: why an absurd policy banning gay men as blood donors has not been changed. *The American Journal of Bioethics* 10 (2): 1–2.

23 Meyer, I.H. (2003). Prejudice, social stress, and mental health in lesbian, gay, and bisexual populations: conceptual issues and research evidence. *Psychological Bulletin* 129 (5): 674–697.

24 Goldberg, N.G. and Gates, G.J. (2010). *Effects of Lifting Blood Donation Bans on Men Who Have Sex with Men*. Williams Institute, UCLA School of Law.

25 Berkman, A. and Zhou, L. (2015). Misinformation, discrimination, and the blood supply: the FDA's role in protecting public health. *American Journal of Public Health* 105 (5): 867–868.

26 Witteck, L. (2016). Giving life: why the FDA should amend its policy on gay blood donation. *Seton Hall Law Review* 46 (4): 1011–1044.

27 Schreiber, G.B., Glynn, S.A., Damesyn, M.A. et al. (2003). Lapsed donors: an untapped resource. *Transfusion* 43 (1): 17–24.

28 Liszewski, W., Terndrup, C., Jackson, N.R. et al. (2017). The beliefs and willingness of men who have sex with men to comply with a one year blood donation deferral policy: a cross-sectional study. *BMC Public Health* 17 (1): 1–8.

29 Grenfell, P., Nutland, W., McManus, S. et al. (2011). Views and experiences of men who have sex with men on the ban on blood donation: a cross sectional survey with qualitative interviews. *BMJ* 343: d5604.

9

Addressing Barriers and Disparities in Clinical Trials: FDA's Diversity Plan

Abstract

This chapter discusses the importance of enhancing diversity in clinical trials and the various barriers and disparities that hinder diverse representation. It begins by highlighting the crucial role of clinical trials in ensuring the safety and effectiveness of medical interventions, and the significance of reflecting the diverse populations that will ultimately receive these treatments. The chapter then delves into the current state of biomedical research, revealing the underrepresentation of racial and ethnic minorities in clinical trials and the factors contributing to these disparities, such as persistent racial disparities in health, limited healthcare access, and mistrust in the healthcare system. The chapter proceeds to outline the legislative and regulatory efforts undertaken by the FDA and Congress to address the issue of diversity in clinical trials, including the passage of various acts and the issuance of guidance documents. It then explores the potential impact of increased diversity on medical outcomes, such as individualized dosing recommendations and the identification of population-specific adverse events. The chapter also discusses the limitations and challenges in enforcing diversity requirements, such as the FDA's lack of statutory authority to enforce its guidance and the evolving nature of racial and ethnic classifications. It then offers strategies to increase access and participation in clinical trials, such as providing financial reimbursement, partnering with community-based organizations, and engaging with primary care providers (PCPs). Furthermore, the chapter proposes incentives and post-approval requirements to promote diversity, including tax credits, fast-track eligibility, and mandatory post-launch real-world data collection. Finally, it concludes by outlining future steps and expanding diversity efforts, emphasizing the need for continued education, outreach, and consideration of other underrepresented groups, such as pregnant women, older people, and people with disabilities.

Keywords   *clinical trial diversity; FDA guidelines; barriers to participation; health disparities; trust in healthcare; legislative efforts; recruitment strategies; underrepresented populations*

Jennifer, a 35-year-old African American woman, was diagnosed with an aggressive form of breast cancer. When her oncologist mentioned the possibility of participating in a clinical trial for a promising new treatment, Jennifer hesitated. She had heard stories of the Tuskegee experiment and other instances of medical mistreatment in her community, leading to a deep-rooted mistrust in the healthcare system. Jennifer ultimately decided not to participate, wondering if the trial would truly prioritize her well-being.

Kamal, a 62-year-old South Asian man, suffered from chronic pain due to osteoarthritis. His primary care physician suggested a clinical trial for a novel pain management device, but Kamal faced several barriers. The trial site was located far from his home, and he lacked reliable transportation. Additionally, the informed consent forms were only available in English, making it difficult for Kamal to fully understand the risks and benefits of participation.

Dr. Emily Nguyen, a researcher at a major university hospital, was designing a clinical trial for a groundbreaking diabetes medication. She recognized the importance of recruiting a diverse participant population to ensure the drug's safety and efficacy across different racial and ethnic groups. However, Dr. Nguyen struggled to connect with community-based organizations and primary care providers serving underrepresented populations, hindering her ability to build trust and increase diverse enrollment in her trial.

9.1 Enhancing Diversity in Clinical Trials: Addressing Barriers and Disparities

Clinical trials are crucial for ensuring the safety, proper labeling, and effectiveness of drugs, biologics, and devices approved by the FDA [1]. It is essential that these trials reflect the diverse populations of patients who will ultimately receive the approved interventions. The outcomes of clinical trials directly impact the treatments and practices available to patient populations, and different stages of clinical trials have varying implications for safety, contraindications, side effects, risks, and efficacy. Moreover, race and ethnicity are important considerations during drug development because factors that affect pharmacokinetics, pharmacodynamics, safety, and efficacy can differ among racial and ethnic groups [2]. These factors include genetic polymorphisms in metabolism or transport pathways, dose-proportionality of pharmacokinetics, steepness of the dose– or exposure–response relationship, therapeutic index, bioavailability, concomitant medications, medical practices, body habitus, and diet. If data demonstrates demographic variance during the clinical trial process, the FDA could make individualized label recommendations for subgroups, enabling providers to better counsel their patients.

However, most biomedical research has failed to keep pace with the increasing diversity of the US population. Clinical trials often do not adequately represent either the general population or the proportion of demographics with the incidence of the diseases the drug, biologic, or device is intended to treat or prevent. An analysis of cancer therapeutics approved by the FDA between 2012 and 2017 found that while clinical trials used to support labeling decisions adequately represented white women, only 27% represented older adults, and a mere 11% met the bar for representation of racial and ethnic groups [3].

Several factors contribute to these disparities. Patient participation in clinical trials is strongly influenced by persistent racial disparities in health, limited healthcare access, and negative encounters with healthcare providers [4]. Studies have shown that the least deprived patients were nearly twice as likely to be referred for early-phase oncology clinical trials, while non-white populations were less likely to be recruited [5]. In a hospital trust in England, non-white minorities were 30% less likely to be recruited than white patients [6]. Lower access rates for clinical trials reflect broader issues with healthcare access stemming from structural and historical problems with people of color's experiences in the healthcare system and social determinants of health [7]. For example, African Americans and other marginalized groups have higher rates of mistrust in academic, healthcare, and research institutions due to historic events such as the Tuskegee experiment [8]. Some communities even perceive that research might benefit white participants or the research institution more than the underrepresented individuals enrolled in the study, or that researchers might misuse information in a way that could jeopardize federal government benefits or impact a family member's immigration status [9]. This mistrust is compounded by a lack of cultural diversity and competence among physicians and differential treatment compared to white people.

Despite the well-documented presence of mistrust within underrepresented populations, some research suggests that these groups are just as willing to participate in clinical trials, indicating that access to clinical trials might be the underlying problem [10]. The FDA notes additional barriers to the participation of racial and ethnic minorities, including inadequate recruitment and retention efforts, high frequencies of study visits, time and resource constraints, transportation difficulties, language and cultural differences, health literacy, religion, limited healthcare system access, and lack of education about clinical trials and what participation entails [11]. Some of these barriers could be addressed through strategic and intentional clinical trial study design to ease the burden of participation, while others may be better suited to targeted outreach and education for providers working with larger proportions of patients from lower-income or diverse populations [5].

> *"It's critical that we increase participation from diverse communities in clinical research and generate representative data to strengthen our science and better inform treatment decisions."*
> Nicole Richie, PhD, Global Head of Health Equity and Population Science at Roche

9.2 Legislative and Regulatory Efforts to Enhance Clinical Trial Diversity

The FDA and Congress have been working to address the underrepresentation of diverse subjects in clinical trials for years, beginning with efforts to promote the evaluation of drug effectiveness based on gender in the 1980s [12]. However, a 1992 report concluded that women were underrepresented in clinical trials, and data was not analyzed for differences in response by sex [13].

In 2012, Congress passed Section 907 of the FDA Safety and Innovation Act, directing the FDA to investigate the inclusion of demographic subgroups in clinical trials and the availability of subgroup safety and efficacy data [14]. The FDA's 2013 report on the demographic makeup of research subjects in clinical trials for 72 drugs, biologics, and Class III devices revealed that while some sponsors adequately recruited subjects reflecting the distribution of disease in the population for age and sex, clinical trials lacked representative participation by racial minorities [15].

Congress enacted the FDA Reauthorization Act of 2017 (FDARA), requiring the FDA to publish guidance on enhancing diversity in clinical trials [16]. The guidance was finalized in 2020, and in 2022, the FDA issued guidance recommending that clinical trial sponsors develop diversity action plans to improve the enrollment of racial minority populations in clinical trials [17]. The guidance required sponsors of any Phase 3 or pivotal drug study or device trial to submit diversity action plans alongside the study protocol. In 2023, Congress enacted the Food and Drug Omnibus Reform Act of 2022 (FDORA), mandating the FDA to issue or update guidance on the format or content of these diversity action plans by the end of the year. The Act provides extensive detail on what the guidance and diversity action plans should cover, largely tracking the FDA's recommendations in the April 2022 guidance [18].

Under the 2022 guidance and FDORA, diversity action plans should include the sponsor's goals for clinical study enrollment, disaggregated by age group, sex, and racial and ethnic characteristics; the rationale for these enrollment goals, including information about the disease or condition and its prevalence or incidence among various demographics; and how the sponsor intends to meet these goals, including demographic-specific outreach and enrollment strategies, inclusion and exclusion practices, and diversity training for study personnel [19].

9.3 Potential Impact of Diversity in Clinical Trials on Medical Outcomes

In the short term, the guidance and FDORA's statutory mandate will continue to focus FDA's attention on racial and ethnic diversity in clinical trials. Directly incorporating diversity into the goals and structures of a clinical trial could have significant medical impact. For instance, additional data may lead to different dosing recommendations for specific racial populations, recommendations for considering alternative therapy for specific populations, additional warnings and precautions for specific racial populations, likelihood of contraindications, or even whether a drug is indicated for specific racial groups and not others. This has already happened in the past when there was enough data to make these determinations. For example, Rosuvastatin has specific dosing for Asians, who had clinically relevant differences in pharmacokinetics [20]. Similarly, research found that Asian ancestry, among other factors, alters response to certain tyrosine kinase inhibitors (TKIs) like gefitinib and erlotinib [21]. This is largely due to the higher incidence of mutations in the epidermal growth factor receptor (EGFR) which these drugs target.

Moreover, population differences in adverse events have also been reported previously for several drugs, leading to the approval or withdrawal of a drug from specific markets. For instance, ibufenac, used in the treatment of rheumatoid arthritis, was never approved in the United States and was withdrawn in the United Kingdom because of hepatotoxicity, although it remained available in Japan because hepatotoxicity was not a concern in that population [22].

9.4 Limitations and Challenges in Enforcing Diversity Requirements

While the FDA's guidance and FDORA are a good first step, the FDA has no ability to enforce the requirements set out in its guidance. The FDA does not fund investigational drug trials; it only assesses them. This means that the FDA has less room to set restrictions on what can and cannot be included compared to the NIH. However, the FDA does have the ability to put clinical trials on hold in some situations where the trial structures do not seem likely to yield the information that the FDA needs to make safety and adequacy determinations. For instance, a law in 2000 gave the FDA the power to put a clinical trial on hold if men or women were excluded due to reproductive potential, although it has never been used [23]. After receiving some of the reports following FDORA, a reasonable next step would be for Congress to require the FDA to consider whether a trial population adequately represents the diversity of the target population for which the drug is intended. Additionally, the FDA can mandate that demographic information be made public across all stages of the trials. Ultimately, it would be even more useful if the FDA had some statutory ability to enforce these requirements, rather than merely considering them when evaluating the data and applications.

Another challenge that faces mandatory increases in diversity across clinical trials is that the current perception of racial and ethnic classification is based on social constructs that evolve over time and whose definitions are not necessarily specific [24]. As these requirements and plans continue, it is important for those designing clinical trials to understand the proper ways to disaggregate data to fully comprehend which populations are affected (e.g. Asians – East Asians? Southeast Asians? South Asians?). Furthermore, because race and ethnicity are usually self-reported, inquiring deeper into what an individual means when they identify could be helpful in obtaining useful data.

9.5 Strategies to Increase Access and Participation in Clinical Trials

The FDA guidance offers several suggestions for increasing access to clinical trials, such as providing financial reimbursement for expenses incurred, offering language access, and partnering with community-based organizations to support participants. When designing trials, supervisors could reexamine inclusion and exclusion criteria to ensure they are appropriate for the specific study. Additionally, they could work to expand trials to more sites or use technology to reach more patients. Research shows that the distance between a patient's home community and the location of health care and clinical research is a barrier – the greater the distance between home communities and where patients are required to be present for involvement, study visits, or exit interviews, the lower the likelihood of participation [25]. To address this, supervisors could consider providing reliable transportation and child care to reduce the opportunity cost of participating.

Strong, trusting relationships with PCPs have been found to have significant impacts on research engagement [26]. One study found that having a PCP was the strongest predictor of clinical trial follow-up among a population of predominantly ethnically underrepresented individuals. This presents an opportunity for clinical trial developers to reach out to physicians and other providers working outside of academic centers to educate them on the clinical trial process, their specific trial, and its relevance to future participants. In turn, this education could lead to referrals and assistance throughout the process.

9.6 Incentives and Post-Approval Requirements to Promote Diversity

To support its guidance, the FDA could introduce additional incentives for creating studies that adequately reflect the communities the drug or device will serve. For instance, studies that achieve the target goals might receive tax credits, fast-track eligibility, reduced fees, and extended market exclusivity. Additionally, the FDA should relax rules on reimbursing minority study participants and cover expenses for transportation, dependent care, and lost wages to ensure that its existing regulations do not hinder researchers' ability to help patients access these opportunities.

If final data or study results fail to reach the diversity goals, the FDA could require a sub-study on a representative population of ethnically identical individuals or mandatory post-launch real-world data collection to assess product safety and efficacy in local populations [27]. This approach is not new; for example, in the past, the FDA required Simeprevier to conduct a post-approval clinical trial to assess the serious risk of increased frequency of adverse events in patients of East Asian ancestry, and Loflupane to conduct a clinical trial that assesses the agreement between imaging rules and diagnostic outcomes among non-Caucasian and Caucasian patients. Incorporating these types of post-approval checks will encourage researchers to design their initial studies correctly from the outset.

9.7 Conclusion: Future Steps and Expanding Diversity Efforts

Moving forward, the FDA will issue additional guidance clarifying specific topics, and submit annual reports to Congress as the program progresses [28]. However, more can be done on both the study design and regulatory sides to address these priorities and make the process easier for study organizers and patients alike [29]. The FDA should use FDORA's requirements and the guidance creation process as another opportunity to educate minority communities about the process and reach out to communities that could benefit from the additional information and access. Furthermore, although race and ethnicity are the primary targets of these policies, there is further space for the inclusion of other underrepresented groups, such as pregnant women, older people, and people with disabilities. As more guidance is drafted and trial supervisors develop their diversity plans, all stakeholders in the clinical trial space need to consider how patients weigh the costs and benefits of participation and find ways to ensure that people of lower socioeconomic groups can afford to join.

Key Policies and Their Impact on Equity in Clinical Trial Diversity

Policy/Initiative	Description	Impact on Equity
Civil Rights Act of 1964	Prohibited racial discrimination in federally funded programs, including medical research	Aimed to reduce racial discrimination, although enforcement has been inconsistent
National Research Act of 1974	Established the National Commission for the Protection of Human Subjects of Biomedical and Behavioral Research, resulting in the Belmont Report	Introduced ethical principles (respect, beneficence, and justice) to protect vulnerable populations in research

Policy/Initiative	Description	Impact on Equity
NIH Revitalization Act of 1993	Mandated the inclusion of women and minorities in NIH-funded clinical research	Increased participation of women and minorities in clinical trials, although gaps remain
FDA Safety and Innovation Act of 2012 (FDASIA)	Required the FDA to evaluate the inclusion of demographic subgroups in clinical trials and report to Congress	Promoted transparency and accountability in the inclusion of diverse populations in clinical trials
FDA's 2016 Guidance on Race and Ethnicity Data Collection	Provided instructions for the standardized collection of race and ethnicity data in clinical trials	Aimed to improve the consistency and quality of demographic data, enhancing the ability to analyze subgroup differences
CMS Coverage for Clinical Trials (2000)	Directed Medicare to cover routine costs for patients participating in clinical trials	Improved access for financially disadvantaged patients, although barriers like transportation and time off work remain
Affordable Care Act (2010)	Established the National Institute on Minority Health and Health Disparities and mandated insurance coverage for clinical trial participation	Expanded access to clinical trials for low-income and minority patients, reducing financial barriers
FDA's 2020 Guidance on Enhancing Diversity	Advised sponsors to include diverse populations by modifying eligibility criteria and improving enrollment practices	Encouraged more inclusive clinical trial designs, although enforcement remains a challenge

References

1 Dabrowska, A. and Thaul, S. (2018). *How FDA Approves Drugs and Regulates Their Safety and Effectiveness*, 1–25. Washington: Congressional Research Service.

2 Chen, M.L. (2006). Ethnic or racial differences revisited: impact of dosage regimen and dosage form on pharmacokinetics and pharmacodynamics. *Clinical Pharmacokinetics* 45: 957–964.

3 Varma, T., Mello, M., Ross, J.S. et al. (2023). Metrics, baseline scores, and a tool to improve sponsor performance on clinical trial diversity: retrospective cross sectional study. *BMJ Medicine* 2 (1): e000395. https://doi.org/10.1136/bmjmed-2022-000395.

4 Murthy, V.H., Krumholz, H.M., and Gross, C.P. (2004). Participation in cancer clinical trials: race-, sex-, and age-based disparities. *JAMA* 291 (22): 2720–2726.

5 Duma, N., Vera Aguilera, J., Paludo, J. et al. (2018). Representation of minorities and women in oncology clinical trials: review of the past 14 years. *Journal of Oncology Practice* 14 (1): e1–e10. https://doi.org/10.1200/JOP.2017.025288.

6 Masood, Y., Bower, P., Waheed, M.W. et al. (2019). Synthesis of researcher reported strategies to recruit adults of ethnic minorities to clinical trials in the United Kingdom: a systematic review. *Contemporary Clinical Trials* 78: 1–10.

7 Tunis, S.R., Stryer, D.B., and Clancy, C.M. (2003). Practical clinical trials: increasing the value of clinical research for decision making in clinical and health policy. *JAMA* 290 (12): 1624–1632.

8 Scharff, D.P., Mathews, K.J., Jackson, P. et al. (2010). More than Tuskegee: understanding mistrust about research participation. *Journal of Health Care for the Poor and Underserved* 21 (3): 879.

9 George, S., Duran, N., and Norris, K. (2014). A systematic review of barriers and facilitators to minority research participation among African Americans, Latinos, Asian Americans, and Pacific Islanders. *American Journal of Public Health* 104 (2): e16–e31. https://doi.org/10.2105/AJPH.2013.301706.

10 Wendler, D., Kington, R., Madans, J. et al. (2006). Are racial and ethnic minorities less willing to participate in health research? *PLoS Medicine* 3 (2): e19.

11 Thakur, N., Lovinsky-Desir, S., Appell, D. et al. (2021). Enhancing recruitment and retention of minority populations for clinical research in pulmonary, critical care, and sleep medicine: an official American Thoracic Society research statement. *American Journal of Respiratory and Critical Care Medicine* 204 (3): e26–e50.

12 Ramamoorthy, A., Araojo, R., Vasisht, K.P. et al. (2023). Promoting clinical trial diversity: a highlight of select US FDA initiatives. *Clinical Pharmacology & Therapeutics* 113 (3): 528–535.

13 Bennett, J.C. (1993). Inclusion of women in clinical trials – policies for population subgroups. *New England Journal of Medicine* 329 (4): 288–292.

14 Lennox, K. (2014). *Substantially Unequivalent: Reforming FDA Regulation of Medical Devices*, 1363. University of Illinois Law Review.

15 Eshera, N., Itana, H., Zhang, L. et al. (2015). Demographics of clinical trials participants in pivotal clinical trials for new molecular entity drugs and biologics approved by FDA from 2010 to 2012. *American Journal of Therapeutics* 22 (6): 435–455.

16 Van Norman, G.A. (2020). Update to drugs, devices, and the FDA: how recent legislative changes have impacted approval of new therapies. *Basic to Translational Science* 5 (8): 831–839.

17 Versavel, S., Subasinghe, A., Johnson, K. et al. (2023). Diversity, equity, and inclusion in clinical trials: a practical guide from the perspective of a trial sponsor. *Contemporary Clinical Trials* 126: 107092.

18 Green, A.K., Trivedi, N., Hsu, J.J. et al. (2022). Despite the FDA's five-year plan, black patients remain inadequately represented in clinical trials for drugs: study examines FDA's five-year action plan aimed at improving diversity in and transparency of pivotal clinical trials for newly-approved drugs. *Health Affairs* 41 (3): 368–374.

19 Adashi, E.Y. and Cohen, I.G. (2023). The FDA initiative to assure racial and ethnic diversity in clinical trials. *The Journal of the American Board of Family Medicine* 36 (2): 366–368.

20 Lee, E., Ryan, S., Birmingham, B. et al. (2005). Rosuvastatin pharmacokinetics and pharmacogenetics in white and Asian subjects residing in the same environment. *Clinical Pharmacology & Therapeutics* 78 (4): 330–341.

21 Touma, J.A., McLachlan, A.J., and Gross, A.S. (2017). The role of ethnicity in personalized dosing of small molecule tyrosine kinase inhibitors used in oncology. *Translational Cancer Research* 6 (Suppl 10).

22 Jasani, M.K., Downie, W.W., Samuels, B.M., and Buchanan, W.W. (1968). Ibuprofen in rheumatoid arthritis. Clinical study of analgesic and anti-inflammatory activity. *Annals of the Rheumatic Diseases* 27 (5): 457.

23 Knepper, T.C. and McLeod, H.L. (2018). When will clinical trials finally reflect diversity? *Nature* 557 (7704): 157–159.

24 Popejoy, A.B. and Fullerton, S.M. (2016). Genomics is failing on diversity. *Nature* 538 (7624): 161–164.

25 Goodman, D.C., Fisher, E., Stukel, T.A., and Chang, C.H. (1997). The distance to community medical care and the likelihood of hospitalization: is closer always better? *American Journal of Public Health* 87 (7): 1144–1150.

26 Murray, B. and McCrone, S. (2015). An integrative review of promoting trust in the patient–primary care provider relationship. *Journal of Advanced Nursing* 71 (1): 3–23.

27 Unger, J.M. (2021). Representativeness in premarketing vs postmarketing US food and drug administration trials. *JAMA Network Open* 4 (4): –e217159.

28 Bibbins-Domingo, K., Helman, A., and Dzau, V.J. (2022). The imperative for diversity and inclusion in clinical trials and health research participation. *JAMA* 327 (23): 2283–2284.

29 Kelsey, M.D., Patrick-Lake, B., Abdulai, R. et al. (2022). Inclusion and diversity in clinical trials: actionable steps to drive lasting change. *Contemporary Clinical Trials* 116: 106740.

10

Strengthening the Safety Net to Mitigate Reproductive Health Inequity After Dobbs

Abstract

The Supreme Court's Dobbs v. Jackson Women's Health decision overturning Roe v. Wade has eliminated federal protections for abortion access, allowing states to ban or severely restrict abortion. This shift will disproportionately impact low-income women, women of color, and other marginalized groups who already face systemic barriers to reproductive healthcare. As these populations see their reproductive autonomy further constrained, safety-net providers like community health centers, family planning clinics, and public hospitals will play a critical role in addressing the fallout. To mitigate the most severe harms, safety-net providers must be reinforced through strategic policies and resource allocation. At the federal level, increased funding is needed for key programs supporting these providers. State Medicaid programs must also expand coverage for pregnant women, new mothers, and their children. Simultaneously, community-informed research is essential to understand the scope of damage done by abortion restrictions and guide equity-focused solutions. This research should be collaborative, interdisciplinary, and centered on the lived experiences of those most affected. Examining disparate impacts across intersecting social strata, evaluating workforce and health system strains, and identifying innovations to promote equity are key priorities. Executing this research agenda will require dedicated funding and authentic community partnerships. Amid this crisis, safety-net providers are poised to play a vital role in blunting the impact on vulnerable populations. However, they cannot do so alone. Reinforcing their capacity through policy initiatives, while building an evidence base through community-engaged research, is critical. Only by leveraging both policy and research in service of equity, can we hope to mitigate the reproductive health harms unleashed by Dobbs. Lives depend on swift and sustained action on both fronts.

Keywords *reproductive health inequity; Dobbs versus Jackson; abortion access; safety-net providers; maternal health disparities; policy interventions; community-informed research; health equity*

Achieving Health Equity: The Role of Law and Policy, First Edition. Y. Tony Yang.
© 2025 John Wiley & Sons Ltd. Published 2025 by John Wiley & Sons Ltd.

> *Jasmine, a Black single mother, just found out she's pregnant. She's worried about how she'll afford prenatal care on her limited income, especially now that the nearby planned parenthood closed down after her state banned abortion. Jasmine wonders if she'll have to forgo additional ultrasounds and genetic screening due to cost.*
>
> *Dr. Patel, an OB-GYN, is leaving her practice in a state that just outlawed abortion. She no longer feels able to provide the full range of care her pregnant patients may need in a crisis. Halfway across the country, Dr. Patel's new employer is struggling to keep up with the surge in demand from out-of-state women seeking abortions.*

10.1 Reproductive Health Inequities Post-Dobbs

The US Supreme Court's landmark 2022 decision in Dobbs v. Jackson Women's Health, which overturned the constitutional right to abortion established nearly 50 years prior in Roe v. Wade, has ushered in a new era of reproductive health in America [1]. The Dobbs ruling eliminated federal protections for abortion access and returned the issue to states to regulate as they see fit. In the wake of this seismic shift, over half the states have enacted laws that ban or severely restrict abortion care [2]. The impact of these new restrictions will not fall evenly on all populations. Low-income women, women of color, and other marginalized groups who already face systemic barriers to healthcare access and quality are likely to suffer the most dire consequences [3].

As states hostile to abortion rights move swiftly to implement bans and limitations, safety-net healthcare providers will find themselves on the frontlines of this new reality, tasked with serving the needs of communities hardest hit by these policy changes. Clinics and organizations that comprise the healthcare safety net, such as community health centers, family planning clinics, public hospitals, and HIV/AIDS service providers, will play an increasingly vital role in addressing the fallout from restricted abortion access. These safety-net providers are the primary source of care for underserved populations who will feel the gravest impacts of state abortion bans, in terms of both unintended pregnancy and other reproductive health challenges [4].

To effectively confront this daunting landscape and mitigate the most severe harms, safety-net providers urgently need reinforcement through strategic policy initiatives and resource allocation. At the same time, community-informed research and data collection must be prioritized to fully understand the scope of damage done by abortion restrictions and light the way toward equity-enhancing solutions. Only by acting decisively to strengthen the healthcare safety net, while simultaneously building an evidence base on the real-world impacts of Dobbs, can we hope to protect the most vulnerable and advance reproductive health equity in a post-Dobbs America [5].

> *"The bans and restrictions on abortions may widen the already stark racial disparities in maternal health, especially since some states do not explicitly have exceptions that allow abortion services when pregnancy is jeopardizing a woman's health."*
>
> Kaiser Family Foundation (2024)

10.2 Maternal Health Inequities Deepen Post-Dobbs

Even prior to the Dobbs decision, the state of maternal health in the United States was one of stark inequity, with women of color bearing the brunt of adverse outcomes. The US maternal mortality rate, which is more than double that of other high-income countries, has been rising in recent years, increasing from 17.4 deaths per 100,000 live births in 2018 to 32.9 deaths per 100,000 in 2021 [6]. Disaggregating this data reveals appalling racial disparities. Black and American Indian/Alaska Native women experienced the sharpest increases in maternal deaths over this period [6].

Shockingly, even prior to Dobbs, maternal mortality rates were higher for every racial/ethnic group in states with more restrictive abortion policies compared to states with fewer restrictions [7]. The structural racism baked into the foundations of American society conspires with gender discrimination and economic inequality to make the mere act of childbearing perilous for far too many. These dire statistics are manifestations of what can be termed the "injuries of inequality" – the physical, psychological, and social tolls exacted by interlocking systems of oppression.

The concept of injuries of inequality provides a useful lens for understanding the disproportionate burden of reproductive health challenges borne by marginalized communities. Injuries of inequality are more than just unfortunate happenstance or the product of individual choices and behaviors. Rather, they are the predictable and preventable outcomes of public policies and institutional practices that create an uneven playing field and stack the deck against certain populations [8].

Discriminatory policies like abortion bans and the long history of reproductive coercion aimed at low-income women and women of color are prime examples of systemic drivers of injuries of inequality [9]. By further restricting bodily autonomy and reproductive freedom, the Dobbs decision has poured fuel on the fire of inequity, virtually ensuring that these injuries will multiply and intensify.

The post-Dobbs fallout will extend far beyond diminished access to abortion care itself. We are already seeing ripple effects that threaten the full spectrum of reproductive and maternal health services [10]. In states with abortion bans, reports are emerging of women being denied medically necessary treatment during pregnancy out of providers' fear of legal liability [11]. Pharmacists are refusing to dispense medications routinely used to manage miscarriage and ectopic pregnancies [12]. Genetic counseling and prenatal screening services are being curtailed. Access to contraception, Sexually Transmitted Infection (STI) testing, and other reproductive health care are being compromised as clinics that provide abortions are forced to close down [13].

Medical training is also suffering, as OB-GYN residency programs in states with abortion bans struggle to ensure their trainees gain adequate experience in essential skills like miscarriage management or emergency uterine evacuation [14]. Applications to OB-GYN and family medicine residency programs have fallen in states enacting abortion restrictions [15]. Providers contemplating practice locations increasingly factor in state reproductive health policies out of concern for their own families' access to care. A brain drain is occurring, with experienced physicians leaving states hostile to abortion and fewer medical graduates choosing to train or practice there. This will inevitably translate into growing provider shortages.

The chilling effects of abortion criminalization are likely to hamper the collection and reporting of reliable data on reproductive health outcomes [16]. Fear of surveillance and prosecution may lead patients to withhold sensitive information from providers [17]. Clinicians may be more circumspect in their documentation [18]. Public health departments may be wary of maintaining registries of data that could be weaponized against those seeking or providing reproductive care. A vicious cycle could ensue, where worsening outcomes remain hidden due to data blind spots, in turn preventing evidence-based policy responses.

Safety Net Policy and Equity Post-Dobbs

Focus Area	Description	Equity Implications
Safety-Net Providers	Community health centers, public hospitals, family planning clinics, and HIV/AIDS clinics serving vulnerable populations	Critical for serving underserved communities disproportionately affected by abortion bans
Federal Funding	Title V, Title X, community health centers, National Health Service Corps, and mental health programs need expansion	Necessary to support safety-net providers in managing increased demands post-Dobbs
Medicaid Policies	Postpartum coverage, pregnancy-related eligibility, continuous enrollment, and support for maternal and infant care	Essential for maintaining coverage and care continuity for mothers and infants
EMTALA (Emergency Medical Treatment and Labor Act)	Federal guidelines to ensure care for pregnancy-related emergencies without state interference	Vital safeguard for ensuring emergency care is provided without legal barriers
EPSDT (Early Periodic Screening, Diagnostic, and Treatment)	Comprehensive coverage for Medicaid-enrolled infants, children, and adolescents, including home visits and community outreach	Support for high-risk cases and adolescent parents to address social risks
Family Planning Coverage	Encouraging states to adopt coverage options including contraception, STI services, and family planning	Expanding access to essential reproductive health services for marginalized populations

All of these dire impacts will fall hardest on communities already facing intersecting oppressions and barriers to care [19]. Low-income women, women of color, rural residents, LGBTQ individuals, immigrants, and people with disabilities are among those most likely to see their reproductive autonomy further constrained and their health jeopardized [20]. Many of these same populations were struggling to access high-quality, culturally responsive reproductive and maternal care even when Roe was the law of the land. Now, they will be fighting an even steeper uphill battle, with fewer resources and recourses.

10.3 The Critical Role of Safety-Net Providers

Given this grim forecast, safety-net providers will be called upon like never before to support the reproductive health and well-being of marginalized communities in a post-Dobbs environment. The healthcare safety net, composed of community health centers, free and charitable clinics, family planning providers, public hospitals, local health departments, and other organizations serving low-income and uninsured populations, has long been a vital source of care for underserved communities. In the aftermath of Dobbs, the safety net will be stretched to the limit as demand for services surges among populations facing new and intensified barriers to reproductive care [21].

Meeting this challenge will require a multipronged effort to shore up safety-net providers with the necessary policy support and resources. At the federal level, Congress must increase funding for key safety-net programs like Title X family planning, Federally Qualified Health Centers, the Ryan White HIV/AIDS Program, and the National Health Service Corps [22]. These funding streams support the staffing, infrastructure, and service delivery capacity of frontline providers who will be caring for those most impacted by state abortion restrictions.

State Medicaid programs also have a pivotal role to play in bolstering the safety net. Medicaid covers nearly half of all births in the United States and an even larger share in many states with abortion bans. Expanding Medicaid coverage for pregnant women, new mothers, and their children must be a top priority [23]. States should take up the new option to extend postpartum Medicaid coverage to a full year, as opposed to just 60 days. The evidence clearly shows that access to postpartum care for a full 12 months improves outcomes for both mothers and infants [24]. Yet to date, many states with the most restrictive abortion laws have failed to adopt this policy.

Income eligibility levels for pregnancy-related Medicaid also need to be raised. Some states with abortion bans maintain very low eligibility thresholds, leaving many low-income women who don't qualify for traditional Medicaid without affordable coverage options. Ensuring continuous eligibility for both pregnant women and children is also critical to prevent churn and coverage losses, especially as pandemic-related protections expire [25].

Strengthening Medicaid coverage of family planning services is another key strategy. Half the states still have not expanded their Medicaid family planning programs to cover individuals not otherwise eligible for Medicaid, which could help mitigate the impact of dwindling abortion access [26]. The scope of coverage should include the full range of FDA-approved contraceptives, as well as STI screening, HPV vaccines, and other preventive reproductive care. Reimbursement rates for these services must be adequate to sustain family planning providers.

Beyond coverage and financing policies, upholding fundamental protections for access to emergency and stabilizing care is paramount. The Emergency Medical Treatment and Labor Act (EMTALA) requires hospitals to provide necessary treatment to stabilize emergency medical conditions regardless of state law [27]. In July 2022, the US Department of Health and Human Services issued guidance affirming EMTALA's applicability to pregnant patients and its preemption of any state abortion restrictions in emergency situations. Several lawsuits are underway challenging EMTALA's scope as it relates to reproductive care (as of 2024) [28]. The outcome of this litigation could have profound implications for access to life-saving treatment for pregnant patients, including ectopic pregnancy, preeclampsia, and miscarriage management.

To implement these federal and state policy supports, safety-net providers will need robust technical assistance, streamlined reporting and compliance processes, and a seat at the table in implementation planning. Collaboration across the sector to share best practices and advocate for needed changes will be essential. So too will be partnerships with grassroots organizations and reproductive justice advocates to ensure programs and services are responsive to community needs.

10.4 Advancing Equity Through Research

Informing these safety-net policy and practice interventions will require a concerted research agenda to elucidate the on-the-ground impacts of shifting abortion access. Understanding in real-time how the Dobbs decision is affecting the health and well-being of marginalized communities is critical to guide an equity-focused response. Investigators in academia, nonprofit institutes, government agencies, and healthcare delivery systems all have a role to play in building this evidence base.

To maximize relevance and impact, research on post-Dobbs reproductive health equity must be intentionally collaborative, interdisciplinary, and community-engaged [29]. The voices and lived experiences of those most directly affected should be centered at all stages of the research process, from conceptualization through dissemination [30]. Community-based organizations are vital thought partners who can ensure research questions reflect priorities on the ground, recruit diverse study participants, contextualize findings, and translate evidence into action.

Examining disparate impacts across racial, ethnic, socioeconomic, and geographic strata will be critical to surface inequities and tailor interventions. The intersectional barriers experienced by groups who sit at multiple social margins must be rigorously captured and meaningfully disaggregated. Studying outcomes and mechanisms holistically, beyond just abortion services to the full continuum of reproductive and maternal care, will yield important insights [31]. So too will longitudinal assessment of ripple effects into other domains like mental health, chronic disease management, child development, and economic security.

Evaluating workforce and health system strains will also be key. How are abortion restrictions affecting the pipeline, training, and distribution of clinicians qualified to provide the full scope of reproductive health services? [32] What practice changes are providers making to limit legal liability, and how are these changes impacting the quality and continuity of care? To what extent are facility closures and service reductions siphoning resources away from other essential public health programs? Creative, mixed-method research designs combining quantitative analysis of surveillance, claims, and clinical data with qualitative assessment of patient and provider experiences will be needed to robustly answer these questions.

Of utmost importance, research must do more than document problems – it should inform solutions. Descriptive studies to monitor shifts in access, utilization, and outcomes must be paired with rigorous evaluations of innovations to mitigate harm and enhance equity. Implementation research to identify effective models for expanding safety-net capacity and community-led quality improvement initiatives should be prioritized [33]. Data must be rapidly disseminated in formats accessible to policymakers, practitioners, and the public, not just siloed in academic journals.

Executing this ambitious research agenda will require dedicated funding streams commensurate with the urgency and scale of the situation [34]. Both government research agencies and private foundations have an important role to play. Flexibilities may be needed in budgets and grant review processes to be maximally responsive to evolving needs and promote authentic community partnership [35]. Incentivizing data harmonization, linkage, and sharing across disparate sources can unlock powerful population-level insights. At the same time, robust privacy safeguards must be in place to prevent data from being misused to target individuals seeking or providing reproductive care.

Throughout the research enterprise, a committed focus on equity, anti-racism, and reproductive justice must be the guiding light. Deliberate efforts to reflect these values in funding priorities, study designs, research teams, and dissemination strategies are paramount. For too long, the reproductive health research agenda has been largely shaped by the interests and assumptions of socially privileged investigators and institutions. Rectifying these epistemic injustices by amplifying marginalized voices, valuing diverse ways of knowing, and sharing power in knowledge production is long overdue.

10.5 Conclusion: Advancing Equity Amid Reproductive Crisis

The Supreme Court's decision in Dobbs v. Jackson Women's Health has unleashed a reproductive health crisis in America that is widening already unacceptable disparities. Access to abortion care is being decimated in many states, with sweeping implications for the full spectrum of sexual and reproductive health services. These policy changes will be disproportionately detrimental to the health and well-being of communities historically oppressed by structural racism, misogyny, economic injustice, homophobia, transphobia, xenophobia, and ableism [36].

Safety-net healthcare providers are poised to play a critical role in blunting the impact of state abortion bans and other restrictions on these vulnerable populations [37]. However, they cannot shoulder this burden alone [38]. Reinforcing the reproductive health safety net through enhanced Medicaid coverage, expanded public health funding, protected access to emergency care, and other targeted policy initiatives is imperative.

Simultaneously, community-engaged research must be catalyzed to rigorously document post-Dobbs inequities and light the way toward effective, equity-promoting interventions [39]. Descriptive and evaluative studies that center the priorities and experiences of marginalized groups, elucidate intersectional impacts across the reproductive life course, and take a holistic view of health and well-being are urgently needed to guide the response.

Only by leveraging both public policy tools to bolster safety-net capacity and research evidence generated in partnership with affected communities can we hope to mitigate the injuries of inequality that are being exacerbated by diminished abortion access [40]. The reproductive health, rights, and dignity of all hang in the balance. Swift, strategic, and sustained action to advance equity on both fronts has never been more important. Lives depend on it.

References

1 Schreiber, C.A., Khabele, D., and Gehrig, P.A. (2023). The Dobbs v Jackson Women's Health Organization Supreme Court Decision – concerns, challenges, and consequences for health care. *JAMA Surgery* 158 (3): 229–230.

2 MacDonald, A., Gershengorn, H.B., and Ashana, D.C. (2022). The challenge of emergency abortion care following the Dobbs ruling. *JAMA* 328 (17): 1691–1692.

3 Zernike, K. (2022). Roe overturned: a comprehensive guide to the Supreme Court decision. *The New York Times*. https://www.nytimes.com/news-event/roe-v-wade-supreme-court-abortion.

4 Donley, G., Chen, B.A., and Borrero, S. (2022). The legal and medical necessity of abortion care amid the COVID-19 pandemic. *Journal of Law and the Biosciences* 7 (1): 1–17. https://doi.org/10.1093/jlb/lsaa013.

5 Planned Parenthood. (2022). What is the safety net and why is it important? https://www.plannedparenthood action.org/issues/health-care-equity.

6 Joseph, K.S., Lisonkova, S., Boutin, A. et al. (2024). Maternal mortality in the United States: are the high and rising rates due to changes in obstetrical factors, maternal medical conditions, or maternal mortality surveillance? *American Journal of Obstetrics and Gynecology* 230 (4): 440–e1.

7 Treder, K.M., Amutah-Onukagha, N., and White, K.O. (2023). Abortion bans will exacerbate already severe racial inequities in maternal mortality. *Women's Health Issues* 33 (4): 328–332.

8 Centers for Disease Control and Prevention (2022). Maternal mortality rates in the United States, 2020. https://www.cdc.gov/nchs/data/hestat/maternal-mortality/2020/maternal-mortality-rates-2020.htm (accessed 29 August 2024).

9 Addante, A.N., Eisenberg, D.L., Valentine, M.C. et al. (2019). The association between state-level abortion restrictions and maternal mortality in the United States, 1995-2017. *Contraception* 100 (4): 281–284. https://doi.org/10.1016/j.contraception.2019.06.008.

10 Bailey, Z.D., Feldman, J.M., and Bassett, M.T. (2021). How structural racism works – racist policies as a root cause of US racial health inequities. *New England Journal of Medicine* 384 (8): 768–773. https://doi. org/10.1056/nejmms2025396.

11 Heisler, M., Mitchell, N., Arey, W. et al. (2024). US abortion bans should not pre-empt the duty to provide life-saving abortion care to pregnant patients in medical emergencies. *The Lancet* 403 (10434): 1318–1321.

12 Rafie, S., Majerczyk, D., Cieri-Hutcherson, N. et al. (2024). Pharmacist dispensing of mifepristone: an opinion of the Women's Health Practice and Research Network of the American College of Clinical Pharmacy. *Journal of the American College of Clinical Pharmacy* 7 (3): 270–278.

13 Knight, A. and Miller, J. (2023). *Prenatal Genetic Testing, Abortion, and Disability Justice.* Oxford University Press.

14 Roberts, D.E. (1999). *Killing the Black Body: Race, Reproduction, and the Meaning of Liberty.* Vintage Books.

15 Famiglietti, C. (2023). Where Have All the OBGYNs Gone? An Investigation Into the Effect of Abortion Restrictions on Availability of Women's Health Providers. https://dune.une.edu/cgi/viewcontent.cgi?article= 1005&context=ph_ile.

16 Dellinger, J., and Pell, S. K. (2024, April 18). The criminalization of abortion and surveillance of women in a post-Dobbs world, Brookings. https://www.brookings.edu/articles/the-criminalization-of-abortion-and-surveillance-of-women-in-a-post-dobbs-world/.

17 Arnold, C. (2022). Doctors weren't considered in Dobbs, but now they're on abortion's legal front lines. *NPR.* https://www.npr.org/sections/health-shots/2022/07/16/1111344635/doctors-werent-considered-in-dobbs-but-now-theyre-on-abortions-legal-front-lines.

18 Guttmacher Institute (2023). State laws and policies: Medication abortion. https://www.guttmacher.org/state-policy/explore/medication-abortion.

19 Alligood-Percoco, N.R. and Yano, J. (2022). The road ahead in obstetrics and gynecology after Dobbs v Jackson. *JAMA* 328 (7): 621–622. https://doi.org/10.1001/jama.2022.13656.

20 Frieden, J. (2022). Match numbers down for ob/gyn, family medicine. *MedPage Today.* https://www.medpagetoday.com/special-reports/exclusives/100581.

21 Chapman, E.N., Kaatz, A., and Carnes, M. (2013). Physicians and implicit bias: how doctors may unwittingly perpetuate health care disparities. *Journal of General Internal Medicine* 28 (11): 1504–1510. https://doi.org/10.1007/s11606-013-2441-1.

22 Health Resources & Services Administration (2022). Bureau of primary health care. https://www.hrsa.gov/about/organization/bureaus/bphc (accessed 29 August 2024).

23 Kaiser Family Foundation (2022). Medicaid postpartum coverage extension tracker. https://www.kff.org/medicaid/issue-brief/medicaid-postpartum-coverage-extension-tracker/ (accessed 29 August 2024).

24 Gordon, S.H., Sommers, B.D., Wilson, I.B., and Trivedi, A.N. (2020). Effects of Medicaid expansion on postpartum coverage and outpatient utilization. *Health Affairs* 39 (1): 77–84. https://doi.org/10.1377/hlthaff.2019.00547.

25 Ranji, U., Bair, Y., and Salganicoff, A. (2022). *Medicaid Coverage of Family Planning Benefits: Findings From a 2021 State Survey*. Kaiser Family Foundation. https://www.kff.org/womens-health-policy/report/medicaid-coverage-of-family-planning-benefits-findings-from-a-2021-state-survey/.

26 Serafi, K., Mann, C., Carrera, M., et al. (2023). Implementing State-Level Policy and Operational Processes That Enhance Access to Medicaid Family Planning Program Services. https://www.manatt.com/insights/white-papers/2023/implementing-state-level-processes-that-enhance-ac.

27 U.S. Department of Health and Human Services (2022). Reinforcement of EMTALA Obligations Specific to Patients who are Pregnant or Experiencing Pregnancy Loss. https://www.hhs.gov/sites/default/files/emergency-medical-care-letter-to-health-care-providers.pdf (accessed 29 August 2024).

28 Heipt, W.S. (2023). EMTALA in a post-Dobbs World: the March towards fetal personhood continues. *Idaho Law Review* 59: 369.

29 Ross, L. and Solinger, R. (2017). *Reproductive Justice: An Introduction*. University of California Press.

30 Lucero, J.E., Wright, K.E., and Reese, A. (2020). Trust development in CBPR partnerships. In: *Community-based Participatory Research for Health: Advancing Social and Health Equity*, 3rde (ed. N.D. Wallerstein, B. Duran, J.G. Oetzel, and M. Minkler), 61–78. Jossey-Bass.

31 Crenshaw, K. (1991). Mapping the margins: Intersectionality, identity politics, and violence against women of color. *Stanford Law Review* 43 (6): 1241–1299. https://doi.org/10.2307/1229039.

32 Howell, E.A., Egorova, N.N., Balbierz, A. et al. (2016). Site of delivery contribution to black-white severe maternal morbidity disparity. *American Journal of Obstetrics and Gynecology* 215 (2): 143–152. https://doi.org/10.1016/j.ajog.2016.05.007.

33 Brownson, R.C., Colditz, G.A., and Proctor, E.K. (ed.) (2017). *Dissemination and Implementation Research in Health: Translating Science to Practice*, 2nde. Oxford University Press.

34 National Institutes of Health. (2022). Research on the health of women of understudied, underrepresented and underreported (U3) populations (admin supp clinical trial optional). https://grants.nih.gov/grants/guide/pa-files/pa-20-222.html (accessed 29 August 2024).

35 Ford, C.L. and Airhihenbuwa, C.O. (2010). Critical race theory, race equity, and public health: toward antiracism praxis. *American Journal of Public Health* 100 (S1): S30–S35. https://doi.org/10.2105/ajph.2009.171058.

36 Light, A.D., Wang, L.F., and Zeymo, A. (2018). Comparison of obstetric outcomes and postpartum utilization in Medicaid and commercial insurance populations. *Maternal and Child Health Journal* 22 (12): 1803–1810. https://doi.org/10.1007/s10995-018-2571-5.

37 Gavin, L., Frederiksen, B., Robbins, C. et al. (2017). New clinical performance measures for contraceptive care: their importance to healthcare quality. *Contraception* 96 (3): 149–157. https://doi.org/10.1016/j.contraception.2017.05.013.

38 Hardeman, R.R., Medina, E.M., and Kozhimannil, K.B. (2016). Structural racism and supporting black lives – the role of health professionals. *New England Journal of Medicine* 375 (22): 2113–2115. https://doi.org/10.1056/nejmp1609535.

39 Dehlendorf, C., Reed, R., Fox, E. et al. (2020). Ensuring our research reflects our values: the role of family planning research in advancing reproductive autonomy. *Contraception* 101 (1): 4–7. https://doi.org/10.1016/j.contraception.2019.11.006.

40 Frieden, T.R. (2014). Six components necessary for effective public health program implementation. *American Journal of Public Health* 104 (1): 17–22. https://doi.org/10.2105/ajph.2013.301608.

11

Advancing Mental Health Equity Through Policies

Abstract

This chapter examines the persistent racial and ethnic disparities in access to and quality of mental health care in the United States and outlines major policy shifts needed to advance mental health equity. The background section highlights the disproportionate burden of untreated mental illness among communities of color and the multiple barriers they face to receiving care, which have only been exacerbated by the COVID-19 pandemic. The chapter then describes the key areas where policy change is needed: expanding and diversifying the mental health workforce; transforming the user navigation experience; scaling up innovative care delivery models; strengthening insurance coverage and payment structures; and investing in upstream prevention and early intervention. Next, the chapter also emphasizes the importance of addressing the social determinants of mental health to make long-term progress on equity. It calls for policies to reduce socioeconomic inequality, build community resilience, and mitigate the impacts of structural racism. The unique role of states as policy laboratories is discussed, with examples of high-impact Medicaid and regulatory levers they can use to spur innovation and extend access to underserved groups. Finally, the chapter underscores the urgency of the current moment, with the pandemic having taken a stark toll on mental health, particularly for youth and people of color. The confluence of new federal funding opportunities, growing bipartisan interest in behavioral health, and heightened public awareness create a window for enacting transformational policy change to bring about a more equitable mental health system. The chapter concludes with a call to action for policymakers to seize this moment, in partnership with advocates and stakeholders, and builds a system of care that can provide accessible, affordable, and culturally responsive mental health services for all.

Keywords   *mental health equity; racial disparities; culturally competent care; workforce diversity; access to care; social determinants; community-based services*

Achieving Health Equity: The Role of Law and Policy, First Edition. Y. Tony Yang.
© 2025 John Wiley & Sons Ltd. Published 2025 by John Wiley & Sons Ltd.

Jamal, a Black teenager, found himself in a cycle of juvenile detention due to untreated depression. With no access to a culturally competent therapist, he struggled alone. His grades plummeted, and his future seemed bleak. When he finally encountered a school-based mental health program, he began to thrive academically and emotionally.

Elena, a Latina mother, juggled multiple jobs to make ends meet, leaving little time for her mental health. Without insurance coverage for mental health services, her anxiety went untreated. A community health worker helped her navigate the system, connecting her to affordable care. This intervention transformed her life, allowing her to care for her family and pursue career goals.

Mr. Lee, an elderly Asian man, was diagnosed with severe depression but faced language barriers in accessing care. His daughter found a mental health clinic with bilingual staff, and for the first time, Mr. Lee received culturally responsive treatment. This support improved his quality of life, highlighting the need for diverse mental health professionals in underserved communities.

11.1 Disparities in Mental Health Care

Racial and ethnic disparities in access to and quality of mental health care in the United States are long-standing, persistent, and well-documented [1]. In 2001, the US Surgeon General's report "Mental Health: Culture, Race, and Ethnicity" found that people of color had less access to mental health services, were less likely to receive needed care, often received poorer quality care, and were underrepresented in mental health research. Two decades later, little has changed [2].

While the prevalence of mental illness is similar across racial and ethnic groups, minorities have a greater burden of disability from mental disorders [3]. This is in large part due to receiving less and lower quality care. For example, a 2022 Kaiser Family Foundation report found that over half of Black adults with moderate to severe symptoms of anxiety and depression did not receive treatment, compared to about one-third of White adults. Lack of insurance coverage, a dearth of culturally competent providers, language barriers, and cultural stigma are among the many barriers minorities face to accessing care [4].

Racial and ethnic minorities also tend to be overrepresented in high-need settings like jails, prisons, and psychiatric hospitals but underrepresented in outpatient treatment services [5]. When in treatment, they often receive a poorer quality of care. For instance, studies have found that compared to White patients with the same symptoms, Black and Latino patients are more likely to be diagnosed with behavior disorders or oppositional defiance disorders than mental disorders (such as depression) and less likely to be offered evidence-based medication [6].

Multiple factors contribute to these disparities at the patient, provider, and system levels [7]. Mistrust of the medical establishment due to historical abuses [8], cultural beliefs about mental illness, and limited diversity in the mental health workforce can all inhibit help-seeking among people of color [9]. Meanwhile, both explicit and implicit provider bias can lead to misdiagnosis and inequitable treatment. More broadly, structural racism – in the form of discriminatory policies and practices that systematically disadvantage people of color – underlies unequal access to the social determinants of mental health like stable housing, quality education, and economic security [10].

The COVID-19 pandemic, which has disproportionately impacted communities of color, has intensified the need for equitable mental health care. The cumulative toll of longstanding inequities compounded by the crises of COVID-19, economic upheaval, and racial injustice has led to increased rates of depression, anxiety, substance use, and suicide among racial and ethnic minorities. Urgent action to transform the mental health care system and advance equity is needed now more than ever [11].

"Mental illness is considered taboo in the African American community. Many of us try to mask our illness or pray it away, which in turn perpetuates stigma."

Mental Health America

11.2 Major Shifts Needed

The Biden administration and Congress have put a spotlight on mental health, proposing initiatives to strengthen the behavioral health workforce, improve care integration, enforce parity laws, and invest in community-based services [12]. States also have important levers they can pull through Medicaid policies, insurance regulations, and grant programs [13]. By seizing this moment and enacting smart policies at the federal and state levels, policymakers have an opportunity to transform the mental health system into one that provides timely, affordable, effective, and culturally responsive care for all who need it. Based on a synthesis of evidence and input from experts, major shifts are needed to improve access and advance equity in the mental health care ecosystem.

First, the mental health workforce needs to be significantly expanded. Even before the pandemic, over a third of Americans lived in areas with shortages of mental health professionals [14]. Racial and ethnic minorities are especially underserved, with few providers who share their cultural background or language. Loan repayment programs and grants can incentivize more diversity in the pipeline of mental health professionals and encourage them to practice in high-need areas. Training programs for peers, community health workers, and lay counselors can also help extend the reach of the existing workforce.

Second, the user navigation experience has to be transformed [15]. Currently, finding affordable mental health care is a daunting and confusing process, especially for those in crisis. People need "no wrong door" to enter the system and get connected to appropriate services. By funding care navigators, creating user-friendly online platforms with up-to-date provider directories, and bringing human-centered design principles to insurance plans, policymakers can make it much easier for people to access care. Particular attention should be paid to meeting the needs of high-risk groups like youth in the child welfare system.

Third, innovative care models that have shown promise need to be scaled up more rapidly [16]. While the integration of behavioral health into primary care has demonstrated positive results in improving access and outcomes, uptake remains low. Mobile crisis teams, clubhouses, and mental health services in non-traditional settings like schools, libraries, and homeless shelters are other impactful innovations that merit expansion. States can use Medicaid waivers and managed care contracting to spur wider adoption of evidence-based models. The federal government should robustly fund demonstration programs and disseminate best practices so effective interventions spread more quickly.

Fourth, insurance coverage and payment models must be strengthened to promote access and quality [17]. Despite parity laws, disparities in insurance coverage for mental health treatment persist, with high out-of-pocket costs deterring many from seeking care. Enforcing parity rules, expanding coverage of new service delivery modes like telehealth and mobile crisis response in Medicare and Medicaid, and shifting to value-based payment can improve access and incentivize quality. Commercial insurers should include a full continuum of crisis services as essential health benefits in all plans.

Fifth, there needs to be much greater investment in prevention and early intervention services [18]. Half of mental health conditions begin by age 14, but the average delay between onset and treatment is 11 years. Policies that support the healthy social–emotional development of children and make it easier to identify and treat mental health issues early on are crucial for promoting lifelong mental wellness and reducing disparities. This includes universal mental health screening, funding school and community-based prevention programs, and integrating infant and maternal mental health into pediatric primary care.

11.3 Addressing Root Causes

While improving access to high-quality treatment is a critical priority, advancing mental health equity in the long run also requires addressing the underlying social determinants that place some populations at higher risk for mental illness in the first place [19]. Decades of research have clearly established the powerful influence of socioeconomic factors like poverty, discrimination, adverse childhood experiences, and neighborhood conditions on mental health. People of color face the compounded burden of experiencing both disproportionate social and economic disadvantages as well as barriers to care when mental health needs arise [20].

As such, policies that reduce inequality, build economic security and mobility, and create health-promoting environments are key to achieving mental health equity [21]. Increasing the supply of affordable housing, expanding job training and employment opportunities, raising the minimum wage, providing paid family and sick leave, and investing in high-quality childcare and early education programs can have positive spillover effects on community mental health. Meanwhile, more research is needed to understand the complex pathways through which structural racism gets "under the skin" to affect psychological well-being and resilience and how to disrupt and buffer against its toxic effects.

The federal government should fully implement the Social Determinants Accelerator Act passed by Congress in 2022, which will provide planning grants and technical assistance to help states and localities develop cross-sector, evidence-based interventions to address social determinants of health [22]. Agencies like the CDC and SAMHSA should strengthen their "health in all policies" approach by building partnerships with leaders in housing, education, justice, transportation, and other sectors to promote mental health. Bringing a racial equity lens to policy analysis and community engagement processes in all of these areas is critical.

Better data collection and more inclusivity in research are also paramount for surfacing the unique challenges facing communities of color and identifying strategies to close disparities [23]. Population health surveys need to oversample historically underrepresented groups and all federally funded research studies on mental health should be required to include diverse study participants and report results disaggregated by race and ethnicity. Building the evidence base for community-defined practices that resonate with the cultural values, beliefs, and lived experiences of different population groups is especially important [24]. By understanding the assets and risk factors for supporting mental well-being within communities of color, interventions can be tailored to their specific needs and priorities.

Key Policy Considerations for Mental Health Equity

Policy Area	Key Points
Expand Mental Health Workforce	Augment loan repayment programs and incentives. Invest in community mental health training. Encourage workforce diversity. Engage retiring providers.
Transform User Navigation Experience	Create shared data systems. Develop digital crisis support platforms. Fund care navigators. Apply human-centered design to insurance.
Catalyze Innovative Models	Promote integrated behavioral and primary care models. Expand mobile crisis response. Implement in-shelter care. Utilize library-based services.
Increase Insurance Coverage	Refine regulatory framework. Eliminate exclusionary policies. Expand telemedicine coverage. Incentivize providers to accept Medicaid.
Reform Payment Systems	Reduce paperwork burden. Support alternative payment models. Facilitate cross-state licensing.
Address Social Determinants of Health	Invest in protective factors like housing and job opportunities. Embed mental health literacy in community organizations. Implement peer support specialist programs.
Federal and State Roles	Leverage Medicaid and Medicare policies. Develop and enforce parity laws. Utilize state-specific innovation through Medicaid waivers and pilot programs.

11.4 States as Laboratories for Innovation

States are uniquely positioned to be laboratories for mental health policy innovation because of their central role in regulating health insurance, licensing health care providers, and overseeing safety net programs [25]. In particular, Medicaid is the single largest payer for mental health services in the United States, giving state Medicaid agencies significant leverage to drive delivery system reform and value-based payment models. State employee health plans can also be powerful market motivators in covering and incentivizing evidence-based mental health prevention and treatment.

One key area where states should focus is enforcing mental health parity and network adequacy standards for both Medicaid and commercial insurance plans [26]. This means ensuring that coverage and access to mental health services are on par with physical health services in terms of cost sharing, utilization management, provider reimbursement, and network participation. Despite the passage of the federal Mental Health Parity and Addiction Equity Act over a decade ago, true parity remains elusive [27]. More resources for state insurance departments to conduct market conduct exams, review plan compliance, and respond to consumer complaints are needed.

Expanding coverage and reimbursement of telehealth services, including audio-only telephone visits, is another high-impact policy states can pursue to improve access, especially in rural and underserved areas [28]. The pandemic prompted many states to issue emergency waivers to allow for greater telehealth flexibilities in Medicaid and private insurance – these should be made permanent with appropriate guardrails for quality and safety. Value-based payment models that incentivize the integration of behavioral health and primary care are also important for sustainability.

Increasing funding for mobile crisis response teams, peer support services, and Certified Community Behavioral Health Clinics can help divert people experiencing acute mental health episodes from costly and traumatic hospitalizations or incarcerations. Authorizing state Medicaid programs to cover these services and provider types, including allowing same-day billing for primary care and behavioral health visits, can expand their availability. Similarly, strengthening school-based mental health services and partnerships between schools and community behavioral health providers should be a priority given the youth mental health crisis exacerbated by the pandemic [29].

Other high-impact Medicaid policy levers that states can pursue [30] include implementing maternal depression screening and referral programs; using Section 1115 waiver authority to pilot alternative payment models for serving high-need populations; ensuring robust coverage of Medications for Addiction Treatment (MAT) and recovery supports for substance use disorders; building a more culturally and linguistically diverse mental health workforce through loan forgiveness and pipeline development programs; expanding mental health consultation in early childhood education settings; and leveraging the option to cover transition services for incarcerated individuals to facilitate continuity of care.

States should actively learn from each other to identify promising practices and policy strategies that can be spread and scaled [31]. The National Academy for State Health Policy and CDC's Public Health Law Program maintain databases tracking state behavioral health legislation and programs that can facilitate cross-pollination. Private foundations and the federal government should provide targeted funding and technical assistance for states to implement evidence-based practices and spur innovation via new waiver authorities or pilot programs.

11.5 Conclusion: Urgency for Mental Health Reform

The devastating impact of the COVID-19 pandemic on the nation's mental health, particularly for young people and people of color, has created new urgency and momentum around strengthening the full continuum of mental health promotion, prevention, and treatment services [32]. Major bipartisan investments in behavioral health services as part of a larger mental health legislative package should be considered, while record funding increases for SAMHSA block grants and new initiatives to improve system capacity and accountability are urgently needed.

This confluence of crises and opportunities presents a unique window for transformational policy change. By enacting the major shifts outlined earlier in this chapter – rapidly expanding and diversifying the mental health workforce; improving care navigation and coordination; scaling innovative models like integrated care and peer services; strengthening enforcement of parity and network adequacy rules while expanding coverage of new modalities; and focusing "upstream" on prevention and eliminating inequities – the United States can create a mental health system that is more accessible, affordable, effective, and equitable. Policies that tackle the social determinants of mental health and provide targeted, culturally responsive support for historically marginalized groups are also essential to achieve population impact.

No single policy is a panacea on its own, but in strategic combination, federal and state actions can dramatically improve the lives of the millions of Americans experiencing mental health and substance use challenges. Achieving equity has to be an explicit goal embedded in policy design, implementation, and evaluation. Policymakers will need to work closely with consumer advocates, professional associations, health plans, employers, and other key constituencies to build broad-based support for a transformative mental health equity agenda.

The science is clear that there is no health without mental health. It is long past time to treat mental health as a core component of overall health and invest in it commensurately and equitably. In the same way, public policies have spurred innovations in biomedical research and medical and surgical care focused attention on mental health can unleash creative solutions to long-standing access and quality challenges. With smart, evidence-based policies and a strong equity framework, we can build a mental health care system that provides healing, hope, recovery, and dignity for all.

References

1 U.S. Department of Health and Human Services (2001). Mental health: culture, race, and ethnicity – a supplement to mental health: a report of the surgeon general. https://www.ncbi.nlm.nih.gov/books/NBK44243/ (accessed 29 August 2024).

2 Perzichilli, T. (2020). The historical roots of racial disparities in the mental health system. *Counseling Today* https://www.counseling.org/publications/counseling-today-magazine/article-archive/article/legacy/the-historical-roots-of-racial-disparities-in-the-mental-health-system.

3 National Alliance on Mental Illness (2020). Identity and cultural dimensions. https://www.nami.org/Your-Journey/Identity-and-Cultural-Dimensions (accessed 29 August 2024).

4 Panchal, N., Kamal, R., Cox, C., and Garfield, R. (2021). *The Implications of COVID-19 for Mental Health and Substance Use.* Kaiser Family Foundation. https://www.kff.org/coronavirus-covid-19/issue-brief/the-implications-of-covid-19-for-mental-health-and-substance-use/.

5 Moore, K.R. and Kressin, N.R. (2021). The affordable care act and disparities in mental health care. *Medical Care Research and Review* 78 (5): 393–405. https://doi.org/10.1177/1077558720954148.

6 Fadus, M.C., Ginsburg, K.R., Sobowale, K. et al. (2020). Unconscious bias and the diagnosis of disruptive behavior disorders and ADHD in African American and Hispanic youth. *Academic Psychiatry* 44: 95–102.

7 Alegria, M., Alvarez, K., Ishikawa, R.Z. et al. (2016). Removing obstacles to eliminating racial and ethnic disparities in behavioral health care. *Health Affairs* 35 (6): 991–999. https://doi.org/10.1377/hlthaff.2016.0029.

8 Whaley, A.L. (2001). Cultural mistrust: an important psychological construct for diagnosis and treatment of African Americans. *Professional Psychology: Research and Practice* 32 (6): 555–562. https://doi.org/10.1037/0735-7028.32.6.555.

9 Kugelmass, H. (2016). "Sorry, I'm not accepting new patients": an audit study of access to mental health care. *Journal of Health and Social Behavior* 57 (2): 168–183. https://doi.org/10.1177/0022146516647098.

10 Bailey, Z.D., Krieger, N., Agénor, M. et al. (2017). Structural racism and health inequities in the USA: evidence and interventions. *The Lancet* 389 (10077): 1453–1463. https://doi.org/10.1016/S0140-6736(17)30569-X.

11 Lund, C. (2018). Improving access to mental health care. *Nature Human Behaviour* 2 (11): 759–760. https://doi.org/10.1038/s41562-018-0449-6.

12 The White House (2021). Biden-Harris Administration Calls for Historic Levels of Funding to Prevent and Treat Addiction and Overdose. https://www.whitehouse.gov/ondcp/briefing-room/2021/05/28/biden-harris-administration-calls-for-historic-levels-of-funding-to-prevent-and-treat-addiction-and-overdose/

13 National Conference of State Legislatures (2021). Mental health. https://www.ncsl.org/research/health/mental-health.aspx (accessed 29 August 2024).

14 Petterson, S., Westfall, J. M., & Miller, B. F. (2020). Projected Deaths of Despair During the Coronavirus Recession. Well Being Trust. https://wellbeingtrust.org/wp-content/uploads/2020/05/WBT_Deaths-of-Despair_COVID-19-FINAL-FINAL.pdf.

15 Brody, D.J., Gu, Q., and Cyffka, A. (2020). Trends in the use of complementary health approaches among adults: United States, 2012-2017. *NCHS Data Brief* 380: 1–8. https://www.cdc.gov/nchs/products/databriefs/db380.htm.

16 Funk, M., Drew, N., and Knapp, M. (2012). Mental health, poverty and development. *Journal of Public Mental Health* 11 (4): 166–185. https://doi.org/10.1108/17465721211289356.

17 Graaf, G. and Snowden, L. (2017). The role of Medicaid in improving the health of communities of color. *American Journal of Public Health* 107 (10): 1592–1594. https://doi.org/10.2105/AJPH.2017.304023.

18 Substance Abuse and Mental Health Services Administration (2019). Ready, set, go, review: screening for behavioral health risk in schools. https://www.samhsa.gov/resource/ebp/ready-set-go-review-screening-behavioral-health-risk-schools.

19 Allen, J., Balfour, R., Bell, R., and Marmot, M. (2014). Social determinants of mental health. *International Review of Psychiatry* 26 (4): 392–407. https://doi.org/10.3109/09540261.2014.928270.

20 Arredondo, P. (2019). *Eliminating Race-based Mental Health Disparities: Promoting Equity and Culturally Responsive Care Across Settings*. New Harbinger Publications.

21 Shim, R.S. and Compton, M.T. (2018). Addressing the social determinants of mental health: if not now, when? If not us, who? *Psychiatric Services* 69 (8): 844–846. https://doi.org/10.1176/appi.ps.201800060.

22 H.R.379 – 117th Congress (2021–2022): Social determinants accelerator act of 2021. https://www.congress.gov/bill/117th-congress/house-bill/379 (accessed 29 August 2024).

23 Krahn, G.L., Walker, D.K., and Correa-De-Araujo, R. (2015). Persons with disabilities as an unrecognized health disparity population. *American Journal of Public Health* 105 (S2): S198–S206. https://doi.org/10.2105/AJPH.2014.302182.

24 Hoagwood, K.E., Peth-Pierce, R., Glaeser, E. et al. (2017). Implementing evidence-based psychotherapies for children and adolescents within complex mental health systems. In: *Evidence-based Psychotherapies for Children and Adolescents*, 3rde (ed. J.R. Weisz and A.E. Kazdin), 466–483. The Guilford Press.

25 Rosenbaum, S. (2011). The Patient Protection and Affordable Care Act: implications for public health policy and practice. *Public Health Reports* 126 (1): 130–135. https://doi.org/10.1177/003335491112600118.

26 Weber, M.C., Segal, M., and Appelbaum, P.S. (2021). Strengthening mental health parity in Medicaid. *Psychiatric Services* 72 (10): 1165–1168. https://doi.org/10.1176/appi.ps.202000630.

27 Hoffman, D.L. and Duffy, E.E. (2021). Ensuring compliance with the mental health parity and addiction equity act. *Journal of Health Politics, Policy and Law* 46 (5): 859–880. https://doi.org/10.1215/03616878-9156083.

28 Mehrotra, A., Huskamp, H.A., Souza, J. et al. (2017). Rapid growth in mental health telemedicine use among rural Medicare beneficiaries, wide variation across states. *Health Affairs* 36 (5): 909–917. https://doi.org/10.1377/hlthaff.2016.1461.

29 Busch, S.H. and Barry, C.L. (2007). Mental health disorders in childhood: assessing the burden on families. *Health Affairs* 26 (4): 1088–1095. https://doi.org/10.1377/hlthaff.26.4.1088.

30 Larrison, C.R., Hack-Ritzo, S., Koerner, B.D. et al. (2011). State budget cuts, health care reform, and a crisis in rural community mental health agencies. *Psychiatric Services* 62 (11): 1255–1257. https://doi.org/10.1176/ps.62.11.pss6211_1255.

31 Pfefferle, S., Spanhel, C., Wyatt, L., and Polgar, M. (2021). States' use of policy levers to promote access to behavioral health services in Medicaid. *Psychiatric Services* 72 (3): 286–293. https://doi.org/10.1176/appi.ps.201900373.

32 Panchal, N., Kamal, R., Cox, C. et al. (2021). *Mental Health and Substance Use Considerations Among Children During the COVID-19 Pandemic.* Kaiser Family Foundation https://www.kff.org/coronavirus-covid-19/issue-brief/mental-health-and-substance-use-considerations-among-children-during-the-covid-19-pandemic/.

Part II

Health Behaviors: Exploring the Influences of Exercise, Diet, and Drug Use

This part delves into policy-driven approaches to influence health behaviors related to physical activity, diet, drug use, and disease prevention, with a focus on health equity. Chapter 12 explores the promotion of physical activity through equitable policies, emphasizing the need for community engagement and urban planning to create inclusive spaces. Chapter 13 addresses the reduction of sugary beverage consumption, discussing regulatory measures like taxes and marketing restrictions aimed at decreasing intake and improving public health. Chapter 14 examines tobacco control efforts, highlighting policies that protect vulnerable communities from the harmful effects of smoking through legislation and cessation programs. Chapter 15 focuses on achieving health equity in response to the drug overdose crisis, advocating for harm reduction strategies, equitable access to treatment, and comprehensive public health interventions. Chapter 16 confronts the HIV/AIDS epidemic, reviewing the progress made, ongoing challenges, and the path forward to end disparities in prevention, treatment, and care. Collectively, these chapters provide a roadmap for addressing key health behaviors through policies that prioritize equity and inclusivity, aiming to improve health outcomes for all populations.

Achieving Health Equity: The Role of Law and Policy, First Edition. Y. Tony Yang.
© 2025 John Wiley & Sons Ltd. Published 2025 by John Wiley & Sons Ltd.

12

Promoting Physical Activity: Policy Strategies for Equity and Engagement

Abstract

This chapter examines the global issue of physical inactivity and the initiatives undertaken to address this public health concern, focusing on promoting equity and inclusivity. It discusses the WHO's Global Action Plan on Physical Activity, which provides policy recommendations to increase physical activity levels worldwide, and delves into the disparities among racial and ethnic minorities, highlighting the need for strategies that address systemic inequities and prioritize community engagement. The chapter presents the CDC's Active People, Healthy Nation initiative, and Health Equity Guide as examples of comprehensive approaches to increasing physical activity levels and incorporating health equity into public health practices. It also explores the role of legal strategies and policy domains in promoting physical activity and addressing inequities. Finally, the chapter addresses the challenges faced in improving physical activity opportunities for young people of color, emphasizing the need for a multifaceted approach involving collaboration between various levels of government, community organizations, and individuals. It concludes by stressing the importance of creating accessible and inclusive spaces, addressing systemic inequities, and fostering a culture of active living to improve the health and well-being of young people of color.

Keywords *physical activity; health equity; community engagement; urban planning; inclusive spaces; systemic inequities; youth of color*

> *Sarah, a 15-year-old African American girl, lives in an urban neighborhood with limited access to safe parks and recreational facilities. Despite her desire to be active, Sarah often finds herself confined to her apartment after school, as her parents worry about her safety in the poorly maintained local park. The lack of accessible, inclusive spaces for physical activity has led to Sarah leading a sedentary lifestyle, putting her at risk for obesity and related health issues.*
>
> *Michael, a city planner in Utah, attended a training session organized by the state's Department of Health in collaboration with transportation planning agencies. The training focused on developing walking trails and bike lanes to improve physical activity levels in the community. Inspired by*

> *the session, Michael worked with local health officials and community leaders to create new "Complete Streets" policies and transportation plans that prioritize walkability without compromising utility, promoting a more active lifestyle for residents.*
>
> *John, a community organizer in Detroit, noticed the stark lack of parks and recreational spaces in his predominantly African American neighborhood. Determined to make a change, he rallied local residents and petitioned the city council, leveraging data on neighborhood walkability and public health. Their collective voice led to the development of new green spaces, transforming vacant lots into vibrant parks that encouraged the community to engage in physical activity.*

12.1 Tackling the Global Inactivity Crisis: WHO's Action Plan for a Healthier World

Physical activity is often overshadowed by more pressing issues in global public health discussions, despite the fact that insufficient physical activity poses significant health risks and is a well-recognized public health concern. To address this issue, various public policy initiatives have been implemented, with the World Health Organization (WHO) setting an ambitious goal to reduce global physical inactivity. In support of this target, the WHO released the Global Action Plan on Physical Activity, which outlines 4 broad objectives and 20 universally applicable policy recommendations [1]. These recommendations aim to increase physical activity levels by addressing the complex interplay of cultural, environmental, and individual factors that contribute to inactivity.

The WHO emphasizes that if physical activity rates continue to decline worldwide without intervention, there will be negative consequences for health systems, the environment, quality of life, and socioeconomic structures. To achieve meaningful change, support from both the public and private sectors is crucial, as well as robust multisectoral partnerships involving corporations, local community groups, NGOs, and individuals. The Global Action Plan acknowledges that nations are at different stages of development and will adopt policy changes based on their unique priorities and at varying rates. This flexibility allows countries to tailor their approaches to promoting physical activity while working towards the common goal of reducing global inactivity levels.

> *"The causes of obesity are varied and complex, but the lack of daily physical activity is an important factor."*
>
> Former CEO of the Robert Wood Johnson Foundation, Risa Lavizzo-Mourey

12.2 Addressing Inequities in Physical Activity: Inclusive Strategies and Community Engagement

Despite the global increase in physical inactivity across all socioeconomic levels, studies indicate that racial and ethnic minorities are disproportionately affected [2]. This disparity stems from systemic inequities, including inadequate urban planning, limited access to parks and public recreation spaces, and poor community engagement [3]. To prevent vulnerable populations from being left behind, most health authorities recognize the need to prioritize equity and inclusivity in plans to increase physical activity rates. As a result, physical activity programs have shifted their focus to addressing social determinants of health rather than solely relying on initiatives that encourage individuals to exercise more [4].

The CDC's Active People, Healthy Nation initiative exemplifies this comprehensive approach, aiming to increase physical activity levels for 27 million Americans by 2027 [5]. The program advocates for the implementation of seven evidence-based strategies, all of which focus on promoting equitable and inclusive access to physical activity opportunities. These strategies encompass a wide range of approaches, including designing communities that encourage physical activity, ensuring access to places where people can engage in physical activity, developing school and youth programs that promote active lifestyles, launching community-wide campaigns to raise awareness about the importance of physical activity, providing social support networks to motivate individuals, offering individualized support to help people overcome barriers to physical activity, and creating prompts that serve as reminders and encouragement for people to engage in regular physical activity. These strategies address various barriers to equal opportunities for physical activity while maintaining a commitment to eradicating disparities for ethnic and racial minorities and low-income individuals. For instance, under "community design," the CDC acknowledges that racial and ethnic minorities and rural residents are less likely to have access to parks and walkable streets. While encouraging the creation of more such spaces, the CDC also recognizes that this process can take months or years and often requires coordination between communities and local and/or state governments. To initiate these projects, the CDC suggests that local community stakeholders organize initiatives like "walk/move audits" to collect data on neighborhood walkability and recreational space, which can be presented to local leaders. Such data-driven solutions have proven effective, as demonstrated by New York City's Department of Parks and Recreation, which invested over $300 million in high-need communities during the 2010s, improving 70 acres of parkland in neighborhoods previously lacking equipment, facilities, and green space [6].

Moreover, the CDC and other policymakers emphasize community engagement as a crucial strategy for improving physical activity levels across racial and ethnic groups [7]. A study found that peer-based interventions, such as walking groups, "contracts" between friends to stay active, and "buddy systems," are particularly effective in boosting activity levels among disadvantaged groups [8]. The CDC encourages communities that have experienced historic disinvestment to empower community members by placing them in positions of influence, enabling them to shape programs and policies. This is especially relevant to land use projects due to the diverse range of interested stakeholders. For example, community leaders may advocate against highway projects that threaten local parks, while emergency service workers may need to provide input on bike lanes and walkable street plans to ensure they accommodate emergency vehicles.

12.3 Implementing Inclusive Health Equity Strategies: CDC Guidelines and Community Examples

The CDC's Health Equity Guide offers a comprehensive framework designed to help public health professionals integrate health equity principles into their practices [9]. The Guide underscores the significance of addressing historical inequities and emphasizes the crucial role of effective communication in achieving this goal. It provides six overarching guidelines for public health communications, which include viewing health disparities through a health equity lens when framing information, employing humanizing language that respects the dignity of individuals (e.g. using "people who are experiencing homelessness" instead of "the homeless") [10], using preferred terms when referring to specific groups, ensuring that health communications products are developed with an inclusive approach, using images only when they are culturally appropriate, clear, and inclusive, and exploring additional resources and references related to health equity communications. By following these guidelines, public health professionals can ensure that the information they convey is not only coherent but also inclusive, thereby reaching a wider audience and fostering a deeper understanding of health equity issues among the general public. Ultimately, the primary goal of the CDC's Health Equity Guide is to enable public health professionals to communicate effectively and inclusively, breaking down barriers and promoting greater health equity for all.

Several communities have incorporated the CDC's recommendations for inclusivity into their health equity and physical activity projects. In 2019, a community organization in Wisconsin utilized CDC funding to revitalize the Chief Niwopet Park, addressing the lack of access to public recreation spaces in the area [11]. As many local residents are members of the Menominee Nation, the new park is strategically located less than a mile from the local tribal school and features the Menominee language, art, and history. The organization intends to construct additional local parks with similar designs. Similarly, the Utah Department of Health collaborated with the state's transportation planning agencies to develop walking trails and bike lanes throughout the state [12]. The project included training sessions for hundreds of local health employees, city planners, and community leaders, resulting in the creation of new "Complete Streets" policies and transportation plans aimed at improving street walkability without compromising utility.

12.4 Leveraging Legal Strategies and Policy Domains to Promote Physical Activity and Address Inequities

Legal and policy experts are exploring ways to use the legal system to support physical activity initiatives, as legal solutions addressing sedentary behavior remain underexplored, even in countries that recognize physical inactivity as a severe issue [13]. However, legal and policy professionals have reported that legislation and regulations related to infrastructure, education, and interagency cooperation can be leveraged to boost physical activity rates. This area is particularly promising because the mechanisms used to encourage physical activity span many regulatory dimensions and include initiatives at the local, state, and federal levels, allowing community leaders to benefit from expert advice on navigating the legal regimes involved.

Scholars from the Australian Prevention Partnership Centre created the Regulatory Approaches to Movement, Physical Activity, Recreation, Transport, and Sport (RAMPARTS) framework, which defines legal strategies and policy domains potentially relevant to physical activity [14]. RAMPARTS suggests 20 policy actions and 7 legal strategies across 4 policy domains for policymakers to explore. These legal strategies (awareness, funding, incentive, standards, authorization, and prohibition) and policy domains (active societies, active environments, active people, and active systems) are deliberately broad, aligning with the WHO Global Action Plan's recognition that public health priorities and solutions will vary based on countries' developmental stages and governance structures.

The RAMPARTS framers hope policymakers will use the tool to guide discussions about regulatory options for promoting physical activity and identify research gaps.

In the United States, ChangeLab Solutions, a nonprofit, offers training to help local leaders leverage different policy areas to improve physical activity rates in their communities [15]. The nonprofit teaches public health advisers, municipal attorneys, and elected officials about the relationships between land use zoning, transportation planning, education laws, and public health. Community leaders can encourage walking instead of driving by investing in trails and mass transit and supporting zoning regulations that increase the number of local grocery stores while limiting fast-food restaurants.

Legal mechanisms created under state and local governments' police power can directly increase opportunities for exercise and recreation. These tools include joint-use agreements, which are contracts between parties that prescribe terms and conditions for shared use of public property, such as sports leagues signing agreements with schools to access fields and playgrounds outside of school hours.

Community leaders can also help develop comprehensive plans that prioritize physical activity. These long-term land use planning tools place restrictions on future development and are increasingly used by local health departments to influence community public health. However, community plans have legal limitations and cannot affect existing land uses or impose binding health standards on businesses, public works projects, or schools. More broadly, legal mechanisms created by states and localities under their police power are subject to strict constitutional limitations.

ChangeLab Solutions also encourages peer and community-tailored strategies for boosting physical activity, with some existing laws supporting local solutions. The Safe, Accountable, Flexible, Efficient Transportation Equity Act includes the Safe Routes to School program, which encourages children to develop active lifestyles by walking or biking to school, while the Volunteer Protection Act provides broad protection from liability for volunteers who help children get safely to school [16].

Lastly, inequities in physical activity can be viewed as a civil rights issue, as the Equal Protection Clause of the 14th Amendment and the Civil Rights Act of 1964 prevent the federal and state governments from discriminating on the basis of race [17]. Activists have gathered data about disparities in access to public recreational facilities and physical education to write civil rights legislation, such as in California, where a group mapped parks across the state and helped draft legislation defining the terms "park poor" and "income poor," setting standards for future measures of process and equity and directing state funding to create parks in low-income areas [18].

Policy Strategies and Equity Considerations for Promoting Physical Activity

Policy Sector	Key Strategy	Equity Consideration
Community Design	Creation and maintenance of sidewalks and parks	Ensuring that facilities are accessible and maintained in all communities, including underprivileged areas
Public Transportation	Support for infrastructure that promotes active transportation, like bus stops that encourage walking	Funding challenges and community prioritization of public transit development
Healthcare	Physical activity counseling as part of routine healthcare	Barriers include lack of reimbursement for counseling and the need for training healthcare providers

(Continued)

Policy Sector	Key Strategy	Equity Consideration
Education	Mandatory physical education in schools	Varying state laws on PE time and intensity; need for comprehensive implementation and monitoring
Workplace	Promoting physical activity through facilities like gyms and incentives for active commuting	Implementing policies that are inclusive and consider diverse employee needs
Public Spaces	Policies that enhance access to public recreational facilities	Focusing on the maintenance and safety of these spaces to ensure they are usable by all community members
Legal Framework	Utilizing legal mechanisms to support physical activity initiatives	Addressing inequities through policies that ensure equal access to facilities across different demographics

12.5 Conclusion: Overcoming Challenges in Promoting Physical Activity for Youth of Color

Despite the successes mentioned above, advocates face significant challenges in improving physical activity opportunities for young people of color due to a lack of public interest [19]. Even as health equity gains more attention, physical activity inequities remain a low priority because policymakers do not perceive them as urgent issues and have yet to fully acknowledge the implications for the environment and broader socioeconomic structures. Further complicating the issue is the fact that effective solutions cannot come from a single regulator or level of government.

Experts agree that people cannot be legally compelled to exercise. Instead, the responsibility falls on policymakers to create opportunities for physical activity, while local communities and individuals must take on the task of encouraging themselves and those around them to engage in physical activity [20]. This can only be achieved through holistic programs that address multiple issues, including access to public recreation, land use and transportation inequities, and community engagement.

To effectively promote physical activity among young people of color, a multifaceted approach is necessary [21]. This approach should involve collaboration between various levels of government, community organizations, and individuals. By working together to create accessible and inclusive spaces for physical activity, addressing systemic inequities, and fostering a culture of active living, communities can make significant strides in improving the health and well-being of young people of color.

References

1 World Health Organization (2019). *Global Action Plan on Physical Activity 2018-2030: More Active People for a Healthier World*. World Health Organization.

2 Crespo, C.J., Smit, E., Andersen, R.E. et al. (2000). Race/ethnicity, social class and their relation to physical inactivity during leisure time: results from the Third National Health and Nutrition Examination Survey, 1988–1994. *American Journal of Preventive Medicine* 18 (1): 46–53.

3 Thornton, C.M., Conway, T.L., Cain, K.L. et al. (2016). Disparities in pedestrian streetscape environments by income and race/ethnicity. *SSM-Population Health* 2: 206–216.

4 Kohl, H. III, Murray, T., and Salvo, D. (2019). *Foundations of Physical Activity and Public Health*. Human Kinetics Publishers.

5 Fulton, J.E., Buchner, D.M., Carlson, S.A. et al. (2018). CDC's active people, Healthy NationSM: creating an active America, together. *Journal of Physical Activity and Health* 15 (7): 469–473.

6 Katz, C. (2013). Power, space, and terror: social reproduction and the public environment. In: *The Politics of Public Space*, 105–121. Routledge.

7 Wallerstein, N., Minkler, M., Carter-Edwards, L. et al. (2015). Improving health through community engagement, community organization, and community building. In: *Health Behavior: Theory, Research and Practice*, 5, 5e (ed. K. Glanz, B.K. Rimer, and K.V. Viswanath), 277–300. Jossey-Bass/Wiley.

8 Thøgersen-Ntoumani, C., Quested, E., Biddle, S.J. et al. (2019). Trial feasibility and process evaluation of a motivationally-embellished group peer led walking intervention in retirement villages using the RE-AIM framework: the residents in action trial (RiAT). *Health Psychology and Behavioral Medicine* 7 (1): 202–233.

9 Calanan, R.M., Bonds, M.E., Bedrosian, S.R. et al. (2023). CDC's guiding principles to promote an equity-centered approach to public health communication. *Preventing Chronic Disease* 20: E57.

10 Palmer, G.L. (2018). People who are homeless are "people" first: opportunity for community psychologist to lead through language reframing. *Global Journal of Community Psychology Practices* 9 (2): 1–16.

11 University of Wisconsin-Madison (2020). Extension team enhances recreation spaces in Menominee County Nation. https://menominee.extension.wisc.edu/files/2021/09/Enhancing-recreation-spaces-in-Menominee-County-Nation.pdf (accessed 28 August 2024).

12 Burbidge, S.K. (2010). Merging long range transportation planning with public health: a case study from Utah's Wasatch Front. *Preventive Medicine* 50: S6–S8.

13 Sallis, J., Bauman, A., and Pratt, M. (1998). Environmental and policy interventions to promote physical activity. *American Journal of Preventive Medicine* 15 (4): 379–397.

14 Nau, T., Smith, B.J., Bauman, A., and Bellew, B. (2021). Legal strategies to improve physical activity in populations. *Bulletin of the World Health Organization* 99 (8): 593.

15 Torres, S. (2020). Health Ambassadors: A Model for Engaging Community Leaders to Promote Better Health. https://repository.usfca.edu/capstone/1076/.

16 Fischer, J.W. and Resources, Science, and Industry Division (2005). *Safe, Accountable, Flexible, Efficient Transportation Equity Act – A Legacy for Users (SAFETEA-LU Or SAFETEA): Selected Major Provisions*. Congressional Research Service, The Library of Congress.

17 Harris, A.P. and Pamukcu, A. (2020). The civil rights of health: a new approach to challenging structural inequality. *UCLA Law Review* 67: 758.

18 García, R. (2013). Social justice and leisure: the usefulness and uselessness of research. *Journal of Leisure Research* 45 (1): 7–22.

19 Day, K. (2006). Active living and social justice: planning for physical activity in low-income, black, and Latino communities. *Journal of the American Planning Association* 72 (1): 88–99.

20 Piercy, K.L., Troiano, R.P., Ballard, R.M. et al. (2018). The physical activity guidelines for Americans. *JAMA* 320 (19): 2020–2028.

21 Floyd, M.F., Taylor, W.C., and Whitt-Glover, M. (2009). Measurement of park and recreation environments that support physical activity in low-income communities of color: highlights of challenges and recommendations. *American Journal of Preventive Medicine* 36 (4): S156–S160.

13

Reducing Sugary Beverage Consumption: Regulatory Measures

Abstract

Sugary drinks, defined as beverages with added sweeteners such as high-fructose corn syrup, sucrose, or fruit juice concentrates, are the primary source of calories and added sugar in the American diet. These drinks are calorie-dense but nutrient-poor, and consuming them does not lead to the same feeling of fullness as eating an equivalent amount of calories from solid food. This becomes particularly problematic when individuals do not compensate for the extra calories by reducing their food intake. Mounting evidence suggests that high-sugar beverages are a significant contributor to premature death and preventable illnesses linked to dietary factors. Despite allocating a substantial portion of its GDP to healthcare, the United States ranks poorly among OECD countries in terms of death rates, with diet-related risks being the leading cause of death. This paradox underscores the costly and inefficient nature of the American healthcare system compared to other nations. Reversing these trends requires a multifaceted approach, but experts agree that improving diet and nutrition, particularly reducing sugar consumption, would have the most significant impact on Americans' physical health. However, the health issues associated with sugary drink consumption disproportionately affect communities of color, which is the focus of this chapter. The following section will explore the disparate impact of sugary drink consumption on communities of color and how manufacturers target these populations. Subsequently, an examination of current laws and policies designed to address the issue and their limitations will be provided. The chapter will then offer recommendations for the future before concluding with a summary of the key points and insights.

Keywords *sugary drinks; health disparities; targeted marketing; public health policies; sugary drink tax; food deserts; school nutrition; agricultural subsidies*

> *James, a middle-aged Black man from an urban neighborhood, noticed an increase in sugary drink ads in his community. Every billboard and bus stop seemed to flaunt colorful, enticing images of sodas, and sweetened beverages. As his own health battles with diabetes worsened, James grew increasingly aware of the targeted marketing strategies that seemed to disproportionately affect his community, urging a lifestyle that contributed to their health issues.*

Achieving Health Equity: The Role of Law and Policy, First Edition. Y. Tony Yang.

> *Samantha, a school teacher in a predominantly Hispanic area, observes her students consuming multiple sugary drinks daily, a norm that worries her. She has attempted to integrate lessons about healthy eating into her curriculum, but the availability and advertising of these beverages overpower her efforts. Samantha's frustration mounts as she sees firsthand the effects of poor diet choices influenced by aggressive marketing tactics and the lack of healthy alternatives in her community.*

13.1 Consequences of Sugary Drink Consumption

Sugary drinks are the primary source of added sugars in the American diet, accounting for nearly one-quarter (24%) of all added sugars consumed by individuals aged 2 and older [1]. These beverages are low in nutrients and do not provide a feeling of fullness despite their calorie content [2]. Excessive consumption of added sugars, particularly from sugary drinks, is associated with an increased risk of weight gain, heart disease, high blood pressure, type 2 diabetes, and tooth decay [3]. Consuming just one additional sugary drink per day can elevate a person's risk of hypertension by 8% and heart disease by 17%. Strong evidence indicates that children and teens who consume sugary drinks have a higher risk of obesity and cavities, while emerging evidence suggests a link to insulin resistance and caffeine-related effects [4].

Although youth consumption of sugary drinks has decreased in recent years, it remains high, with children consuming an average of 133 calories and adults consuming 138 calories from these beverages daily [5]. Approximately one in six children aged 2–5 consume a regular soda, and one in four consume a fruit drink each day [6]. Adult consumption of sugary drinks is also concerning, with half of adults in the United States consuming a sugary drink on a given day [7]. Men are more likely to consume these beverages than women (53.6% versus 45.1%) and are also more prone to drinking two or more sugary drinks in a single day. The economic impact of missed work due to sugary drink-related diseases, such as obesity, high blood pressure, and diabetes, is estimated to cost the nation tens of billions of dollars annually [8].

13.2 Factors Driving Sugary Drink Consumption Disparities in Communities of Color

This section explores the various factors contributing to the disproportionate impact of sugary drink consumption on communities of color. It examines disparities in consumption rates among racial and ethnic groups, the role of targeted marketing by sugary drink manufacturers, and the influence of limited access to healthy food options in minority neighborhoods.

13.2.1 Sugary Drink Consumption Disparities Among Racial and Ethnic Groups

A recent publication has highlighted striking disparities in sugary drink consumption between white people and people of color [9]. On average, men and women of color consume more calories per day from sugary drinks compared to their white and Asian counterparts. In fact, sugary drinks account for more than 8% of the total daily calorie intake for black men and women, a significantly higher percentage than other populations. Additionally, Alaska Native adults are three times more likely to consume three or more sugary drinks per day compared to white adults [10]. These disparities are also evident in child-age populations.

Latinx and black children under the age of two consume more sugary drinks than white children and are more than twice as likely to be obese [11]. Furthermore, Alaska Native children have a significantly higher likelihood (63%) of consuming at least one sugary drink per day compared to white children (37%) and children of other races (42%) [12]. Children from low-income families across all races, although minority populations are more likely to be low income than whites, are twice as likely to consume sugary drinks compared to children from high-income families [13]. These findings underscore the urgent need to address the disproportionate impact of sugary drink consumption on communities of color and low-income populations.

13.2.2 Targeted Marketing of Sugary Drinks to Minority Youth

Targeted marketing, a strategy used by companies to identify and promote products to specific consumer groups, has been employed by sugary drink manufacturers to reach minority youths [14]. Studies have shown that this pervasive marketing of unhealthy foods contributes to increased consumption, particularly among children and young people. In 2018, sugary drink advertising expenditure surpassed $1 billion, with black and Hispanic youths being the primary targets of these campaigns, which may explain the higher sugary drink consumption rates among minority youths compared to their white counterparts [15]. One study revealed that black children were exposed to twice as many sugary drink ads as white children, with these products being among the most frequently advertised on black-targeted television [15].

Soda companies target minority youths for two reasons: they view them as a growth market (a market with increasing demands for their product) and as trendsetters for white children. Additionally, companies focus on children because they believe that developing brand loyalty at a young age will persist into adulthood and be passed on to future generations. Sugary drink manufacturers often feature black and Hispanic celebrities in their advertisements to appeal to minority youths [15]. For example, Mountain Dew, a PepsiCo brand, ranked first in the number of ads viewed by youth and featured professional basketball players and other teen-oriented appeals [15]. Similarly, Coca-Cola targeted the Hispanic youth market with Powerade, securing endorsements from the US Women's National Soccer Team. PepsiCo's Gatorade, marketed primarily to black and Hispanic youths, ranked third in ads viewed on Spanish-language television, with black teens seeing 2.8 times as many Gatorade ads as white teens [15].

13.2.3 Limited Access to Healthy Options in Minority Neighborhoods

Food deserts, regions with limited access to affordable and healthful food options, also contribute to the increased sugary drink consumption among minority populations [16]. These food deserts often result from low-income levels or the need to travel farther to find healthy food choices [17]. Poor, urban neighborhoods are more likely to be food deserts, lacking supermarkets and farmers' markets where individuals can purchase healthy foods [18]. Instead, residents are often limited to fast food locations or other options that typically offer more processed and unhealthy food choices.

While a neighborhood's income level certainly influences the presence of food deserts, research from 2014 revealed that racial composition also plays a significant role [17]. When comparing black and Hispanic neighborhoods with white neighborhoods that have similar poverty rates, the black and Hispanic neighborhoods had fewer large supermarkets, which translate to fewer options for purchasing healthy foods. Instead, food deserts are characterized by an abundance of corner stores, fast-food restaurants, and bodegas that sell unhealthy beverages [19]. Children living in food deserts tend to purchase these unhealthy beverages from stores near their schools, potentially increasing their daily caloric intake by approximately 350 calories in urban areas [20].

> *"We have solid evidence that keeping intake of free sugars to less than 10% of total energy intake reduces the risk of overweight, obesity, and tooth decay. Making policy changes to support this will be key if countries are to live up to their commitments to reduce the burden of noncommunicable diseases."*
>
> Dr. Francesco Branca, Director of WHO's Department of Nutrition for Health and Development

13.3 Limitations of Current Policies Addressing Sugary Drink Consumption

The primary policy approach to improving healthy eating habits focuses on information and education, with an emphasis on food labeling [21]. While evidence suggests that labels can influence consumer behavior, the effects are relatively small [22]. Moreover, this strategy places the responsibility for healthier diets on an individual's ability to make informed choices, ignoring the complex determinants of dietary habits, such as targeted advertising. Despite the focus on information and education, obesity, diabetes, and other diet-related illness rates have continued to rise [23].

Sugary drink manufacturers have made public commitments to improving public health, such as the Balance Calories Initiative, which aims to reduce caloric intake from sugary drinks by 20% over the next 5 years [24]. A Coca-Cola spokesperson stated that the company is taking steps to reduce sugar consumption through smaller soda cans and more low- and no-calorie beverage options. However, critics question the sincerity of these statements, citing the billion dollars spent on advertising and the 41% increase in advertising for sugared soda over the past 5 years. Recent events have brought social justice and equity issues to light, with PepsiCo's CEO addressing systemic racism in an op-ed. Critics argue that the most effective way for PepsiCo to improve black lives would be to stop engaging in targeted marketing involving minority youths.

Some jurisdictions have introduced taxes on sugary drinks to reduce consumption. The first such tax was implemented in Berkeley, California in 2014, and studies have shown that these taxes can effectively reduce consumption [25]. For example, Philadelphia's tax of $0.015 per ounce of a sweetened beverage reduced adult consumption of sugared soda by more than ten times per month and led to a 30% decrease in overall sugary drink consumption [26]. However, research also suggests that local taxes have limitations [27]. Most studies show that taxes on sugary drinks are regressive, disproportionately affecting low-income earners. In Berkeley and Philadelphia, taxes were more likely to be passed on to consumers in low-income neighborhoods, as residents had a reduced ability to shop outside city limits to avoid the tax. Supermarket owners in Philadelphia warned that stores might have to close due to customers choosing to shop in suburbs to avoid the tax [28].

Public reactions to sugary drink taxes can also change quickly depending on how the tax revenue is used [29]. Cook County, Illinois, used its sugary drink tax primarily to cover a multimillion dollar budget shortfall, with public health improvement as a secondary benefit [30]. After the tax revenue was used solely for budgetary purposes, opponents criticized the measure, claiming it had nothing to do with health and everything to do with revenue. The sugary drink tax in Cook County was ultimately repealed 5 months after its implementation.

Sugary Drinks: Policy Recommendations and Equity Considerations

Policy Recommendations	Equity Considerations
Tax on Sugary Drinks	• Targeting sugary drinks aims to reduce sugar consumption, which is higher among lower-income families and communities of color • Revenue from the tax should be used for public health in underserved communities
Doubling Support for Community Health Centers (CHCs)	• CHCs primarily serve low-income, Black, Hispanic, and other minority populations, improving access to essential health services
Improve School Meals	• Providing free, nutritious school meals to all students, particularly benefiting children from low-income families
Invest in Nutrition Research	• Establish a National Institute of Nutrition to focus on the impact of nutrition on chronic health conditions, addressing disparities in health outcomes
Reform Agricultural Subsidies	• Shift subsidies from unhealthy foods to healthier options, benefiting low-income and minority communities who are disproportionately affected by diet-related diseases

13.4 Policy Strategies for Reducing Sugary Drink Consumption

This section discusses various policy strategies aimed at reducing sugary drink consumption, including implementing a national sugary drink tax, promoting healthier school meals, and reallocating agricultural subsidies to support the production of healthier foods.

13.4.1 A National Sugary Drink Tax: Recommendations and Considerations

A national tax on sugary drinks remains the primary recommendation for reducing consumption, despite potential limitations. Experts suggest that a nationwide tax would be more effective than local taxes, which individuals can avoid by traveling to neighboring jurisdictions. The success of Mexico's national tax on sugary drinks, which led to a 5.5% drop in consumption in the first year and a 9.7% decrease in the second year, serves as an example [31]. The American Heart Association (AHA) has proposed a tiered tax based on a product's sugar and corn syrup content, with the highest tax rate ($0.02/ounce) applied to drinks with the highest sugar content (20 g/8 ounce serving) [32].

While a national sugary drink tax would be regressive from a purely economic perspective, its impact on overall welfare is less clear [33]. If young people reduce their consumption of sugary drinks, they may experience lifelong benefits. Predictions suggest that a national tax could reduce cardiovascular disease rates for black and Hispanic Americans by 15,000 per million [34]. Based on reasonable assumptions, a national tax could save 500,000 lives, cut healthcare costs by $100 billion, and raise around $5 billion annually [35]. If the tax revenue is earmarked for public health measures, it would prevent criticisms similar to those faced by the Cook County tax.

Any tax legislation would need to clearly define which beverages are subject to the tax. A baseline definition for sugary drinks includes all nonalcoholic beverages with any added caloric sweetener, including those intended to be mixed into an alcoholic drink [36]. The legislation would also need to specify exemptions from the tax, such as medically necessary beverages, infant formula, 100% fruit and vegetable juices, and natural and common sweeteners not in beverages (e.g. maple syrup, honey, table sugar) [37].

13.4.2 Promoting Healthier School Meals and Reallocating Agricultural Subsidies

Improving the quality of food and drinks consumed by children at school is another effective strategy for reducing the harmful effects of sugary drink consumption [38]. Schoolchildren, particularly those from low-income families, consume between one-third and one-half of their meals at school. The National School Lunch Program provides approximately five billion meals annually to lower-income students. The city of Boston serves as a model, offering free school meals to all students, regardless of income level, and preparing meals using real foods in on-site kitchens, rather than reheating processed food shipped by food conglomerates [39].

Since the passage of the US Farm Bill in 1973, over $200 billion in subsidies have supported the production of certain foods, including corn [40]. Despite growing health concerns, corn production has continued to rise. A significant portion of these subsidized commodities is transformed into unhealthy foods and high-calorie juices or other drinks sweetened with corn sweeteners. Experts argue that the true beneficiaries of these subsidies are not farmers, but rather large agricultural and food corporations. They advocate for the reallocation of subsidies from the US Farm Bill to support the development of healthier foods.

13.5 Conclusion: A Comprehensive Approach to Reducing Sugary Drink Consumption

To improve public health, it is crucial for Americans to reduce their consumption of sugary drinks. However, this task is particularly challenging for communities of color, which face significantly disparate impacts from sugary drink consumption compared to their white counterparts. From childhood through adulthood, the average person of color is substantially more likely to consume one or more sugary drinks than the average white person. This increased consumption can be attributed to factors such as targeted advertising by sugary drink manufacturers aimed at minority youth and the prevalence of food deserts in low-income communities, which primarily consist of people of color, where access to healthful foods is limited.

Various jurisdictions have implemented policy initiatives to improve public health by reducing the demand for sugary drinks. While policies focused on improving food education can have some impact, they are insufficient when compared to the influence of factors like targeted advertising in driving increased sugary drink consumption. Several counties and cities have also introduced "sin taxes" on sugary drinks, which have been effective in reducing consumption. However, the burden of these taxes falls disproportionately on low-income individuals.

Despite the challenges associated with taxing sugary drinks, a national tax appears to be the most effective policy for reducing demand. Although the tax would have a greater impact on low-income individuals from a purely economic standpoint, this analysis overlooks the other benefits derived from a national tax. These benefits include significant health improvements for individuals who reduce their sugary drink consumption and increased revenue that the government can allocate toward public health initiatives. In addition to a national tax, improving both access to and the quality of school meals should be a priority in all jurisdictions. Finally, federal government subsidies should be directed toward producers of healthy foods, rather than those that exacerbate the public health issues described above.

References

1 Malik, V.S., Popkin, B.M., Bray, G.A. et al. (2010). Sugar-sweetened beverages, obesity, type 2 diabetes mellitus, and cardiovascular disease risk. *Circulation* 121 (11): 1356–1364. https://doi.org/10.1161/CIRCULATIONAHA.109.876185.

2 Vos, M.B., Kaar, J.L., Welsh, J.A. et al. (2017). Added sugars and cardiovascular disease risk in children: a scientific statement from the American Heart Association. *Circulation* 135 (19): e1017–e1034. https://doi.org/10.1161/CIR.0000000000000439.

3 Vartanian, L.R., Schwartz, M.B., and Brownell, K.D. (2007). Effects of soft drink consumption on nutrition and health: a systematic review and meta-analysis. *American Journal of Public Health* 97 (4): 667–675. https://doi.org/10.2105/AJPH.2005.083782.

4 Marshall, T.A., Levy, S.M., Broffitt, B. et al. (2003). Dental caries and beverage consumption in young children. *Pediatrics* 112 (3 Pt 1): e184–e191. https://doi.org/10.1542/peds.112.3.e184.

5 Bleich, S.N., Wang, Y.C., Wang, Y., and Gortmaker, S.L. (2009). Increasing consumption of sugar-sweetened beverages among US adults: 1988-1994 to 1999-2004. *The American Journal of Clinical Nutrition* 89 (1): 372–381. https://doi.org/10.3945/ajcn.2008.26883.

6 Ogden, C.L., Kit, B.K., Carroll, M.D., and Park, S. (2011). Consumption of sugar drinks in the United States, 2005-2008. *NCHS Data Brief* 71: 1–8.

7 Park, S., Xu, F., Town, M., and Blanck, H.M. (2016). Prevalence of sugar-sweetened beverage intake among adults – 23 states and the District of Columbia, 2013. *MMWR. Morbidity and Mortality Weekly Report* 65 (7): 169–174. https://doi.org/10.15585/mmwr.mm6507a1.

8 Finkelstein, E.A., DiBonaventura, M., Burgess, S.M., and Hale, B.C. (2010). The costs of obesity in the workplace. *Journal of Occupational and Environmental Medicine* 52 (10): 971–976. https://doi.org/10.1097/JOM.0b013e3181f274d2.

9 Bleich, S.N., Vercammen, K.A., Koma, J.W., and Li, Z. (2018). Trends in beverage consumption among children and adults, 2003-2014. *Obesity (Silver Spring, Md.)* 26 (2): 432–441. https://doi.org/10.1002/oby.22056.

10 Elwan, D., de Schweinitz, P., and Wojcicki, J.M. (2016). Beverage consumption in an Alaska Native village: a mixed-methods study of behaviour, attitudes and access. *International Journal of Circumpolar Health* 75: 29905. https://doi.org/10.3402/ijch.v75.29905.

11 Taveras, E.M., Gillman, M.W., Kleinman, K. et al. (2010). Racial/ethnic differences in early-life risk factors for childhood obesity. *Pediatrics* 125 (4): 686–695. https://doi.org/10.1542/peds.2009-2100.

12 Chi, D.L., Coldwell, S.E., Mancl, L. et al. (2019). Alaska native children do not prefer sugar-sweetened fruit drinks to sugar-free fruit drinks. *Journal of the Academy of Nutrition and Dietetics* 119 (6): 984–990. https://doi.org/10.1016/j.jand.2019.02.007.

13 Han, E. and Powell, L.M. (2013). Consumption patterns of sugar-sweetened beverages in the United States. *Journal of the Academy of Nutrition and Dietetics* 113 (1): 43–53. https://doi.org/10.1016/j.jand.2012.09.016.

14 Harris, J.L., Schwartz, M.B., and Brownell, K.D. (2010). Marketing foods to children and adolescents: licensed characters and other promotions on packaged foods in the supermarket. *Public Health Nutrition* 13 (3): 409–417. https://doi.org/10.1017/S1368980009991339.

15 Harris, J.L. (2020). Targeted food marketing to black and hispanic consumers: the tobacco playbook. *American Journal of Public Health* 110 (3): 271–272. https://doi.org/10.2105/AJPH.2019.305518.

16 Walker, R.E., Keane, C.R., and Burke, J.G. (2010). Disparities and access to healthy food in the United States: a review of food deserts literature. *Health & Place* 16 (5): 876–884. https://doi.org/10.1016/j.healthplace.2010.04.013.

17 Bower, K.M., Thorpe, R.J. Jr., Rohde, C., and Gaskin, D.J. (2014). The intersection of neighborhood racial segregation, poverty, and urbanicity and its impact on food store availability in the United States. *Preventive Medicine* 58: 33–39. https://doi.org/10.1016/j.ypmed.2013.10.010.

18 Larson, N.I., Story, M.T., and Nelson, M.C. (2009). Neighborhood environments: disparities in access to healthy foods in the U.S. *American Journal of Preventive Medicine* 36 (1): 74–81. https://doi.org/10.1016/j.amepre.2008.09.025.

19 Borradaile, K.E., Sherman, S., Vander Veur, S.S. et al. (2009). Snacking in children: the role of urban corner stores. *Pediatrics* 124 (5): 1293–1298. https://doi.org/10.1542/peds.2009-0964.

20 Briefel, R.R., Wilson, A., and Gleason, P.M. (2009). Consumption of low-nutrient, energy-dense foods and beverages at school, home, and other locations among school lunch participants and nonparticipants. *Journal of the American Dietetic Association* 109 (2 Suppl): S79–S90. https://doi.org/10.1016/j.jada.2008.10.064.

21 Roberto, C.A., Swinburn, B., Hawkes, C. et al. (2015). Patchy progress on obesity prevention: emerging examples, entrenched barriers, and new thinking. *Lancet (London, England)* 385 (9985): 2400–2409. https://doi.org/10.1016/S0140-6736(14)61744-X.

22 Brownell, K.D. and Frieden, T.R. (2009). Ounces of prevention – the public policy case for taxes on sugared beverages. *The New England Journal of Medicine* 360 (18): 1805–1808. https://doi.org/10.1056/NEJMp0902392.

23 Nestle, M. and Jacobson, M.F. (2000). Halting the obesity epidemic: a public health policy approach. *Public Health Reports (Washington, D.C.: 1974)* 115 (1): 12–24. https://doi.org/10.1093/phr/115.1.12.

24 Bogart, L.M., Castro, G., and Cohen, D.A. (2019). A qualitative exploration of parents', youths' and food establishment managers' perceptions of beverage industry self-regulation for obesity prevention. *Public Health Nutrition* 22 (5): 805–813. https://doi.org/10.1017/S1368980018003865.

25 Falbe, J., Thompson, H.R., Becker, C.M. et al. (2016). Impact of the Berkeley excise tax on sugar-sweetened beverage consumption. *American Journal of Public Health* 106 (10): 1865–1871. https://doi.org/10.2105/AJPH.2016.303362.

26 Zhong, Y., Auchincloss, A.H., Lee, B.K., and Kanter, G.P. (2018). The short-term impacts of the Philadelphia beverage tax on beverage consumption. *American Journal of Preventive Medicine* 55 (1): 26–34. https://doi.org/10.1016/j.amepre.2018.02.017.

27 Powell, L.M., Chriqui, J.F., Khan, T. et al. (2013). Assessing the potential effectiveness of food and beverage taxes and subsidies for improving public health: a systematic review of prices, demand and body weight outcomes. *Obesity Reviews: An Official Journal of the International Association for the Study of Obesity* 14 (2): 110–128. https://doi.org/10.1111/obr.12002.

28 Cawley, J., Frisvold, D., Hill, A., and Jones, D. (2019). The impact of the Philadelphia beverage tax on purchases and consumption by adults and children. *Journal of Health Economics* 67: 102225. https://doi.org/10.1016/j.jhealeco.2019.102225.

29 Thomas-Meyer, M., Mytton, O., and Adams, J. (2017). Public responses to proposals for a tax on sugar-sweetened beverages: a thematic analysis of online reader comments posted on major UK news websites. *PLoS One* 12 (11): e0186750. https://doi.org/10.1371/journal.pone.0186750.

30 Powell, L.M. and Leider, J. (2020). Evaluation of changes in beverage prices and volume sold following the implementation and repeal of a sweetened beverage tax in cook county, Illinois. *JAMA Network Open* 3 (12): e2031083. https://doi.org/10.1001/jamanetworkopen.2020.31083.

31 Colchero, M.A., Rivera-Dommarco, J., Popkin, B.M., and Ng, S.W. (2017). In Mexico, evidence of sustained consumer response two years after implementing a sugar-sweetened beverage tax. *Health Affairs (Project Hope)* 36 (3): 564–571. https://doi.org/10.1377/hlthaff.2016.1231.

32 Labarthe, D.R., Goldstein, L.B., Antman, E.M. et al. (2016). Evidence-based policy making: assessment of the American Heart Association's strategic policy portfolio: a policy statement from the American Heart Association. *Circulation* 133 (18): e615–e653.

33 Long, M.W., Gortmaker, S.L., Ward, Z.J. et al. (2015). Cost effectiveness of a sugar-sweetened beverage excise tax in the U.S. *American Journal of Preventive Medicine* 49 (1): 112–123. https://doi.org/10.1016/j.amepre.2015.03.004.

34 Wang, Y.C., Coxson, P., Shen, Y.M. et al. (2012). A penny-per-ounce tax on sugar-sweetened beverages would cut health and cost burdens of diabetes. *Health Affairs (Project Hope)* 31 (1): 199–207. https://doi.org/10.1377/hlthaff.2011.0410.

35 Chouinard, H.H., Davis, D.E., LaFrance, J.T., and Perloff, J.M. (2007). Fat taxes: big money for small change. *Forum for Health Economics & Policy* 10 (2). De Gruyter.

36 Chriqui, J.F., Chaloupka, F.J., Powell, L.M., and Eidson, S.S. (2013). A typology of beverage taxation: multiple approaches for obesity prevention and obesity prevention-related revenue generation. *Journal of Public Health Policy* 34 (3): 403–423. https://doi.org/10.1057/jphp.2013.17.

37 Taber, D.R., Chriqui, J.F., Perna, F.M. et al. (2012). Weight status among adolescents in States that govern competitive food nutrition content. *Pediatrics* 130 (3): 437–444. https://doi.org/10.1542/peds.2011-3353.

38 Terry-McElrath, Y.M., O'Malley, P.M., and Johnston, L.D. (2015). Foods and beverages offered in US public secondary schools through the National School Lunch Program from 2011-2013: early evidence of improved nutrition and reduced disparities. *Preventive Medicine* 78: 52–58. https://doi.org/10.1016/j.ypmed.2015.07.010.

39 Stern, A.L., Levine, S., Richardson, S.A. et al. (2023). Improving school lunch menus with multi-objective optimisation: nutrition, cost, consumption and environmental impacts. *Public Health Nutrition* 26 (8): 1715–1727. https://doi.org/10.1017/S1368980023000927.

40 Do, W.L., Bullard, K.M., Stein, A.D. et al. (2020). Consumption of foods derived from subsidized crops remains associated with cardiometabolic risk: an update on the evidence using the National Health and Nutrition Examination Survey 2009-2014. *Nutrients* 12 (11): 3244. https://doi.org/10.3390/nu12113244.

14

Promoting Health Equity via Tobacco Control

Abstract

The chapter delves into the complex relationship between tobacco use and health disparities, particularly among vulnerable communities such as minority and low-income populations. It begins by highlighting the disproportionate impact of tobacco-related health problems on these communities, despite an overall decrease in tobacco use. The chapter examines the factors contributing to this disparity, including targeted advertising by tobacco companies, limited access to health services and cessation resources, and the use of tobacco as a coping mechanism for stress related to racism and prejudice. It then explores various strategies for policy interventions to foster health equity, such as implementing smoke-free laws, investing in anti-tobacco education and cessation programs, increasing the cost of tobacco products, regulating sales, raising the minimum age for purchases, and strengthening enforcement. The chapter emphasizes the importance of a comprehensive approach that addresses the unique needs of each community and monitors the impact of policies to prevent unintended consequences. It also discusses the need for investment in tobacco control programs and the promotion of community buy-in. The chapter concludes by stressing the importance of a multilayered approach involving federal, state, and local authorities, healthcare providers, private actors, and the community itself to achieve equity in tobacco control interventions and establish tobacco-free communities.

Keywords *tobacco control; health equity; vulnerable communities; smoke-free laws; targeted advertising; cessation programs; policy interventions; tobacco-related disparities*

> *Tara, a 45-year-old mother living in a low-income neighborhood in Chicago, frequently visits her local convenience store. The store, like many in her community, is inundated with tobacco advertisements. From colorful posters offering discounted cigarette packs to window signs advertising flavored cigars, the tobacco industry has left its mark. For Tara, the choice to smoke was never really a conscious one; it was just a part of life, something she started in her teenage years, influenced by the environment around her.*

> *James, a city councilman from San Francisco, has been at the forefront of initiating tobacco control policies in the city. Witnessing the effects of tobacco on communities first-hand, especially those that are marginalized, he champions the cause of implementing smoke-free zones and regulating the sale of e-cigarettes. James recalls an emotional testimony from a high school student about the allure of flavored vaping products and how rampant their use had become in schools, strengthening his resolve.*

14.1 Tobacco-Related Disparities

Tobacco use, the leading cause of preventable death in the United States, remains a critical health issue, particularly in vulnerable communities [1]. Despite a general decrease in tobacco use and an increased understanding of its harmful effects, certain communities continue to suffer disproportionately from tobacco-related health problems [2]. This is particularly evident in minority and low-income communities, which often lack the protections needed to mitigate these harms, leading to a wider health disparity between high and low socioeconomic status of the communities. Comprehensive tobacco control policies have the potential to reduce these health disparities [3]. Given the clear correlation between an individual's socioeconomic status, their environment, and the prevalence of tobacco use, it is essential that tobacco control laws and policies are designed with a focus on the communities' most vulnerable to tobacco-related harm [4].

The Cancer Action Network asserts that tobacco use continues to be the leading cause of preventable death in the United States [5]. While its prevalence has declined in higher-income communities, certain populations remain particularly vulnerable, and this vulnerability perpetuates existing health disparities. Social determinants like education, income, and environmental factors are significant contributors to the risk and effects of tobacco use. As a result, communities with higher smoking rates face uneven health outcomes since they are more susceptible to tobacco-related health issues [6].

Health equity signifies the equal opportunity for everyone to attain their best health, regardless of their social, economic, or environmental circumstances. However, higher tobacco use rates within low-income communities and communities of color often obstruct this pursuit of health equity. The conditions in which people live and die are often shaped by political, social, and economic forces [7]. These factors also influence the unequal distribution of power, income, goods, services, and access to vital resources like healthcare and education. Differences in tobacco use among specific populations correlate with the risk of morbidity, mortality, tobacco-related illnesses, and secondhand smoke exposure. Hence, social and environmental circumstances significantly impact an individual's likelihood of smoking and their exposure to secondhand smoke.

> *"Communities of color, especially Black Americans, have higher rates of tobacco use than their white counterparts. This discrepancy isn't a mere coincidence but a direct result of targeted advertising by tobacco companies."*
>
> The American Lung Association

Multiple factors account for the higher incidence of tobacco use in these vulnerable communities. One factor is tobacco advertising itself. Though there have been recent upticks in electronic cigarettes amongst teens and young adults, tobacco use has become less popular over the past 50 years. This has left the tobacco industry searching for populations to keep their companies in business. Unfortunately, they have looked to marginalized communities to fill that void. Tobacco companies often exploit low-income and minority communities with aggressive marketing, competitive pricing, and other strategies, making tobacco initiation and cessation increasingly challenging [8]. They deliberately target Black Americans, young individuals, low-income communities, and LGBTQ+ communities with their marketing [9]. Predatory advertising tactics include hosting promotions at music events, retail stores, and media platforms associated with Black communities. They also offer discounted prices in these areas, making their products more appealing to low-income and price-sensitive youth. Furthermore, tobacco companies have introduced flavored and mentholated products, which can make initial experiences with tobacco less harsh and potentially more addictive.

Another factor that accounts for the higher incidence of tobacco use in vulnerable communities is stress. The Centers for Disease Control and Prevention found that over a quarter of Americans who smoke cigarettes report severe psychological distress [10]. Scholars, such as David R. Williams and Selina A. Mohammed, have found that racism and prejudice take a profound toll on health [11]. Racism and prejudiced encounters also place individuals in situations that could prompt them to cope with stress in unhealthy ways. Studies have found that individuals who experience racial/ethnic harassment are twice as likely to use tobacco daily [12]. Other studies have found that self-reported racial/ethnic discrimination is associated with substance abuse later in life [13]. Individuals who live in chronically stressful environments are more likely to utilize substances such as tobacco [14]. The impact of racism on stress increases the risk of health problems from tobacco use among racial minorities by exacerbating stress levels.

Research indicates that these strategies have a "devastating impact" on Black communities, as tobacco use is the leading cause of preventable death among Black Americans [15]. Smoking and tobacco use are associated with higher rates of cancer, heart disease, and stroke and can increase the risk of serious illness from COVID-19. Exposure to secondhand smoke also has grave health consequences – placing family members and other community members at risk of illness. Combined with factors like limited access to health services and tobacco cessation resources, the use of tobacco in these communities significantly hampers health equity. It is worth noting that some minority communities, such as indigenous populations, utilize tobacco in sacred religious practices. Public health and health equity professionals must be mindful of the importance of these cultural and religious practices, while also providing communities with multifaceted support [16]. The contributing factors to high tobacco prevalence in these communities are interlinked, creating a vicious cycle of tobacco use and health disparity. Therefore, it's essential that tobacco control policies take a comprehensive approach, addressing all the contributory elements to tobacco use in vulnerable communities, thus mitigating health disparities.

14.2 Strategies for Policy Interventions to Foster Health Equity

Experts recommend a combination of tobacco control laws and policies to mitigate tobacco use and foster health equity in vulnerable communities [17]. The most potent strategies are detailed below.

14.2.1 Implementation of Smoke-Free Laws

Smoke-free laws serve to make smoking less socially acceptable while also curtailing exposure to secondhand smoke [18]. By restricting where and when individuals can smoke, these laws influence tobacco use in two fundamental ways. First, they adjust the environmental context, making smoking inconvenient and less socially acceptable. Over time, these laws promote healthier choices, such as abstaining from smoking, as the default behavior. Such normalization could instigate significant behavioral and societal changes within communities. Some experts suggest that this cessation of smoking could potentially be "contagious," creating a positive ripple effect on younger generations. Second, smoke-free laws reduce the prevalence of secondhand smoking, leading to improved overall community health, including the health of nonsmokers and children, who are often vulnerable to the harmful effects of tobacco smoke.

14.2.2 Investment in Anti-tobacco Education and Ad Campaigns

Tobacco companies often direct their marketing efforts toward vulnerable communities, leveraging sophisticated advertising techniques to appeal to these groups [19]. Over the years, there have been several instances of regulatory changes aimed at controlling the promotion of tobacco products. For example, the ban on cigarette advertising on television and radio in many countries was a landmark effort to reduce the exposure of the general populace, and especially youth, to tobacco promotion.

However, despite such interventions, the tobacco lobby has wielded significant influence, even shaping legislative decisions in ways favorable to their interests. While some measures, such as graphic warning labels and restrictions on advertising near schools, have shown positive outcomes, the industry often finds loopholes or alternate channels to continue their aggressive marketing. For instance, they might increase their presence on social media or employ subtle product placements in popular culture, bypassing traditional restrictions.

Counteracting these advertisements with information about the negative consequences of tobacco use can help neutralize the influence of the tobacco industry. Studies indicate that consistent, targeted, and culturally sensitive anti-tobacco ad campaigns can lead to a decline in smoking rates among vulnerable populations [20]. Thus, refining and reinforcing regulations around tobacco promotion is a critical and ongoing need.

Anti-tobacco ad campaigns and educational initiatives can empower individuals, particularly youth who have yet to encounter tobacco products, to make informed decisions against tobacco use. It is also essential for congressional accountability to be in place, ensuring that regulations effectively curtail aggressive marketing tactics and prioritize public health over corporate interests.

14.2.3 Investment in Tobacco Cessation Programs

Due to the addictive nature of tobacco products, quitting is often challenging for users [21]. Tobacco cessation treatments provide the necessary support for individuals wanting to quit, but these treatments can be prohibitively expensive, especially for individuals from low socioeconomic backgrounds. By investing in affordable and accessible tobacco cessation programs, communities can ensure that those desiring to quit have the necessary resources.

14.2.4 Increase in the Cost of Tobacco Products

An increase in the cost of tobacco products can serve as a deterrent for users [22]. Price-sensitive groups may be less inclined to continue tobacco use if the cost is prohibitive. Furthermore, higher prices could dissuade youth from initiating tobacco use. Profits derived from tobacco taxes can be redirected into anti-tobacco education and other tobacco control resources.

14.2.5 Regulation of Tobacco Product Sales

Experts suggest implementing regulations and limitations on the sale of tobacco products [23]. The number of tobacco retail stores correlates with increased smoking rates. Limiting the number of retailers through licensing regulations can reduce the accessibility of tobacco. Certain products, such as e-cigarettes, menthol cigarettes, and other flavored tobacco products, are used to target vulnerable communities. These products are designed to attract new users and can be particularly addictive [24]. Restricting the sale of such products may contribute to a decline in tobacco use. Cities like San Francisco and Chicago have already enacted such bans and restrictions, providing a blueprint for other communities considering similar policies.

14.2.6 Raising the Minimum Age for Tobacco Purchases

Some experts suggest raising the minimum age for purchasing tobacco products from 18 to 21 to limit access for underage individuals [25], akin to alcohol restrictions. While this might not entirely prevent illegal sales and access, it would create an additional barrier for young individuals looking to purchase tobacco products. Moreover, raising the minimum purchase age would limit the effectiveness of tobacco advertising targeting underage youth. After many years of state and local action to again raise the age to 21, a US nationwide standard of 21 as the minimum legal sale age for all tobacco products, including e-cigarettes, was enacted in 2020 [26].

14.2.7 Strengthening Enforcement

Increased enforcement of existing tobacco control laws, such as minimum age and smoke-free laws, is suggested by experts [27]. This includes placing the onus on retailers to prevent sales to underage individuals and ramping up enforcement to ensure compliance. Over time, improved enforcement can contribute to changing societal attitudes toward tobacco use and reducing its prevalence. While there is no singular solution to address the myriad environmental, educational, health, generational, and behavioral factors contributing to tobacco use and health disparities, a comprehensive implementation of these varied tobacco control strategies could effectively improve health equity.

14.3 Strategizing Policy Implementation to Enhance Health Equity

Tobacco control measures have proven effective: since their increase in 1964, there's been a decline in smokers and in advertising for tobacco products [28]. However, this general decline overlooks communities with a higher prevalence of smoking. Strategic and comprehensive implementation of tobacco control is crucial to address the unique needs of these communities. Comprehensive programs can reduce tobacco use across various racial, ethnic, and socioeconomic groups. However, it is vital for policymakers to customize policies to community needs and monitor their impact to prevent unintentionally creating new health disparities.

14.3.1 The Comprehensive Approach

An equity-focused approach to tobacco control aims to address the socio-environmental factors contributing to high tobacco use in specific communities, thereby preventing health disparities [29]. Tobacco control policies have been unevenly adopted and enforced across the country, leading to geographic tobacco-related disparities [30]. To address these disparities, coordinated efforts focused on reducing tobacco use and exposure are necessary. The strategies discussed earlier should be employed together to provide a comprehensive approach that prevents young individuals from starting tobacco, discourages current users, counteracts tobacco companies' messaging, and supports current users who struggle to quit independently.

Before implementing major policy changes, a thorough analysis of potential health effects on certain communities is necessary. Using data to understand how policies will affect communities at high risk for tobacco use enables more efficient resource allocation. It is crucial to monitor the implementation and effectiveness of tobacco control programs to ensure they do not unintentionally create new disparities. Community assessments can guide the design of a comprehensive control program and aid in evaluating the program's effectiveness.

14.3.2 Minimizing Unintended Consequences

Improperly implemented tobacco control policies may yield unintended consequences [31]. For instance, as discussed earlier, taxing tobacco or increasing its price can foster cultural change and discourage smoking. High tobacco prices deter low-income individuals and young people from smoking due to cost barriers. However, policymakers should be aware of the addictive nature of tobacco when implementing such taxes. Low-income smokers may struggle to access costly cessation treatments, resulting in a greater proportion of their incomes spent on cigarettes than high-income smokers, exacerbating the disparity. These programs should exist in tandem. Implementing them separately could have grave consequences, such as mass withdrawal.

When raising tobacco product prices, the increase should apply universally to prevent users from switching to cheaper alternatives. Policymakers should simultaneously escalate tobacco education campaigns and fund tobacco control programs while increasing tobacco prices. Making tobacco cessation treatments more affordable improves accessibility and liberates income otherwise spent on tobacco products and related medical expenses.

14.3.3 Promoting Investment in Tobacco Control

Administrative and operational costs associated with tobacco control programs can be burdensome, particularly for resource-limited communities [32]. Funds from the Tobacco Multistate Settlement Agreement, tobacco taxes, and government healthcare programs could be harnessed to implement and maintain these programs. It's worth noting that populations experiencing health disparities make up a significant portion of healthcare costs [33]. Advocates should highlight that investing in tobacco control programs could eliminate tobacco-related disparities, decrease healthcare costs, and result in substantial state savings.

Tobacco use is a significant risk factor for other community and public health issues [34]. To foster community buy-in for tobacco control programs, awareness of the connection between tobacco use and other community problems should be raised. This awareness could attract new partners and strengthen support for the initiatives. To ensure equal protection, tobacco control policies should be consistently implemented across socioeconomic strata. This consistency will help reduce tobacco-related disparities, discourage tobacco use, and enhance health equity.

14.4 Conclusion: Achieving Equity in Tobacco Control

Achieving equity in tobacco control interventions is paramount to ensuring that all populations, regardless of socioeconomic status, have the opportunity to benefit from the reduction in tobacco use and exposure to secondhand smoke. Implementing such interventions through a health-equity framework is pivotal, yet the roles and responsibilities of various stakeholders need to be distinctly articulated.

At the federal level, policymakers can establish comprehensive guidelines and regulations for tobacco control. They can set mandates for standardized labeling, advertising restrictions, and pricing policies that account for health equity. Federal agencies can also allocate funds to research and support the implementation of national tobacco control initiatives. State and local governments should tailor tobacco control policies to address the unique needs of their communities. This may include imposing taxes on tobacco products, implementing smoke-free laws, and initiating public health campaigns to educate citizens. Local authorities can actively engage in monitoring and enforcing these regulations, ensuring that interventions are effective and equitable. Healthcare providers play a critical role in tobacco control by incorporating smoking cessation programs and counseling as part of routine care. They can collaborate with communities to understand the specific barriers faced by individuals in accessing these resources and work toward eliminating them. Private actors, including NGOs and community organizations, can complement public efforts by advocating for tobacco control, conducting outreach programs, and offering support services. These entities can often provide a grassroots perspective, ensuring that interventions are culturally sensitive and equitable. Engaging communities in designing and implementing tobacco control interventions ensures that the strategies employed are culturally competent and address the specific needs of the population. Community leaders can act as liaisons between policymakers and the public, ensuring that interventions are not only accepted but also effective.

In conclusion, for tobacco control interventions to be genuinely equitable and impactful, a multilayered approach involving federal, state, and local authorities, healthcare providers, private actors, and the community itself is essential. A concerted effort to invest in long-term, equity-focused tobacco control programs can significantly improve health outcomes and contribute to the establishment of tobacco-free communities. By clarifying the roles and responsibilities at each level, we can ensure a coordinated and effective approach to mitigating the disparities tied to tobacco use and fostering health equity.

Policies to Advance Equity in Tobacco Control

Policy	Details	Rationale
Banning Menthol Cigarettes	Proscribe the sale of mentholated tobacco products	Menthol cigarettes are disproportionately used by African American smokers, contributing to higher rates of tobacco-related health issues in this group
Improving Data Collection	Enhance data collection systems to adequately represent the diversity within Asian American, Native Hawaiian, and Pacific Islander communities	Better data collection will help identify specific needs and tailor tobacco control programs to effectively reach these diverse populations
Involving Local Communities	Include local communities in policymaking processes and allocate financial resources to community organizations	Involving communities ensures policies are relevant and supported, empowering them to advocate for health equity
Targeted Cessation Programs	Develop culturally and linguistically tailored tobacco prevention and cessation programs for specific populations	Culturally relevant programs are more effective in addressing the unique challenges faced by diverse communities
Integrating Tobacco Cessation in Mental Health	Make tobacco cessation a part of mental health treatment strategies	People with mental illness have higher smoking rates and face greater challenges in quitting, requiring integrated support
Expanding LGBT-Specific Programs	Create and support tobacco cessation programs specifically designed for LGBT populations	LGBT individuals smoke at significantly higher rates, and targeted programs can address specific social and cultural factors influencing their smoking
Regional and State Efforts	Focus on regional and state policies to address the unequal burden of tobacco-related diseases, particularly in Southern and Midwestern states	Addressing regional disparities ensures that populations in areas with less stringent tobacco control measures receive adequate protection and support
Restricting Tobacco Marketing	Implement policies to restrict predatory tobacco marketing practices targeting marginalized communities	Limiting targeted marketing can reduce the exposure and influence of tobacco advertisements on vulnerable populations
Taxation Policies	Increase tobacco taxes in low-income and rural areas to reduce smoking prevalence	Higher tobacco taxes are effective in reducing smoking rates, particularly among price-sensitive low-income populations
Equitable Treatment and Support	Ensure equal treatment for all groups (horizontal equity) and provide additional support for marginalized groups (vertical equity)	Addressing both horizontal and vertical equity helps create a fairer and more effective public health response to tobacco use disparities

References

1 Cornelius, M.E., Wang, T.W., Jamal, A. et al. (2020). Tobacco product use among adults – United States, 2019. *MMWR. Morbidity and Mortality Weekly Report* 69 (46): 1736–1742.

2 Fagan, P., King, G., Lawrence, D. et al. (2004). Eliminating tobacco-related health disparities: directions for future research. *American Journal of Public Health* 94 (2): 211–217.

3 Center for Public Health Systems Science, Brossart, L., Moreland-Russell, S., and Andersen, S. (2015). *Best Practices User Guide: Health Equity in Tobacco Prevention and Control*, 77. Center for Public Health Systems Science.

4 Garrett, B.E., Dube, S.R., Babb, S., and McAfee, T. (2015). Addressing the social determinants of health to reduce tobacco-related disparities. *Nicotine & Tobacco Research: Official Journal of the Society for Research on Nicotine and Tobacco* 17 (8): 892–897.

5 Cwalina, S.N., Ihenacho, U., Barker, J. et al. (2023). Advancing racial equity and social justice for Black communities in US tobacco control policy. *Tobacco Control* 32 (3): 381–384.

6 Fagan, P., Moolchan, E.T., Lawrence, D. et al. (2007). Identifying health disparities across the tobacco continuum. *Addiction* 102: 5–29.

7 Navarro, V. and Shi, L. (2001). The political context of social inequalities and health. *Social Science & Medicine (1982)* 52 (3): 481–491.

8 Kong, A.Y. and Henriksen, L. (2022). Retail endgame strategies: reduce tobacco availability and visibility and promote health equity. *Tobacco Control* 31 (2): 243–249.

9 Stevens, P., Carlson, L.M., and Hinman, J.M. (2004). An analysis of tobacco industry marketing to lesbian, gay, bisexual, and transgender (LGBT) populations: strategies for mainstream tobacco control and prevention. *Health Promotion Practice* 5 (3 Suppl): 129S–134S.

10 CDC (2023). *Current Cigarette Smoking Among Adults in the United States*. Centers for Disease Control and Prevention https://www.cdc.gov/tobacco/data_statistics/fact_sheets/adult_data/cig_smoking/index.htm (last visited 11 August 2023).

11 Williams, D.R. (2018). Stress and the mental health of populations of color: advancing our understanding of race-related stressors. *Journal of Health and Social Behavior* 59: 466. Williams, D.R. and Mohammed, S.A. (2009). Discrimination and racial disparities in health: evidence and needed research. *Journal of Behavioral Medicine* 32:20.

12 Bennett, G.G. et al. (2005). Perceived racial/ethnic harassment and tobacco use among African American young adults. *American Journal of Public Health* 95: 238.

13 Gibbons, F.X. et al. (2004). Perceived discrimination and substance use in African American parents and their children: a panel study. *Journal of Personality and Social Psychology* 86: 517.

14 Jackson, J.S., Knight, K.M., and Rafferty, J.A. (2010). Race and unhealthy behaviors: chronic stress, the HPA axis, and physical and mental health disparities over the life course. *American Journal of Public Health* 100: 933.

15 Kong, A.Y. and King, B.A. (2021). Boosting the tobacco control vaccine: recognizing the role of the retail environment in addressing tobacco use and disparities. *Tobacco Control* 30 (e2): e162–e168.

16 Truth Initiative(2017). In a good way: indigenous commercial tobacco control practices. https://keepitsacred.itcmi.org/wp-content/uploads/2015/02/InAGoodWay_finalWeb-1.pdf).

17 Okuyemi, K.S., Reitzel, L.R., and Fagan, P. (2015). Interventions to reduce tobacco-related health disparities. *Nicotine & Tobacco Research: Official Journal of the Society for Research on Nicotine and Tobacco* 17 (8): 887–891.

18 Yang, T., Abdullah, A.S., Li, L. et al. (2013). Public place smoke-free regulations, secondhand smoke exposure and related beliefs, awareness, attitudes, and practices among Chinese urban residents. *International Journal of Environmental Research and Public Health* 10 (6): 2370–2383.

19 Baig, S.A., Pepper, J.K., Morgan, J.C., and Brewer, N.T. (2017). Social identity and support for counteracting tobacco company marketing that targets vulnerable populations. *Social Science & Medicine* 1982 (182): 136–141.

20 Cruz, T.B., Rose, S.W., Lienemann, B.A. et al. (2019). Pro-tobacco marketing and anti-tobacco campaigns aimed at vulnerable populations: a review of the literature. *Tobacco Induced Diseases* 17: 68.

21 Kozlowski, L.T., Wilkinson, D.A., Skinner, W. et al. (1989). Comparing tobacco cigarette dependence with other drug dependencies. Greater or equal 'difficulty quitting' and 'urges to use,' but less 'pleasure' from cigarettes. *JAMA* 261 (6): 898–901.

22 McLaughlin, I., Pearson, A., Laird-Metke, E., and Ribisl, K. (2014). Reducing tobacco use and access through strengthened minimum price laws. *American Journal of Public Health* 104 (10): 1844–1850.

23 Chapman, S. and Freeman, B. (2009). Regulating the tobacco retail environment: beyond reducing sales to minors. *Tobacco Control* 18 (6): 496–501.

24 Mejia, A.B. and Ling, P.M. (2010). Tobacco industry consumer research on smokeless tobacco users and product development. *American Journal of Public Health* 100 (1): 78–87.

25 Winickoff, J.P., Hartman, L., Chen, M.L. et al. (2014). Retail impact of raising tobacco sales age to 21 years. *American Journal of Public Health* 104 (11): e18–e21.

26 Kim, S.C.J., Martinez, J.E., Liu, Y., and Friedman, T.C. (2021). US Tobacco 21 is paving the way for a tobacco endgame. *Tobacco Use Insights* 14: 1179173X211050396.

27 Jacobson, P.D. and Wasserman, J. (1999). The implementation and enforcement of tobacco control laws: policy implications for activists and the industry. *Journal of Health Politics, Policy and Law* 24 (3): 567–598.

28 Cokkinides, V., Bandi, P., McMahon, C. et al. (2009). Tobacco control in the United States – recent progress and opportunities. *CA: A Cancer Journal for Clinicians* 59 (6): 352–365.

29 Mentis, A.A. (2017). Social determinants of tobacco use: towards an equity lens approach. *Tobacco Prevention and Cessation* 3: 7.

30 Doogan, N.J., Roberts, M.E., Wewers, M.E. et al. (2017). A growing geographic disparity: rural and urban cigarette smoking trends in the United States. *Preventive Medicine* 104: 79–85.

31 Burgess, D.J., Fu, S.S., and van Ryn, M. (2009). Potential unintended consequences of tobacco-control policies on mothers who smoke: a review of the literature. *American Journal of Preventive Medicine* 37 (2 Suppl): S151–S158.

32 Kahende, J.W., Loomis, B.R., Adhikari, B., and Marshall, L. (2009). A review of economic evaluations of tobacco control programs. *International Journal of Environmental Research and Public Health* 6 (1): 51–68.

33 Braveman, P. (2006). Health disparities and health equity: concepts and measurement. *Annual Review of Public Health* 27: 167–194.

34 Reddy, K.S., Yadav, A., Arora, M., and Nazar, G.P. (2012). Integrating tobacco control into health and development agendas. *Tobacco Control* 21 (2): 281–286.

15

Tackling the Overdose Crisis Through Equitable Harm Reduction Policies

Abstract

This chapter provides a comprehensive overview of the opioid overdose epidemic in the United States, emphasizing the need for an equity-centered, harm reduction approach to address this complex public health crisis. The chapter begins by highlighting the magnitude of the epidemic and its disproportionate impact on communities of color and low-income populations, underscoring the role of structural inequities in perpetuating these disparities. It then outlines key strategies for tackling the crisis, including expanding access to naloxone, providing safer use supplies and services, increasing access to evidence-based treatment, and addressing the social determinants of health. The chapter also stresses the importance of reforming the criminal justice system, combating stigma and misconceptions surrounding substance use and addiction, and enhancing data collection and oversight to ensure an equitable and effective response. Throughout, the chapter emphasizes the critical role of community-based organizations and the need to center the voices and experiences of impacted communities in the design and implementation of interventions. The chapter concludes with a powerful call to action, urging policymakers to leverage resources, such as opioid settlement funds, to support bold, compassionate, and equity-focused initiatives that prioritize harm reduction, dismantle barriers to care, and invest in the social safety net, ultimately building a future in which all individuals have the opportunity to live healthy, fulfilling lives.

Keywords *overdose crisis; harm reduction; health equity; naloxone access; criminal justice reform; structural inequities; community-based programs; substance use disorder treatment*

> *Jaden, a Black man in his early 30s, lost his job and struggled with addiction. Living in a neighborhood with limited healthcare services, he found it nearly impossible to access treatment. His community, riddled with stigma and lacking resources, offered little support. As overdose rates climbed, James felt trapped, knowing that a lack of equitable harm reduction services was costing lives, including those of his friends and neighbors.*

> *Naomi, a single mother in her mid-20s, faced the harsh reality of the opioid crisis in her low-income community. Despite her efforts to stay clean, the criminalization of drug use left her with a record that barred her from stable employment and housing. Each day was a battle against relapse, with minimal access to medications for addiction treatment and an unforgiving system that offered more punishment than help.*

15.1 The Need for an Equity-Centered, Harm Reduction Approach

The United States is facing an opioid overdose epidemic of unparalleled magnitude. Since 1999, more than one million people have lost their lives to drug overdoses, with opioids accounting for an increasingly significant share of these deaths [1]. In 2022 alone, over 100,000 individuals died from drug overdoses [2], making it the leading cause of injury-related mortality in the country, surpassing both motor vehicle accidents and gun violence. Among these deaths, more than 83,000 involved opioids, with fentanyl [3], a highly potent synthetic opioid, being the primary driver of the rising death toll, particularly among Americans aged 18–49.

However, this public health crisis cannot be attributed solely to the overprescribing of opioids or the proliferation of fentanyl in the illicit drug market. Instead, it is deeply rooted in a complex web of structural inequities, including racism, poverty, lack of access to healthcare, and the criminalization of drug use. The overdose epidemic has had a disproportionate impact on communities of color and low-income populations, reflecting the profound disparities that shape health outcomes in the United States. For example, despite similar rates of opioid use across racial groups, Black and Indigenous communities have experienced a more rapid increase in opioid overdose deaths in recent years compared to white populations [4].

These disparities are perpetuated by a range of factors, including unequal access to healthcare and addiction treatment services. An estimated 8.3 million Black and Latino residents reside in "pharmacy deserts," limiting their access to life-saving medications such as naloxone and buprenorphine [5]. Moreover, despite comparable rates of substance use disorders, Black and Hispanic individuals are more likely to encounter barriers to accessing high-quality treatment, as evidenced by studies showing that they receive medication for opioid use disorder (MOUD) for shorter durations than white patients [6].

The criminalization of drug use has also played a significant role in exacerbating the harms associated with the opioid crisis, particularly for communities of color. Punitive drug policies have led to the disproportionate incarceration of Black and Hispanic individuals, who are far more likely to be arrested, prosecuted, and imprisoned for drug-related offenses than their white counterparts, despite similar rates of drug use [7]. This not only perpetuates racial inequities but also increases the risk of overdose and other negative health outcomes for individuals with substance use disorders, as access to evidence-based treatment and harm reduction services is often severely limited or nonexistent in carceral settings.

To effectively address this multifaceted challenge, policymakers must adopt a comprehensive, equity-focused approach that prioritizes harm reduction strategies, expands access to evidence-based treatment, and addresses the social determinants of health that shape patterns of substance use and overdose risk.

At the heart of this response should be a commitment to harm reduction, an evidence-based public health strategy that aims to minimize the negative consequences associated with drug use, such as overdose, HIV/AIDS, and hepatitis C, while providing compassionate, non-judgmental support to individuals struggling with substance use disorders. Rather than insisting on abstinence as the only acceptable goal, harm reduction meets people where they are and helps them stay safe and healthy, regardless of their drug use status.

Harm reduction approaches have been shown to be highly effective in reducing overdose deaths and other drug-related harms. For instance, a study found that community-based naloxone distribution through syringe exchange programs resulted in a 65% reduction in overdose fatalities over a six-month period [8]. Similarly, research has demonstrated that establishing overdose prevention centers (OPCs), where individuals can use drugs under medical supervision, can significantly reduce overdose deaths and increase access to addiction treatment and other health and social services [9].

"There were 54.1 fatal drug overdoses for every 100,000 Black men in the United States in 2020. That was similar to the rate among American Indian or Alaska Native men (52.1 deaths per 100,000 people) and well above the rates among White men (44.2 per 100,000) and Hispanic men (27.3 per 100,000)."
John Gramlich, Associate Director at Pew Research Center

15.2 Expanding Access to Naloxone

One of the most effective harm reduction interventions is the community-based distribution of naloxone, a life-saving medication that can reverse an opioid overdose. Research has shown that when naloxone is made widely available and community members are trained on how to use it, overdose deaths decrease significantly [10]. Policymakers should prioritize expanding access to naloxone, particularly for individuals at high risk of overdose and their social networks. This can be achieved through Opioid Education and Naloxone Distribution (OEND) programs, syringe exchange programs, and partnerships with trusted community organizations that serve people who use drugs.

To ensure an adequate supply of affordable naloxone, states should consider establishing bulk purchasing funds, which would allow them to negotiate reduced prices and guarantee a consistent supply of this life-saving medication. Massachusetts' Municipal Naloxone Bulk Purchase Trust Fund provides a promising model, enabling the state to purchase naloxone at a wholesale price and sell it to cities and towns at a heavily discounted rate.

15.3 Providing Safer Use Supplies and Services

In addition to naloxone, a comprehensive harm reduction approach should include the provision of safer use supplies and services. Distributing sterile syringes, safer smoking supplies, and drug-checking technologies can significantly reduce the risk of overdose, HIV/AIDS, hepatitis C, and other health complications associated with drug use. Policymakers should support community-based organizations in providing these essential supplies and services, while also working to remove legal and policy barriers to their distribution.

Establishing OPCs, also known as supervised consumption sites, is another promising harm reduction strategy. OPCs provide a safe, hygienic space for individuals to use drugs under medical supervision, reducing the risk of overdose death and connecting people to addiction treatment and other health and social services. While legal and political barriers currently prevent the operation of OPCs in the United States, policymakers should explore opportunities to pilot these life-saving interventions, learning from the success of such facilities in Canada, Europe, and Australia.

15.4 Expanding Access to Evidence-Based Treatment

Medications for Addiction Treatment (MAT), such as methadone and buprenorphine, are the gold standard for treating opioid use disorder. Numerous studies have shown that MAT can reduce the risk of overdose, minimize the severity of relapses, and decrease incarceration rates for drug-related crimes [11]. However, access to MAT remains limited due to a combination of stigma, regulatory barriers, lack of provider training, and inadequate insurance coverage, particularly for low-income and marginalized populations.

To expand access to MAT, policymakers should work to eliminate burdensome regulations, such as the X-waiver requirement for buprenorphine prescribing, which limit the number of providers able to offer this life-saving treatment [12]. They should also make permanent the temporary flexibilities implemented during the COVID-19 pandemic, such as allowing take-home doses of methadone and telemedicine evaluations, which have expanded access to care for countless individuals [13].

Expanding Medicaid coverage is another critical step in ensuring equitable access to addiction treatment. Medicaid is the largest payer for MAT, and states that have expanded Medicaid under the Affordable Care Act have seen significant increases in access to substance use disorder treatment [14]. Policymakers should work to eliminate bureaucratic obstacles to Medicaid enrollment and ensure comprehensive coverage for all FDA-approved forms of MAT.

For individuals involved in the criminal justice system, access to MAT is often nonexistent or severely limited, despite the high prevalence of opioid use disorder in this population. Policymakers should ensure that all individuals who are arrested, detained, or incarcerated have access to naloxone, MAT, and related care, as well as robust reentry support upon release. This should include funding for pilot programs that provide MAT in criminal justice settings and evaluating their effectiveness in reducing overdose risk and recidivism [15].

15.5 Addressing Structural Determinants and Promoting Health Equity

While expanding access to harm reduction services and evidence-based treatment is essential, it is not enough to fully address the overdose crisis. To achieve lasting change, policymakers must also confront the structural determinants that shape patterns of substance use and overdose risk, including racism, poverty, housing instability, and lack of access to education and employment opportunities.

The overdose crisis has disproportionately impacted communities of color and low-income populations, reflecting the deep-rooted inequities that permeate American society. Black and Hispanic individuals, for example, face significant barriers to accessing substance use disorder treatment, including lack of insurance coverage, stigma, and mistrust of the healthcare system rooted in a long history of discrimination and abuse [16]. Addressing these disparities requires a concerted effort to dismantle the systemic racism that permeates our health care, criminal justice, and social service systems [17].

15.6 Investing in Community Development

One key strategy for promoting health equity is investing in community development programs that address the social and economic conditions that contribute to substance use and overdose risk. This includes initiatives focused on affordable housing, job training and employment support, trauma-informed mental health services, child care and family support, and other crucial social safety net programs. Critically, these programs should not be preconditioned on abstinence from drug use, which only serves to perpetuate barriers to access and support [18].

Policymakers should also prioritize funding for community-based organizations that are rooted in the communities they serve and have a deep understanding of the unique challenges and strengths of those communities [19]. These organizations are often best positioned to provide culturally responsive, trauma-informed services that address the intersecting needs of individuals and families impacted by substance use and overdose.

15.7 Reforming the Criminal Justice System

The criminalization of drug use has had a devastating impact on communities of color, exacerbating the harms associated with substance use and creating barriers to treatment and support [20]. Despite similar rates of drug use across racial and ethnic groups, Black and Hispanic individuals are far more likely to be arrested, prosecuted, and incarcerated for drug-related offenses than their white counterparts. This not only perpetuates racial inequities but also increases the risk of overdose and other negative health outcomes for individuals with substance use disorders.

To address these disparities, policymakers must work to reform the criminal justice system and shift toward a public health approach to drug use. This includes depenalizing drug possession, implementing alternatives to incarceration for individuals with substance use disorders, and investing in community-based crisis response teams that can address drug-related emergencies with a focus on harm reduction and treatment rather than punishment [21].

Policymakers should also support efforts to expunge or seal criminal records for individuals with past drug-related convictions, which can create significant barriers to housing, employment, and other essential services. Removing these barriers is crucial for promoting long-term recovery and reducing the risk of relapse and overdose [22].

15.8 Addressing Stigma and Misconceptions

Stigma and misconceptions surrounding substance use and addiction treatment pose significant barriers to effective care and support. Despite the overwhelming evidence that addiction is a complex medical condition requiring compassionate, evidence-based treatment, many individuals with substance use disorders continue to face blame, shame, and discrimination from healthcare providers, policymakers, and the general public.

To address these challenges, policymakers should invest in national and state-level campaigns to educate the public and healthcare providers about the nature of addiction, the effectiveness of harm reduction and MAT, and the importance of a non-judgmental, equity-focused response to the overdose crisis. These campaigns should be developed in partnership with people who use drugs and individuals in recovery, ensuring that messaging is accurate, respectful, and resonant with the communities most impacted by substance use and overdose [23].

Policymakers should also support efforts to integrate substance use disorder education into medical and nursing school curricula, as well as ongoing training for healthcare providers. This education should emphasize the importance of harm reduction, the evidence base for MAT, and the role of trauma and structural inequities in shaping patterns of substance use and overdose risk [24].

15.9 Enhancing Data Collection and Oversight

To ensure that the response to the overdose crisis is equitable and effective, policymakers must invest in robust data collection and oversight mechanisms. This includes requiring the collection and reporting of race, ethnicity, and other demographic data in all aspects of the response, from naloxone distribution to MAT access to overdose fatalities. This data should be used to identify disparities, track progress, and inform targeted interventions to address gaps in care and support [25].

Policymakers should also establish independent oversight bodies to monitor the implementation of opioid settlement funds and hold stakeholders accountable for their use [26]. These bodies should include representatives from impacted communities, harm reduction and treatment providers, and public health experts, ensuring a diverse range of perspectives and expertise [27].

Finally, policymakers should support community-based participatory research that engages people who use drugs and individuals in recovery in the design, implementation, and evaluation of overdose prevention and treatment interventions. This approach not only ensures that interventions are responsive to the needs and priorities of impacted communities but also helps to build trust and collaboration between researchers, service providers, and the communities they serve [28].

15.10 Conclusion: Leveraging Resources and Centering Equity in the Fight Against the Opioid Crisis

The opioid overdose crisis is a complex, multifaceted challenge that demands an equally comprehensive and nuanced response [29]. By prioritizing harm reduction, expanding access to evidence-based treatment, addressing structural determinants of health, and centering the voices and experiences of impacted communities, policymakers can chart a path toward a more just, equitable, and effective approach to this devastating public health emergency.

The road ahead is not easy, but the stakes could not be higher. With over a million lives lost to overdose in the past two decades and countless more hanging in the balance, the time for bold, compassionate, and equity-focused action is now. By leveraging opioid settlement funds and other resources to support community-based interventions [30], dismantle barriers to care [31], and invest in the social safety net [17], we can build a future in which all individuals, regardless of their drug use status or socioeconomic background, have the opportunity to live healthy, fulfilling lives [32]. It is a future worth fighting for, and one that we cannot afford to let slip away [33].

Policy and Equity Considerations for Overdose Prevention

Policy Area	Objective	Equity and Stigma Considerations	Aligned Policies	Implementation Strategies	Potential Indicators
Community Distribution of Naloxone	Increase naloxone availability and usage	• Reduce stigma through education and training • Prioritize distribution in underserved and high-risk communities	• FDA approval of OTC naloxone • State laws permitting naloxone dispensing in pharmacies and by community organizations	• Bulk purchasing programs • Training for naloxone administration • Partnerships with community-based organizations	• Number of naloxone doses distributed and used • Number of jurisdictions allowing naloxone distribution
Legalizing Drug Checking Equipment	Enhance drug safety and reduce overdose risk	• Address stigma through public education • Ensure accessibility in marginalized communities	• State laws legalizing fentanyl test strips (FTS) and other drug checking equipment	• Support FTS distribution with evidence-based practices • Establish training programs for FTS use • Engage community champions to advocate for policy changes	• Number of jurisdictions legalizing drug checking equipment • Reduction in HCV rates • Community support metrics for harm reduction services
Establishing Syringe Services Programs (SSPs)	Reduce the spread of infectious diseases and support harm reduction	• Provide non-stigmatizing access to healthcare services • Focus on high-need areas	• State laws authorizing SSPs • Federal funding support for SSPs	• Implement SSPs in both urban and rural areas • Collect data to inform policy and program improvements • Provide comprehensive services including naloxone distribution, vaccinations, and peer support.	• Number of SSPs established and maintained • Decrease in new HIV/HCV infections • Number of people accessing SSP services
Enhancing Substance Use Peer Support Programs	Integrate peer support in healthcare settings to aid recovery	• Reduce stigma through lived experience • Ensure accessibility in rural and underserved areas	• Medicaid reimbursement for peer support services • Federal support for peer programs and research	• Develop training and certification programs for peer support specialists • Embed peers in healthcare and community settings • Create a phone line for rural access	• Number of certified peer support specialists • Evaluation data on peer program effectiveness • Medicaid reimbursement data

References

1 Spencer, M. R., Miniño, A. M., & Warner, M. (2022). Drug overdose deaths in the United States, 2001–2021. NCHS Data Brief No. 457.

2 Centers for Disease Control and Prevention (2022). Drug overdose deaths in the U.S. top 100,000 annually. https://www.cdc.gov/nchs/pressroom/nchs_press_releases/2021/20211117.htm (accessed 28 August 2024).

3 National Institute on Drug Abuse (2021). Fentanyl DrugFacts. https://www.drugabuse.gov/publications/drugfacts/fentanyl (accessed 28 August 2024).

4 Substance Abuse and Mental Health Services Administration (2020). The opioid crisis and the Black/African American population: an urgent issue. https://store.samhsa.gov/product/opioid-crisis-and-blackafrican-american-population-urgent-issue/pep20-05-02-001.

5 Qato, D.M., Daviglus, M.L., Wilder, J. et al. (2014). 'Pharmacy deserts' are prevalent in Chicago's predominantly minority communities, raising medication access concerns. *Health Affairs* 33 (11): 1958–1965. https://doi.org/10.1377/hlthaff.2013.1397.

6 Lagisetty, P.A., Ross, R., Bohnert, A. et al. (2019). Buprenorphine treatment divide by race/ethnicity and payment. *JAMA Psychiatry* 76 (9): 979–981. https://doi.org/10.1001/jamapsychiatry.2019.0876.

7 Mitchell, O. and Caudy, M.S. (2015). Examining racial disparities in drug arrests. *Justice Quarterly* 32 (2): 288–313. https://doi.org/10.1080/07418825.2012.761721.

8 Walley, A.Y., Xuan, Z., Hackman, H.H. et al. (2013). Opioid overdose rates and implementation of overdose education and nasal naloxone distribution in Massachusetts: interrupted time series analysis. *BMJ* 346: f174. https://doi.org/10.1136/bmj.f174.

9 Marshall, B.D.L., Milloy, M.-J., Wood, E. et al. (2011). Reduction in overdose mortality after the opening of North America's first medically supervised safer injecting facility: a retrospective population-based study. *The Lancet* 377 (9775): 1429–1437. https://doi.org/10.1016/S0140-6736(10)62353-7.

10 Wagner, K.D., Bovet, L.J., Haynes, B. et al. (2016). Training law enforcement to respond to opioid overdose with naloxone: impact on knowledge, attitudes, and interactions with community members. *Drug and Alcohol Dependence* 165: 22–28.

11 Strange, C.C., Manchak, S.M., Hyatt, J.M. et al. (2022). Opioid-specific medication-assisted therapy and its impact on criminal justice and overdose outcomes. *Campbell Systematic Reviews* 18 (1): e1215.

12 Davis, C.S. and Carr, D. (2017). Legal changes to increase access to naloxone for opioid overdose reversal in the United States. *Drug and Alcohol Dependence* 157: 112–120. https://doi.org/10.1016/j.drugalcdep.2016.08.621.

13 Huskamp, H.A., Busch, A.B., Souza, J. et al. (2018). How is telemedicine being used in opioid and other substance use disorder treatment? *Health Affairs* 37 (12): 1940–1947. https://doi.org/10.1377/hlthaff.2018.05134.

14 Wen, H., Hockenberry, J.M., Borders, T.F., and Druss, B.G. (2017). Impact of Medicaid expansion on medicaid-covered utilization of buprenorphine for opioid use disorder treatment. *Medical Care* 55 (4): 336–341. https://doi.org/10.1097/MLR.0000000000000703.

15 Green, T.C., Clarke, J., Brinkley-Rubinstein, L. et al. (2018). Postincarceration fatal overdoses after implementing medications for addiction treatment in a statewide correctional system. *JAMA Psychiatry* 75 (4): 405–407. https://doi.org/10.1001/jamapsychiatry.2017.4614.

16 Bauer, G.R. (2014). Incorporating intersectionality theory into population health research methodology: challenges and the potential to advance health equity. *Social Science & Medicine* 110: 10–17. https://doi.org/10.1016/j.socscimed.2014.03.022.

17 Dasgupta, N., Beletsky, L., and Ciccarone, D. (2018). Opioid crisis: no easy fix to its social and economic determinants. *American Journal of Public Health* 108 (2): 182–186. https://doi.org/10.2105/AJPH.2017.304187.

18 Ashford, R.D., Curtis, B., and Brown, A.M. (2018). Peer-delivered harm reduction and recovery support services: initial evaluation from a hybrid recovery community drop-in center and syringe exchange program. *Harm Reduction Journal* 15 (1): 52. https://doi.org/10.1186/s12954-018-0258-2.

19 Wallerstein, N.B. and Duran, B. (2006). Using community-based participatory research to address health disparities. *Health Promotion Practice* 7 (3): 312–323. https://doi.org/10.1177/1524839906289376.

20 Mitchell, S.G., Kelly, S.M., Brown, B.S. et al. (2009). Uses of diverted methadone and buprenorphine by opioid-addicted individuals in Baltimore, Maryland. *The American Journal on Addictions* 18 (5): 346–355. https://doi.org/10.3109/10550490903077820.

21 Schiff, D.M., Drainoni, M.-L., Bair-Merritt, M. et al. (2016). A police-led addiction treatment referral program in Gloucester, MA: implementation and participants' experiences. *Journal of Substance Abuse Treatment* 82: 41–47. https://doi.org/10.1016/j.jsat.2016.09.003.

22 Bukten, A., Stavseth, M.R., Skurtveit, S. et al. (2017). High risk of overdose death following release from prison: variations in mortality during a 15-year observation period. *Addiction* 112 (8): 1432–1439. https://doi.org/10.1111/add.13803.

23 Luoma, J.B., Twohig, M.P., Waltz, T. et al. (2007). An investigation of stigma in individuals receiving treatment for substance abuse. *Addictive Behaviors* 32 (7): 1331–1346. https://doi.org/10.1016/j.addbeh.2006.09.008.

24 van Boekel, L.C., Brouwers, E.P.M., van Weeghel, J., and Garretsen, H.F.L. (2013). Stigma among health professionals towards patients with substance use disorders and its consequences for healthcare delivery: systematic review. *Drug and Alcohol Dependence* 131 (1): 23–35. https://doi.org/10.1016/j.drugalcdep.2013.02.018.

25 Marsh, J.C., Park, K., Lin, Y.-A., and Bersamira, C. (2018). Gender differences in trends for heroin use and nonmedical prescription opioid use, 2007-2014. *Journal of Substance Abuse Treatment* 87: 79–85. https://doi.org/10.1016/j.jsat.2018.01.001.

26 Bicket, M.C., McQuade, B., and Brummett, C.M. (2021). Opioid settlement funds – do not neglect patients with pain. *JAMA Health Forum* 2 (8): e211765. American Medical Association.

27 Pauly, B., Goldstone, I., McCall, J. et al. (2007). The ethical, legal and social context of harm reduction. *The Canadian Nurse* 103 (8): 19–23.

28 Wallerstein, N. and Duran, B. (2010). Community-based participatory research contributions to intervention research: the intersection of science and practice to improve health equity. *American Journal of Public Health* 100 (S1): S40–S46. https://doi.org/10.2105/AJPH.2009.184036.

29 Volkow, N.D. and Collins, F.S. (2017). The role of science in addressing the opioid crisis. *New England Journal of Medicine* 377 (4): 391–394. https://doi.org/10.1056/NEJMsr1706626.

30 Keane, C., Egan, J.E., and Hawk, M. (2018). Effects of naloxone distribution to likely bystanders: results of an agent-based model. *International Journal of Drug Policy* 55: 61–69. https://doi.org/10.1016/j.drugpo.2018.02.008.

31 Ti, L. and Ti, L. (2015). Leaving the hospital against medical advice among people who use illicit drugs: a systematic review. *American Journal of Public Health* 105 (12): e53–e59. https://doi.org/10.2105/AJPH. 2015.302885.

32 Barry, C.L., Huskamp, H.A., and Goldman, H.H. (2010). A political history of federal mental health and addiction insurance parity. *The Milbank Quarterly* 88 (3): 404–433. https://doi.org/10.1111/j.1468-0009.2010.00605.x.

33 Saloner, B., McGinty, E.E., Beletsky, L. et al. (2018). A public health strategy for the opioid crisis. *Public Health Reports* 133 (1_suppl): 24S–34S. https://doi.org/10.1177/0033354918793627.

16

Confronting the HIV/AIDS Epidemic: Progress, Challenges, and the Path Forward

Abstract

The chapter delves into the multifaceted landscape of HIV/AIDS, providing a comprehensive examination of its historical context, epidemiological trends, and the ongoing challenges in managing the disease. It begins with an exploration of the early years of the HIV/AIDS epidemic, highlighting the significant milestones in medical research and public health responses that have shaped our current understanding and approach to the disease. The chapter then transitions to a detailed analysis of the epidemiology of HIV, discussing patterns of transmission, demographic disparities, and the socioeconomic factors influencing the spread of the virus. Central to the chapter is an evaluation of the various prevention and treatment strategies that have been implemented over the years. This includes a discussion on antiretroviral therapy (ART) and its impact on reducing morbidity and mortality, as well as the role of pre-exposure prophylaxis (PrEP) in preventing new infections. The effectiveness of harm reduction approaches, such as needle exchange programs and safe sex education, is also scrutinized. The chapter further addresses the critical issue of health disparities and the inequities in access to HIV care and treatment. It examines the intersectionality of race, gender, and socioeconomic status in shaping the experiences of individuals living with HIV, and the structural barriers that hinder equitable access to healthcare services. Policy initiatives and public health interventions aimed at reducing these disparities are reviewed, highlighting successful models and identifying areas needing improvement. In addition, the chapter discusses the social and ethical dimensions of HIV/AIDS, including stigma, discrimination, and the rights of people living with HIV. The importance of community engagement, advocacy, and the role of nongovernmental organizations in supporting affected populations are emphasized. Finally, the chapter may conclude by discussing current efforts to end the HIV/AIDS epidemic, including global and national strategies, ongoing research, and the importance of addressing social and structural barriers to HIV prevention and treatment. The chapter may also emphasize the need for continued advocacy, education, and collaboration to achieve the goal of ending the HIV/AIDS epidemic worldwide.

Keywords   *HIV/AIDS epidemic; health disparities; stigma and discrimination; antiretroviral therapy (ART); pre-exposure prophylaxis (PrEP); needle exchange programs; structural determinants; criminalization of HIV*

Achieving Health Equity: The Role of Law and Policy, First Edition. Y. Tony Yang.
© 2025 John Wiley & Sons Ltd. Published 2025 by John Wiley & Sons Ltd.

> *John, a young gay man, hesitated to get tested for HIV, fearing discrimination and stigma. He had heard stories of people losing their jobs and facing rejection from loved ones after disclosing their HIV status. John knew he needed to prioritize his health, but the societal barriers seemed insurmountable.*
>
> *Michael, an activist and long-term survivor of HIV, witnessed firsthand the devastating impact of the epidemic in the 1980s. Despite the challenges he faced, Michael found strength in advocating for better treatment options, increased funding for research, and the destigmatization of HIV/ AIDS. His tireless efforts paved the way for a more compassionate and proactive response to the epidemic.*

16.1 Ending the HIV Epidemic: Addressing Social Disparities and Ensuring Access

Since the 1980s, HIV/AIDS has claimed the lives of over 700,000 Americans [1]. The United States has made significant progress in managing the HIV epidemic, including the approval of several effective HIV medications, the allocation of federal funding for HIV/AIDS research and treatment, and the development of three national HIV/AIDS strategies [2]. However, the country has consistently failed to address the relationship between social and structural determinants of health, resulting in the best HIV prevention and treatment resources remaining inaccessible to many US minority residents, marginalized groups, and inhabitants of certain regions [3]. To end the HIV epidemic in the United States, it is imperative that the nation eradicates laws and regulations that perpetuate HIV-related stigma and discrimination. Furthermore, tailored policies must be implemented to ensure that vulnerable populations have ready access to HIV testing, prevention methods, and treatment solutions. These changes are crucial for the country to successfully combat the HIV epidemic and protect the health of all its citizens.

16.2 Addressing Social Determinants: Key to Ending HIV Inequities

Black people, Latinos, and men who have sex with men (MSM) are disproportionately affected by HIV with infection rates significantly higher than those of white people [4]. Despite popular misconceptions attributing these disparities to promiscuity or high-risk behavior, the reality is that HIV/AIDS infections and related health complications are strongly linked to systemic wealth and health inequities [5]. The same groups facing socioeconomic challenges due to systemic inequities are also vulnerable to health inequities, such as limited access to HIV testing, prevention methods, and treatment options.

The Center for American Progress emphasizes the importance of considering social determinants of health when shaping HIV policy [6]. These determinants, which are tied to wealth and minority status, include factors such as residential segregation and housing discrimination. Living in low-income, under-resourced neighborhoods with limited access to HIV testing and treatment increases the risk of infection, particularly due to the communicable nature of HIV. It suggests that fair and affordable housing policies could lead to better health outcomes for these communities.

HIV-related inequities are also experienced geographically, with the Southern United States facing the highest rates of new HIV infections and HIV-related deaths [7]. This is largely due to policy decisions, such as the failure to expand Medicaid in several Southern states, leaving a significant portion of HIV-positive individuals uninsured and unable to afford regular medical visits and treatment. Additionally, Southern states are more likely to have abstinence-only education and less likely to fund HIV prevention programs, hindering awareness and perpetuating misinformation. The stigma surrounding HIV in the South further discourages individuals from seeking testing and treatment.

The failure to address social determinants of health has caused new HIV transmission rates to plateau, as HIV diagnosis and treatment are crucial in preventing its spread [8]. In 2016, while 86% of HIV-infected people in the United States were diagnosed, only 64% were receiving care, and a mere 53% had achieved viral suppression, the point at which HIV becomes undetectable and nontransmittable. Experts believe that the United States must develop targeted policies to improve the diagnosis-to-viral suppression pipeline in order to effectively curb the HIV epidemic [9].

16.3 Effective HIV Prevention: Education, Access, and Comprehensive Strategies

HIV infections in the United States have decreased significantly since the 1980s, with improvements in health outcomes for some disproportionately affected groups [10]. However, Black, Latino, and white gay and bisexual men, along with Black women, continue to be infected at above-average rates, indicating ongoing disparities in access to HIV treatment and prevention resources.

Experts emphasize the importance of educating the public about HIV transmission and prevention, as knowledge gaps perpetuate stigma and hinder protective measures. The 2021 National HIV/AIDS Strategy recommends comprehensive health and sex education, specifically advising against abstinence-only programs, which ignore the reality of sexual activity among youth and fail to equip them with necessary information [11].

The Centers for Disease Control and Prevention (CDC) advocates for social media campaigns promoting condoms as a safe, affordable, and effective method of preventing HIV and other sexually transmitted diseases [12]. Free condom distribution programs are a low-cost way for the government to prevent HIV spread, particularly among sexually active teens who have shown decreased condom use and low HIV testing rates.

PrEP can reduce the risk of HIV infection through sex by over 90%, but public awareness remains low [13]. Despite federal guidelines recommending PrEP for high-risk individuals, its use is limited due to the need for a prescription and high costs. The United States lacks comprehensive policies to provide PrEP access to uninsured, low-income individuals who would benefit most from the medication.

Needle sharing accounts for a significant portion of HIV infections, and needle exchange programs have proven effective in reducing transmission rates [14]. However, some conservative governments oppose these programs, and federal assistance cannot be used to purchase sterile needles or syringes for injecting illegal drugs, creating barriers to effective implementation.

ART and highly active antiretroviral therapy can transform HIV into a manageable chronic condition and prevent transmission through viral suppression [15]. The National HIV/AIDS Strategy emphasizes the importance of making these treatments widely available as a crucial component of HIV prevention efforts.

> *"Estimates suggest 94% of White people who could benefit from PrEP have been prescribed it, but only 13% of Black and 24% of Hispanic/Latino people who could benefit have been prescribed PrEP."*
> National Center for HIV, Viral Hepatitis, STD, and TB Prevention, Centers for Disease Control and Prevention (2023)

16.4 Government Response: Progress and Persistent Challenges in HIV Policy

The 2021 National HIV/AIDS Strategy aims to synthesize the government's HIV treatment and prevention efforts for more comprehensive support [16]. However, current laws and policies remain insufficient in reaching those most in need, and the government's slow initial response allowed HIV/AIDS stigma to persist, resulting in harmful regulations that perpetuate legal discrimination based on HIV status.

The government's delayed action under President Ronald Reagan led to AIDS becoming the leading cause of death for adults aged 25–44 by 1995 [17]. HIV activists pushed for a response, leading to new medications, funding, and policy measures. Currently, Medicare, Medicaid, and the Ryan White HIV/AIDS Program are the largest sources of HIV-related relief [18]. Despite the program's success in helping patients achieve viral suppression, it has faced criticism for outcome disparities based on race and gender [19].

Federal statutes such as the Americans with Disabilities Act (ADA), the Rehabilitation Act, and the Affordable Care Act (ACA) have helped combat HIV by eliminating insurance prohibitions for pre-existing conditions and expanding Medicaid in many states [20]. For many people with HIV, lack of health insurance and limited access to care have been major barriers to effectively managing their condition. The coverage expansion provided by the ACA will be a crucial step in supporting those with the highest incident rates of HIV/AIDS. Additionally, the ACA will promote increased HIV/AIDS testing by integrating these tests into routine care services for women. However, the ACA may also have unintended consequences for community-based organizations that have been essential providers of care for people living with HIV/AIDS. While the ACA has increased support for community-based organizations offering healthcare services, many organizations serving those with HIV/AIDS focus on providing social services rather than medical ones [21]. As biomedical interventions for HIV/AIDS continue to expand, it is crucial to ensure that nonmedical community-based organizations offering HIV/AIDS testing and counseling services continue to receive adequate funding to engage with the community. These centers often serve as the first point of access for people of color and act as a pipeline to care for those who test positive. Therefore, it is essential to sustain the vital work of community-based organizations alongside the expanded medical services provided under the ACA.

The Trump administration's opposition to the ACA undercut the government's commitment to fighting the HIV epidemic by reducing healthcare access for marginalized populations [22]. Policies stigmatizing or punishing people based on HIV status, such as military enlistment restrictions and deployment limitations, have been criticized for discouraging testing and contradicting the reality that HIV-positive individuals who achieve viral suppression can lead full lives. These policies have also faced legal challenges, with a federal district court ruling that an HIV discrimination rule for the Air Force likely violated the Equal Protection Clause [23].

Furthermore, until 2015, MSM were barred from donating blood due to concerns about HIV. In 2020, the FDA revised its guidance to allow donations from MSM who have not had sexual contact with another man within 3 months. Experts have criticized this policy as irrational and stigmatizing, arguing that it unfairly singles out gay and bisexual men and perpetuates the myth that sexual orientation alone increases infection risk, while providing no practical benefit since donated blood is always screened for HIV. In 2023, the FDA finalized its updates to the blood donation guidelines for MSM. The new guidelines eliminate categorical deferrals based on sexual orientation and implement individualized risk assessments for all potential donors [24].

16.5 Dismantling HIV Discrimination: Reforming Laws and Addressing Stigma

The government has recognized the need for legal and policy protections to prevent HIV/AIDS discrimination, but stigmatization remains a significant problem that has exacerbated the HIV epidemic and infiltrated US law and policy [25]. Despite enacting protections from certain types of HIV discrimination, the government needs to focus on large-scale efforts aimed at correcting misinformation and reversing harmful effects on communities. The United States continues to allow states to criminalize the act of infecting another person with HIV, which heavily undermines efforts to normalize HIV testing and treatment.

At the federal level, the ADA and Rehabilitation Act prevent discrimination based on HIV status in various areas, including employment, public accommodations, public services, healthcare, and housing [26]. However, these laws have proven insufficient in ensuring equal healthcare services for HIV-positive individuals. In response, the government passed the Barrier-Free Health Care Initiative in 2012, but its success remains unclear [27].

Individual states can still discriminate against HIV-positive people through criminal laws [28]. As of 2023, 35 states criminalized actions taken by people with HIV such as having sex without disclosing one's HIV-positive status to a partner. Some states use general criminal laws to punish HIV transmission, charging people with assault or homicide for infecting others. These laws and policies cause significant public health damage by discouraging HIV testing and perpetuating false narratives about the risks of sex with HIV-positive individuals, rather than educating the public about prevention measures such as condoms and PrEP. Criminalizing HIV transmission also wrongly characterizes HIV as a "weapon" and illogically singles out HIV from other infectious diseases, despite the lack of evidence that these laws deter HIV-positive people from having sex.

HIV-related criminal laws disproportionately affect marginalized people, such as sex workers and people of color, who are already at higher risk of HIV [29]. Each iteration of the National HIV/AIDS Strategy has encouraged states to reform or repeal these laws, with the 2021 strategy calling for strengthened enforcement of civil rights laws to protect vulnerable groups [11]. The CDC emphasizes that scientific understanding of HIV has significantly changed in the past 40 years, and laws and regulations that do not reflect this new knowledge should be eliminated.

16.6 Conclusion: Addressing HIV/AIDS Inequities, Ensuring Care for All

Despite successive US governments reiterating their commitment to ending the HIV epidemic, they have failed to make the necessary changes to law and policy that would decriminalize HIV status and guarantee quality, life-saving care to at-risk individuals [30]. While medical advances and improved outcomes are commendable, the government will never eradicate HIV without directly addressing the connection between infection and social determinants of health. Policies focused solely on behavioral solutions will not penetrate the deeply rooted racial and regional wealth and healthcare disparities [31]. The government must acknowledge that marginalized groups bear the brunt of the HIV/AIDS crisis and dedicate policy, funding, and research toward solutions aimed at making HIV manageable for all individuals in the United States, regardless of their socioeconomic status or background [32]. Only by recognizing and addressing the systemic inequities that perpetuate the epidemic, the nation can truly make progress toward ending HIV/AIDS [33].

Key Policy Recommendations and Equity Considerations in HIV/AIDS Care

Category	Policy Recommendations	Equity Aspects
General Strategies	• Collaborate across funding sources • Improve coordination among agencies • Expand healthcare coverage under the Affordable Care Act	• Addressing social determinants of health • Increasing transparency and community involvement • Enhancing healthcare access for underserved populations
Funding and Resources	• Redistribute HIV/AIDS funding to high-burden areas • Modify the housing assistance funding formula • Pass antidiscrimination housing laws	• Addressing the impact on communities of color • Ensuring stable housing for people with HIV • Preventing housing discrimination for gay and transgender individuals
Research and Data	• Increase funding for research on HIV/AIDS and health equity • Study HIV risk in prisons	• Understanding structural factors and unique challenges faced by incarcerated populations and communities of color
Education and Prevention	• Provide comprehensive health education • Provide free condoms	• Ensuring access to health information and prevention resources, especially in affected communities
Criminal Justice	• Increase HIV prevention in prisons • Promote care linkage after release	• Addressing high HIV rates among incarcerated people, who are often from Black and Latino communities • Ensuring continuous care post-release
HIV Exposure Laws	• Repeal or reform HIV criminalization laws • Support voluntary HIV status disclosure	• Reducing stigma and preventing the criminalization of HIV-positive individuals • Encouraging disclosure to improve health outcomes

References

1 Centers for Disease Control and Prevention (2021). HIV surveillance report, 2019: vol. 32. U.S. Department of Health and Human Services. https://www.cdc.gov/hiv/pdf/library/reports/surveillance/cdc-hiv-surveillance-report-2019-vol-32.pdf (accessed 28 August 2024).

2 U.S. Department of Health and Human Services (2021). What is ending the HIV epidemic in the U.S.? https://www.hiv.gov/federal-response/ending-the-hiv-epidemic/overview (accessed 28 August 2024).

3 Pellowski, J.A., Kalichman, S.C., Matthews, K.A., and Adler, N. (2013). A pandemic of the poor: social disadvantage and the U.S. HIV epidemic. *American Psychologist* 68 (4): 197–209. https://doi.org/10.1037/a0032694.

4 Goldstein, R.H., Streed, C.G., and Cahill, S.R. (2017). Being PrEPared – preexposure prophylaxis and HIV disparities. *New England Journal of Medicine* 379 (14): 1293–1295. https://doi.org/10.1056/NEJMp1804306.

5 Adimora, A.A., Ramirez, C., Schoenbach, V.J., and Cohen, M.S. (2014). Policies and politics that promote HIV infection in the Southern United States. *AIDS* 28 (10): 1393–1397. https://doi.org/10.1097/QAD.0000000000000225.

6 Center for American Progress (2010). The role of social determinants in promoting health and health equity. https://www.americanprogress.org/issues/healthcare/reports/2010/12/15/8793/the-role-of-social-determinants-in-promoting-health-and-health-equity/ (accessed 28 August 2024).

7 Reif, S., Safley, D., McAllaster, C. et al. (2017). State of HIV in the US deep south. *Journal of Community Health* 42 (5): 844–853. https://doi.org/10.1007/s10900-017-0325-8.

8 HIV.gov (2021). U.S. statistics. https://www.hiv.gov/hiv-basics/overview/data-and-trends/statistics (accessed 28 August 2024).

9 Hall, H.I., Brooks, J.T., and Mermin, J. (2019). Can the United States achieve 90-90-90? *Current Opinion in HIV and AIDS* 14 (6): 464–470. https://doi.org/10.1097/COH.0000000000000578.

10 Centers for Disease Control and Prevention (2024). Fast Facts: HIV in the US by Race and Ethnicity. https://www.cdc.gov/hiv/data-research/facts-stats/race-ethnicity.html

11 Office of National AIDS Policy (2021). *National HIV/AIDS Strategy for the United States 2022-2025*. White House. https://www.whitehouse.gov/wp-content/uploads/2021/11/National-HIV-AIDS-Strategy.pdf.

12 Centers for Disease Control and Prevention (2020). Condom effectiveness. https://www.cdc.gov/condomeffectiveness/index.html (accessed 28 August 2024).

13 Choopanya, K., Martin, M., Suntharasamai, P. et al. (2013). Antiretroviral prophylaxis for HIV infection in injecting drug users in Bangkok, Thailand (the Bangkok Tenofovir study): a randomised, double-blind, placebo-controlled phase 3 trial. *The Lancet* 381 (9883): 2083–2090. https://doi.org/10.1016/S0140-6736(13)61127-7.

14 Jones, L., Pickering, L., Sumnall, H. et al. (2008). *A Review of the Effectiveness and Cost-Effectiveness of Needle and Syringe Programmes for Injecting Drug Users*. Centre for Public Health, Liverpool John Moores University. https://www.drugsandalcohol.ie/12952/1/NICE_NSP_Evidence_Review_Full_Report.pdf.

15 Panel on Antiretroviral Guidelines for Adults and Adolescents (2021). Guidelines for the Use of Antiretroviral Agents in Adults and Adolescents with HIV. Department of Health and Human Services. https://clinicalinfo.hiv.gov/sites/default/files/guidelines/documents/adult-adolescent-arv/guidelines-adult-adolescent-arv.pdf.

16 The White House (2021). National HIV/AIDS strategy. https://www.whitehouse.gov/wp-content/uploads/2021/11/National-HIV-AIDS-Strategy.pdf (accessed 28 August 2024).

17 Kaiser Family Foundation (2019). The HIV/AIDS epidemic in the United States: the basics. https://www.kff.org/hivaids/fact-sheet/the-hivaids-epidemic-in-the-united-states-the-basics/ (accessed 28 August 2024).

18 Health Resources and Services Administration (2021). Ryan White HIV/AIDS program. https://hab.hrsa.gov/about-ryan-white-hivaids-program/about-ryan-white-hivaids-program (accessed 28 August 2024).

19 Ginossar, T., Oetzel, J., Van Meter, L. et al. (2019). The Ryan white HIV/AIDS program after the patient protection and affordable care act full implementation: a critical review of predictions, evidence, and future directions. *Topics in Antiviral Medicine* 27 (3): 91–100.

20 Blumenthal, D., Collins, S.R., and Fowler, E.J. (2020). The Affordable Care Act at 10 years—Its coverage and access provisions. *The New England Journal of Medicine* 382 (10): 963–969.

21 Weaks, F. (2021). Health care reform: exploring health-related quality of life of HIV/AIDS patients in Baltimore post implementation of the affordable care act. *Journal of Healthcare, Science and the Humanities* 11 (1): 193–203.

22 Cahill, S.R., Baker, K., Deutsch, M.B. et al. (2017). Inclusion of sexual orientation and gender identity in stage 3 meaningful use guidelines: a huge step forward for LGBT health. *LGBT Health* 4 (2): 106–110. https://doi.org/10.1089/lgbt.2016.0218.

23 Roe v. Department of Defense, 359 F. Supp. 3d 382 (E.D. Va. 2019). https://casetext.com/case/roe-v-shanahan.

24 Food and Drug Administration (2023). FDA Finalizes Move to Recommend Individual Risk Assessment to Determine Eligibility for Blood Donations. https://www.fda.gov/news-events/press-announcements/fda-finalizes-move-recommend-individual-risk-assessment-determine-eligibility-blood-donations

25 Mahajan, A.P., Sayles, J.N., Patel, V.A. et al. (2008). Stigma in the HIV/AIDS epidemic: a review of the literature and recommendations for the way forward. *AIDS* 22 (Suppl 2): S67–S79. https://doi.org/10.1097/01.aids.0000327438.13291.62.

26 Harsono, D., Galletly, C.L., O'Keefe, E., and Lazzarini, Z. (2020). Criminalization of HIV exposure: a review of empirical studies in the United States. *AIDS and Behavior* 21 (1): 27–50. https://doi.org/10.1007/s10461-016-1540-5.

27 Pendo, E. and Iezzoni, L. (2020). The role of law and policy in achieving healthy people's disability and health goals around access to health care, activities promoting health and wellness, independent living and participation, and collecting data in the United States. Legal Studies Research Paper 2020-11.

28 Centers for Disease Control and Prevention (2014). HIV-specific criminal laws. https://www.cdc.gov/hiv/policies/law/states/exposure.html (accessed 28 August 2024).

29 Hernández-Romieu, A.C., Siegler, A.J., Sullivan, P.S. et al. (2014). How often do condoms fail? A cross-sectional study exploring incomplete use of condoms, condom failures and other condom problems among black and white MSM in southern USA. *Sexually Transmitted Infections* 90 (8): 602–607. https://doi.org/10.1136/sextrans-2014-051581.

30 Barré-Sinoussi, F., Karim, S.S.A., Albert, J. et al. (2013). Towards an HIV cure: a global scientific strategy. *Nature Reviews Immunology* 12 (8): 607–614. https://doi.org/10.1038/nri3262.

31 Millett, G.A., Peterson, J.L., Flores, S.A. et al. (2012). Comparisons of disparities and risks of HIV infection in black and other men who have sex with men in Canada, UK, and USA: a meta-analysis. *The Lancet* 380 (9839): 341–348. https://doi.org/10.1016/S0140-6736(12)60899-X.

32 Earnshaw, V.A. and Chaudoir, S.R. (2009). From conceptualizing to measuring HIV stigma: a review of HIV stigma mechanism measures. *AIDS and Behavior* 13 (6): 1160–1177. https://doi.org/10.1007/s10461-009-9593-3.

33 Beyrer, C., Baral, S.D., van Griensven, F. et al. (2012). Global epidemiology of HIV infection in men who have sex with men. *The Lancet* 380 (9839): 367–377. https://doi.org/10.1016/S0140-6736(12)60821-6.

Part III

Social and Economic Factors: Education, Income, Rurality, and Structural Racism

This part addresses the intersection of social and economic factors with health equity, focusing on the impacts of education, income, rurality, and structural racism. Chapter 17 examines legal measures to address food insecurity during COVID-19 and beyond, highlighting policies to ensure nutritional equity. Chapter 18 promotes access to early care and education through anti-racist policies, emphasizing the importance of equitable early childhood programs. Chapter 19 advocates for enacting paid family leave to promote health equity, detailing its benefits for marginalized communities. Chapter 20 discusses enhancing health equity for rural, remote, and tribal populations through targeted policies and increased access to healthcare services. Chapter 21 addresses the impact of medical debt on marginalized communities, proposing reforms to alleviate financial burdens. Chapter 22 explores preserving diversity in healthcare amidst the Supreme Court's affirmative action ruling, analyzing its implications for health equity. Chapter 23 reforms the public charge rule to improve immigrant health equity, ensuring access to necessary services without fear of repercussions. Chapter 24 promotes the Health in All Policies (HiAP) approach, integrating health considerations into policymaking across sectors. Chapter 25 advocates for repealing state preemption laws to enhance local health equity initiatives. Chapter 26 highlights achieving health and economic equity through broadband access and policy. Chapter 27 expands vaccine equity through strategic policy measures. Chapter 28 emphasizes the importance of disaggregating data to reveal the diversity and disparities within the AAPI population, guiding targeted interventions. These chapters collectively provide a comprehensive roadmap for addressing the social and economic determinants of health equity.

17

Addressing Food Insecurity: Strengthening Assistance Programs and Promoting Equity

Abstract

This chapter explores the critical issue of food insecurity in the United States, focusing on its impact on health risks, the exacerbation of systemic inequities during the COVID-19 pandemic, and the federal government's response through various food assistance programs. The chapter begins by defining food insecurity and highlighting its disproportionate impact on communities of color, as well as the additional risks posed by the pandemic. It then delves into the federal nutrition safety net, examining the adaptations made to food assistance programs for adults, children, and the elderly during the COVID-19 crisis. The chapter also discusses the challenges faced by the current food assistance system in adequately addressing the needs of food-insecure families and proposes strategies for enhancing these programs amidst the ongoing difficulties. These strategies include evaluating programs for equity and efficiency, improving SNAP by tackling barriers and benefit adequacy, and implementing expert recommendations to strengthen food assistance. The chapter concludes with a powerful call to action, emphasizing the need for transformative changes in the food assistance landscape to create a more resilient and equitable future for all Americans. By learning from the lessons of the pandemic and taking decisive steps to reform and invest in food assistance programs, policymakers and society as a whole can work toward ensuring that no one goes hungry in our communities.

Keywords   *food insecurity; COVID-19 impact; SNAP benefits; federal assistance programs; nutritional equity; school meal programs; pandemic relief; social determinants of health*

> *Amidst the COVID-19 pandemic, Sarah, a single mother who lost her job due to lockdowns, found herself struggling to put food on the table for her two young children. Despite her best efforts, she faced barriers in accessing SNAP benefits, leaving her family food insecure and at risk of health complications.*
>
> *Robert, a 68-year-old retiree living on a fixed income, relied on the Commodity Supplemental Food Program to supplement his diet with nutritious food. When the pandemic struck, Robert feared for his health and well-being, as the disruptions to food assistance programs threatened his access to the vital resources he needed to maintain his health.*

Achieving Health Equity: The Role of Law and Policy, First Edition. Y. Tony Yang.
© 2025 John Wiley & Sons Ltd. Published 2025 by John Wiley & Sons Ltd.

> *Lisa, a school cafeteria worker, witnessed firsthand the impact of school closures on children who depended on free and reduced-price meals. As she worked tirelessly to distribute meals to students in need, Lisa recognized the critical role that school meal programs play in combating food insecurity and ensuring the well-being of vulnerable children.*

17.1 Food Insecurity, Health Risks, and COVID-19: Exposing Systemic Inequities

The United States Department of Agriculture (USDA) defines low food security as "reduced diet quality, variety, or desirability of diet," while very low food security is characterized by "multiple indications of disrupted eating patterns and reduced food intake" [1]. In contrast, food security refers to having both physical and economic access to adequate food to meet dietary needs and maintain a healthy lifestyle. Food insecurity is associated with numerous health risks and poor nutrition, disproportionately affecting communities of color, which means that minority groups are more likely to experience the negative health consequences of food insecurity [2].

The COVID-19 pandemic poses an additional risk for individuals experiencing food insecurity [3]. Food insecurity and lack of proper nutrition are "associated with several chronic illnesses that place individuals at higher risk of experiencing COVID-19 with severe complications" [4]. Diet-related chronic diseases, such as heart disease, diabetes, and obesity, are all linked to serious COVID-19 outcomes [5]. Not only does COVID-19 pose a significant threat to food-insecure families, but it has also increased the rates of food insecurity due to inadequate federal and state government responses to the pandemic, which failed to meet the heightened demands of people in need of food assistance [6].

Federal efforts to support those in need through emergency funding and stimulus checks were insufficient in helping families pay for food during the pandemic [7]. The government attempted to implement short-term solutions to address food assistance problems, such as providing benefits to families with children who receive free and reduced meals. However, administrative and distribution issues rendered these programs ineffective or suboptimal [8]. The COVID-19 pandemic exposed pre-existing problems with federal food and nutrition programs, which were further exacerbated during the crisis.

> *"The lack of access to proper nutrition is not only fueling obesity, it is leading to food insecurity and hunger among our children."*
>
> U.S. Secretary of Agriculture, Tom Vilsack

17.2 Federal Food Assistance

The federal nutrition safety net encompasses a range of laws and programs administered by the federal government to ensure access to healthy food for all Americans [9]. These food assistance programs address various aspects of food insecurity, including affordability, distribution, and nutritional value. While designed to promote nutritional well-being, some of these programs may not provide adequate relief to food-insecure families [10]. As will be discussed in the following sections, these programs target different age groups, each with their own unique nutritional needs and challenges.

17.2.1 SNAP and Temporary Relief Efforts

Food-insecure adults under the age of 60 have access to some federal food assistance programs, but their benefits are often restricted based on income [11]. The primary federal food assistance program for adults is the Supplemental Food and Nutrition Program (SNAP). During the COVID-19 pandemic, the government provided additional resources to help adults access food [12].

SNAP helps eligible individuals purchase food at authorized food retailers. Unlike some programs, SNAP is available to people in various life stages. The USDA determines SNAP eligibility based on income, and eligible individuals must go through a lengthy application and verification process to receive benefits. Recipients must also periodically be recertified to continue participating in the program.

SNAP is intended to supplement the cost of healthy, budget-conscious groceries, not to be the sole source of a recipient's food budget. The federal government uses the Thrifty Food Plan to determine SNAP benefits, but critics argue that it is not a realistic measure of the cost of a healthy diet and that the maximum allotments are insufficient [13].

Despite being one of the most accessible food assistance programs across age groups, some eligible individuals do not apply for SNAP due to the stigma of receiving benefits [14]. Additionally, some eligible immigrants may choose not to apply out of fear of impacting their future citizenship status. The inflexible recertification process may also be a barrier.

During the COVID-19 pandemic, the federal government temporarily increased SNAP benefits by 15% for eligible recipients, but this increase did not apply to households already receiving the maximum allotments [15]. In 2021, President Biden's economic relief expanded the temporary increase to those with maximum SNAP benefits.

As SNAP benefits are supplemental, they are not intended to cover all of a family's monthly food expenses. However, during the pandemic, unemployment rates spiked, and states struggled to process unemployment claims, leaving struggling families in dire financial situations and exacerbating food insecurity [16]. Without income from work or other social safety nets, SNAP benefits were insufficient for purchasing healthy food.

Beyond SNAP, the federal government directed additional resources to address the increased need for food assistance during the COVID-19 pandemic. The Emergency Food Assistance Program helped supplement the availability of free, nutritional food by increasing the availability of no-cost food at food banks and other nonprofits, and by supporting farmers through direct food purchases [17]. Similarly, the USDA's Agricultural Marketing Service partnered with food distributors to purchase and deliver more than $6 billion in fresh produce, dairy, and food boxes to those in need [18]. These temporary programs were funded through COVID-19 relief discretionary programs and are not a permanent solution for food insecurity.

In addition to other temporary programs during the pandemic, both the Trump and Biden administrations provided stimulus checks. However, these one-time payments are likely insufficient to make a sustainable difference for food-insecure families who may also be struggling with rent, utilities, mortgages, and other living expenses [19].

17.2.2 Food Assistance Programs for Children and the Elderly

Several programs exist to help children experiencing food insecurity. One of the most common is the Free and Reduced Price School Meals (FARM) program, which has been shown to positively correlate with diet quality, food security, and academic performance [20]. Many children depend on school meals, and during the COVID-19 pandemic, school closures had a severe impact on these children.

In response, school districts and childcare centers made efforts to mitigate COVID-19 transmission while providing meals to go. This was a challenge, as over half of all jurisdictions administering USDA food service programs gave their operators less than 72 hours of notice between school closure announcements and the beginning of alternative meal distribution. Financial hurdles and the need to implement distribution processes that minimized disease transmission required significant innovation from the operators [21].

When schools closed, Congress authorized Pandemic Electronic Benefits Transfer (P-EBT), which provided families with benefits equal to the value of the school meals missed due to school closures [22]. Although providing P-EBT benefits to families in need was invaluable, the rollout was challenging, as agencies responsible for administering benefits did not have the infrastructure in place to handle the administrative burden of the program. The government also increased P-EBT benefits for the duration of the COVID-19 national emergency, including the summer months, to ensure children had access to food [23].

An additional effort to assist students whose access to school meals was interrupted during the pandemic was Meals to You, a public–private partnership focused on distributing food to rural children in need [24]. Although the program is small, it was able to distribute nearly 40 million meals during the first six months of the COVID-19 pandemic. If determined to be successful, it could be used as a model for rural food distribution on a larger scale.

Another common program addressing food insecurity for children is Women, Infants, and Children (WIC), which serves women who are pregnant and/or lactating and children up to five years old at nutrition risk [25]. During the pandemic, Congress established a task force on food delivery models in WIC to reduce in-person contact for recipients. Additionally, the WIC Fruit and Vegetable Cash Value Voucher was temporarily increased to encourage the consumption of healthy foods.

The elderly have unique nutritional needs and are particularly vulnerable during the pandemic. Specific public and private programs are designed to support and care for the elderly, especially those who may have limited access to food. Meals on Wheels is one such private organization that organizes meal delivery to the elderly [26]. The Older Americans Act, reauthorized in 2020 at the start of the pandemic, included administrative and delivery flexibilities for Meals on Wheels to support seniors in need. Subsequent stimulus packages have included supplemental funds to support the increased enrollment in Meals on Wheels. The Commodity Supplemental Food Program also addresses elderly nutritional health by helping to improve the health of low-income people ages 60 and older by supplementing their diets with nutritional food.

17.3 Strategies for Enhancing Food Assistance Programs Amidst Challenges

The current federal safety net and food assistance programs face challenges in adequately addressing the needs of food-insecure families [27]. Limited resources hinder efforts to ensure that healthy food is affordable and accessible for those who need it most. Additionally, there is a lack of comprehensive research on best practices for tackling food insecurity during and beyond the COVID-19 pandemic. To better serve food-insecure individuals, the system must be strengthened and adapted to meet the unique challenges posed by the pandemic and its aftermath. Addressing food insecurity offers numerous benefits, including "increased food expenditures, mitigated declines in calorie intake, improved food insecurity, and reduced Medicaid cost growth." By investing in solutions that prioritize the needs of vulnerable populations, we can work toward a more equitable and resilient food system for all.

17.3.1 Evaluating Food Assistance Programs for Equity and Efficiency

Experts recommend investing in the assessment of temporary programs implemented during COVID-19 to better understand which ones should be extended, expanded, or made permanent [28]. By investing in research, the government can prevent resource waste and promote the effective use of programs that address food insecurity. If successful, these temporary programs can serve as models for permanent improvements. Without careful planning and an assessment of program benefits, there may be overlap or waste among competing programs. To ensure that vulnerable children and families receive the maximum benefit from nutritional programs, resources should be used strategically.

First, assessments should focus on identifying the strengths and shortcomings of existing programs. The data collected should be used to determine which programs should be permanently extended and if and how struggling programs can be improved. Strategic resource allocation is crucial for effectively addressing food insecurity and nutritional needs across various populations. These assessments should also evaluate "whether, and to what extent, [USDA] programs and policies perpetuate systemic barriers to opportunities and benefits for people of color and other underserved groups." As previously noted, food insecurity disproportionately affects communities of color and racial minorities. Assessments can be a valuable tool in identifying the reasons behind this trend, enabling policymakers to address the issue effectively.

Policy Approaches and Equity Considerations in Food Systems

Policy Area	Key Policies and Approaches	Equity Considerations
Food Justice	• Promoting urban agriculture • Supporting farmworkers' rights • Ensuring access to land for food cultivation	Focuses on the human rights aspect, addressing the structural barriers that prevent equitable food access, particularly for marginalized communities
Food Sovereignty	• Advocating for local food production by small producers • Prioritizing community control over resources like land and water	Centers on self-determination and community control, aiming to empower local and Indigenous communities
Ending Food Apartheid	• Addressing systemic racism in food access • Recognizing and dismantling the policies that lead to geographically and racially linked disparities in food access	Calls attention to the deliberate policy choices that create inequities, urging solutions that address the root causes of food inaccessibility
General Policy Approaches	• Implementing zoning laws that support local food systems • Encouraging community participation in food policy development • Investing in research to guide policy improvements	Emphasizes inclusivity and the need for community-driven solutions that reflect the specific needs and conditions of diverse populations

17.3.2 Improving SNAP: Tackling Barriers and Benefit Adequacy

SNAP was particularly crucial during the COVID-19 pandemic when an increasing number of families relied on the benefits to purchase food while they were unemployed and unable to access unemployment benefits [29]. The federal government acknowledged the importance of this vital program, as evidenced by the temporary benefit increases to subsidize the cost of food. However, even with the temporary extensions, families still struggled to provide healthy meals. Experts suggest revising the Thrifty Food Plan to better reflect the cost of a healthy diet and recommend implementing a long-term increase in SNAP benefits, which would help support nutritional diets under normal conditions [30].

In addition to reforming the financial benefits of SNAP, there are opportunities to improve the administrative processes to better accommodate the needs of eligible recipients. Administrative barriers and social stigmas discourage food-insecure people from taking advantage of the program. These issues were highlighted during the pandemic when administering agencies lacked the infrastructure to efficiently implement the program to match the spike in need for benefits, and inflexible requirements prevented eligible people from receiving SNAP benefits. Moreover, the social stigma associated with using SNAP benefits in public can discourage people who are ashamed of using government benefits from seeking help. Offering online SNAP purchasing could protect the privacy of food-insecure individuals and help them access food.

Each additional step and requirement enrollees face in the SNAP application process increases cost and decreases participation in the program. To qualify for SNAP, households must go through a lengthy interview process and provide extensive documentation. The SNAP recertification process makes it difficult for working parents with childcare responsibilities to fit the inflexible interview times into their schedules. A streamlined process available online and offline would improve access to the program. Reforming the application and recertification process would remove barriers to accessing SNAP benefits.

Eligibility restrictions for SNAP are viewed as unfair or counterproductive. For example, low-income Americans applying for SNAP are ineligible if they have money in savings accounts or other assets. Able-bodied adults without dependents cannot receive more than three months of SNAP in a three-year period. There are also work requirements to receive SNAP benefits, and during difficult economic times like the pandemic, job opportunities may not be available. The current SNAP program imposes a lifetime ban for individuals with drug felony convictions. Experts say that this creates a barrier for reintegration and "undermines the food security of many Americans." The eligibility and work requirements may have unintended consequences on self-sufficiency and other social costs. Policymakers should consider reforming SNAP to address these issues.

17.3.3 Strengthening Food Assistance: Expert Recommendations

Experts suggest a range of other reforms to strengthen food assistance programs during COVID-19 and beyond [31]. These include promoting programs for communities in need, providing technical assistance for groups who require help applying for benefits, and investing more in WIC. Additionally, cutting state matching requirements for SNAP and authorizing public–private partnerships between state and tribal governments to deliver healthy food to families in need could further improve access to food assistance.

Providing additional funding to US territories that are not part of the SNAP program is another important consideration. Experts also recommend assessing how programs not directly related to food security, such as the Child Tax Credit and minimum wage laws, may impact food security. Supporting state innovations for food and nutrition assistance programs and prioritizing the role of nutrition programs in addressing both food and nutrition insecurity are also crucial steps.

Moreover, experts suggest taking food insecurity into account for future immigration reforms and creating an administrative solution to coordinate federal food and nutrition agencies. Expanding eligibility for food and nutritional programs is another key recommendation to ensure that more individuals and families in need can access these vital resources.

By implementing these reforms and recommendations, policymakers can work toward strengthening the food assistance safety net, reducing barriers to access, and ultimately improving food security for vulnerable populations during the ongoing pandemic and beyond.

17.4 Conclusion: Transforming Food Assistance for a Resilient Future

Food insecurity was a pervasive issue long before the COVID-19 pandemic, but the public health emergency exposed and exacerbated the existing administrative and food security challenges. As we move forward, it is crucial that we learn from the lessons of the pandemic and take decisive action to strengthen our food assistance programs and infrastructure.

The government must prioritize putting processes and systems in place that enable the rapid scaling up of programs and services during emergency situations. This will ensure that vulnerable populations can access the support they need when they need it most.

Moreover, a comprehensive assessment of existing food assistance programs is essential to identify areas for improvement and reform. By reducing barriers to accessing healthy food and promoting food security, we can build a more resilient and equitable society.

We must transform our food assistance landscape and create a system that truly serves the needs of all individuals and families, regardless of their circumstances. Let us work together to implement the necessary reforms and invest in the programs that will ensure no one goes hungry in our communities. The well-being and prosperity of our nation depend on our commitment to addressing food insecurity head-on.

References

1 United States Department of Agriculture (2023). Definitions of food security. https://www.ers.usda.gov/topics/food-nutrition-assistance/food-security-in-the-u-s/definitions-of-food-security/ (accessed 28 August 2024).

2 Gundersen, C. and Ziliak, J.P. (2015). Food insecurity and health outcomes. *Health Affairs* 34 (11): 1830–1839.

3 Morales, D.X., Morales, S.A., and Beltran, T.F. (2021). Racial/ethnic disparities in household food insecurity during the COVID-19 pandemic: a nationally representative study. *Journal of Racial and Ethnic Health Disparities* 8: 1300–1314.

4 Wolfson, J.A. and Leung, C.W. (2020). Food insecurity and COVID-19: disparities in early effects for US adults. *Nutrients* 12 (6): 1648.

5 Nagata, J.M., Seligman, H.K., and Weiser, S.D. (2021). Perspective: the convergence of coronavirus disease 2019 (COVID-19) and food insecurity in the United States. *Advances in Nutrition* 12 (2): 287–290.

6 Laborde, D., Martin, W., and Vos, R. (2020). *Poverty and Food Insecurity Could Grow Dramatically as COVID-19 Spreads*. Washington, DC: International Food Policy Research Institute (IFPRI).

7 Ziliak, J.P. (2021). Food hardship during the COVID-19 pandemic and great recession. *Applied Economic Perspectives and Policy* 43 (1): 132–152.

8 Kinsey, E.W., Kinsey, D., and Rundle, A.G. (2020). COVID-19 and food insecurity: an uneven patchwork of responses. *Journal of Urban Health* 97: 332–335.

9 Gundersen, C., Hake, M., Dewey, A., and Engelhard, E. (2021). Food insecurity during COVID-19. *Applied Economic Perspectives and Policy* 43 (1): 153–161.

10 Rosenbaum, D. and Neuberger, Z. (2020). *President's 2021 Budget Would Cut Food Assistance for Millions and Radically Restructure SNAP*. Washington, DC: Center for Budget and Policy Priorities. https://bit.ly/ 2WdrFSl.

11 Keith-Jennings, B., Nchako, C., and Llobrera, J. (2021). *Number of Families Struggling to Afford Food Rose Steeply in Pandemic and Remains High, Especially Among Children and Households of Color*. Center on Budget and Policy Priorities.

12 Fleischhacker, S. and Bleich, S.N. (2021). Addressing food insecurity in the United States during and after the COVID-19 pandemic: the role of the federal nutrition safety net. *Journal of Food Law & Policy* 17: 98.

13 Carlson, S., Llobrera, J., and Keith-Jennings, B. (2019). *More Adequate SNAP Benefits Would Help Millions of Participants Better Afford Food*. Center on Budget and Policy Priorities.

14 Gundersen, C., Waxman, E., and Crumbaugh, A.S. (2019). An examination of the adequacy of Supplemental Nutrition Assistance Program (SNAP) benefit levels: impacts on food insecurity. *Agricultural and Resource Economics Review* 48 (3): 433–447.

15 Bryant, A. and Follett, L. (2022). Hunger relief: a natural experiment from additional SNAP benefits during the COVID-19 pandemic, 100224. *The Lancet Regional Health – Americas* 10.

16 Bitler, M., Hoynes, H.W., and Schanzenbach, D.W. (2020). *The Social Safety Net in the Wake of COVID-19 (No. w27796)*. National Bureau of Economic Research.

17 Jablonski, B.B., Casnovsky, J., Clark, J.K. et al. (2021). Emergency food provision for children and families during the COVID-19 pandemic: examples from five US cities. *Applied Economic Perspectives and Policy* 43 (1): 169–184.

18 Baldwin, K., Williams, B.R., Sichko, C., Tsiboe, F., Toossi, S., Jones, J.W., Turner, D., & Raszap Skorbiansky, S. (2023). U.S. agricultural policy review, 2022 (Report No. EIB-260). U.S. Department of Agriculture, Economic Research Service. doi: 10.32747/2023.8134363.ers

19 Mgomezulu, W.R., Edriss, A.K., Machira, K., and Pangapanga-Phiri, I. (2023). Towards sustainability in the adoption of sustainable agricultural practices: implications on household poverty, food and nutrition security. *Innovation and Green Development* 2 (3): 100054.

20 Cohen, J.F., Hecht, A.A., McLoughlin, G.M. et al. (2021). Universal school meals and associations with student participation, attendance, academic performance, diet quality, food security, and body mass index: a systematic review. *Nutrients* 13 (3): 911.

21 McLoughlin, G.M., McCarthy, J.A., McGuirt, J.T. et al. (2020). Addressing food insecurity through a health equity lens: a case study of large urban school districts during the COVID-19 pandemic. *Journal of Urban Health* 97: 759–775.

22 Bauer, L., Pitts, A., Ruffini, K., and Schanzenbach, D.W. (2020). *The Effect of Pandemic EBT on Measures of Food Hardship. The Hamilton Project.* Washington, DC: Brookings Institution.

23 Fern, S.E., Kimbro, R.T., Hill, M.E., and Hughes, C.C. (2023). Emergency food support preference and usage during COVID-19: a neighborhood study of low-income black mothers? Use of school-based food distribution and P-EBT. *American Journal of Public Health* 113 (S3): S227–S230.

24 Ryan, B.J., Telford, V., Brickhouse, M. et al. (2024). Strengthening food systems resilience before, during and after disasters and other crises. *Journal of Homeland Security and Emergency Management* 21 (1): 71–97.

25 Busch, S., Andersen, J.A., Willis, D.E. et al. (2023). Association of the COVID-19 pandemic with women, infants, and children (WIC) receipt among pregnant individuals: United States, 2016–2022. *American Journal of Public Health* 113 (S3): S240–S247.

26 Henning-Smith, C., Tuttle, M., Tanem, J. et al. (2024). Social isolation and safety issues among rural older adults living alone: perspectives of Meals on Wheels programs. *Journal of Aging & Social Policy* 36 (2): 282–301.

27 Saloner, B., Gollust, S.E., Planalp, C., and Blewett, L.A. (2020). Access and enrollment in safety net programs in the wake of COVID-19: a national cross-sectional survey. *PLoS One* 15 (10): e0240080.

28 World Health Organization (2020). *Investing in and Building Longer-Term Health Emergency Preparedness During COVID-19 Pandemic: Interim Guidance for WHO member states (No. WHO/2019-nCoV/Emergency_ Preparedness/Long_term/2020.1).* World Health Organization.

29 Siddiqi, S.M., Cantor, J., Dastidar, M.G. et al. (2021). SNAP participants and high levels of food insecurity in the early stages of the COVID-19 pandemic. *Public Health Reports* 136 (4): 457–465.

30 Young, S.K. and Stewart, H. (2022). US fruit and vegetable affordability on the thrifty food plan depends on purchasing power and safety net supports. *International Journal of Environmental Research and Public Health* 19 (5): 2772.

31 Serchen, J., Atiq, O., Hilden, D., and Health and Public Policy Committee of the American College of Physicians (2022). Strengthening food and nutrition security to promote public health in the United States: a position paper from the American College of Physicians. *Annals of Internal Medicine* 175 (8): 1170–1171.

18

Promoting Access to Early Care and Education: Anti-Racist Policies

Abstract

The chapter explores the complex relationship between education and health, focusing on the inequities present in the education system and their impact on the well-being of children, particularly those from minority communities. It begins by highlighting the disparities in funding and resources between predominantly white and minority school districts, as well as the disproportionate presence of police in majority–minority schools, which can lead to negative outcomes for students. The chapter then delves into the importance of early care and education (ECE), discussing the benefits of high-quality ECE for children, families, and society as a whole, while also addressing the barriers that hinder communities of color from accessing these services. It examines federal programs such as Head Start, Early Head Start, and the Child Care Development Fund (CCDF), which aim to provide support for low-income families, but face challenges in terms of access, eligibility, and funding. The chapter also touches upon additional federal programs and grants that have been implemented in response to the COVID-19 pandemic. It concludes by emphasizing the need to address structural issues in childcare provision, such as the availability of childcare slots, the compensation and qualifications of early childhood educators, and the hours during which care is available. The chapter calls for a multi-faceted approach involving federal, state, and local authorities, as well as private actors, to enhance long-term outcomes for families and children, ensuring a coherent and effective strategy that addresses immediate childcare needs and lays the foundation for the holistic development of future generations.

Keywords *early care and education (ECE); childcare access; racial inequities; head start program; child care development fund (CCDF); workforce compensation; federal assistance programs; quality childcare*

> *Maya, a young black mother, struggling to find affordable and high-quality childcare for her two-year-old daughter, Aria, while she completes her degree.*
>
> *Mr Ramirez, an immigrant childcare provider who faces biases against families of color and is hesitant to accept the Child Care Development Fund because of added requirements.*
>
> *Aisha, an Asian American childcare worker, who despite having a bachelor's degree in early childhood education, struggles with low wages and the high cost of living.*

Achieving Health Equity: The Role of Law and Policy, First Edition. Y. Tony Yang.
© 2025 John Wiley & Sons Ltd. Published 2025 by John Wiley & Sons Ltd.

18.1 Early Care and Education

Education is a well-known social determinant of health. Education is associated with factors such as increased uptake in preventative care and reduced probability of death. Furthermore, health is critical for effective learning. Children who are malnourished or are ill can be impeded in their learning [1]. However, it also is a site for stark inequities [2]. Schools located in predominately minority school districts receive $23 billion less than predominately white school districts, even when they serve the same number of students [3]. Additionally, schools in majority–minority communities are more likely to have a police presence within the school – which numerous studies have shown lead to increases in arrests, are correlated with higher rates of suspension and expulsion, and perpetuate racial inequalities in school discipline [4]. It is worth acknowledging that the benefits of education on health are tied to income. However, economic inequities do disproportionately impact racial and ethnic groups, which can keep them from having resources for health services [5]. While the judiciary and federal policies developed programs intended to rectify racially prejudiced policies impacting Black families, they have also perpetuated inadvertently and propagated systemic racism. Schools are still largely segregated, even though formal avenues for segregation have been outlawed [6]. Beyond these targeted initiatives, many federal programs aim to assist economically disadvantaged children and families, with Black families often falling within these demographics due to systemic disadvantages.

The dialogue on childcare and early childcare typically revolves around licensed childcare centers or home-based care providers. Despite the low wages of childcare workers, this sector's high-quality care can have an immediate and long-term impact. Numerous studies underscore the benefits of high-quality ECE for Black children and children from impoverished backgrounds [7]. High-quality ECE promotes better physical health, kindergarten readiness, critical family support, and increased health equity [8]. Participation in high-quality ECE has been associated with positive school outcomes, economic stability, higher earnings, improved physical and mental health, and increased societal responsibilities [9].

ECE also significantly impacts parents, potentially enabling them to stay in the workforce. Certain ECE programs support parents' participation in employment, training, and educational activities, thereby increasing their earning potential. Equitable access to high-quality preschool can alleviate financial burdens on Black families by reducing ECE tuition fees. Moreover, investment in ECE translates to long-term governmental savings. For every $1 invested in ECE programs, societal savings are estimated to be $8.60 over a child's lifetime [10].

However, several obstacles hinder communities of color from accessing early childcare. Primarily, quality childcare is costly, especially in high living cost areas, owing to significant labor inputs required for care provision. As such, parents may be forced to opt for lower-quality providers, economize elsewhere, or one parent might decide to quit employment for childcare. Secondly, residential neighborhoods affect childcare accessibility. Areas with higher poverty rates and limited resources influence childcare markets, thereby impacting the ability to provide quality, accessible care [11]. For example, Black families are less likely to have local childcare centers, and the available ones may be unaffordable. Though Black families are more likely to exist in nuclear family structures, they are also more likely to spread their resources to support those families [12]. A family's structure can also affect their access to care, with dual-income families potentially better equipped to handle the financial impact of childcare and adjust if care is needed outside traditional hours. Lastly, the nature of employment can pose a barrier, due to the need for care at non-traditional times or because seasonal work does not meet benefit eligibility requirements.

18.2   Head Start and Early Head Start

Established as part of the response to the 1960s Civil Rights Movement, Head Start is a federal program designed to circumvent discriminatory regional policies that prevented resources from reaching Black families [13]. Administered by 1700 public and private nonprofit and for-profit grantees, these programs offer services to over a million children and pregnant women.

Funds are distributed annually to state, territorial, or tribal governments, based on the number of current and anticipated grantees. Grantees directly receive the funding, and they maintain discretion over service design as long as they adhere to national performance standards. The flexible design enables grantees to link parents to educational or employment services and facilitate children's developmental screenings and vaccinations. Furthermore, Head Start programs also strive to connect children to health insurance (Medicaid or Children's Health Insurance Program [CHIP]) and medical and dental services [14].

However, Head Start faces a significant challenge – it cannot serve all eligible children, and the program's impact varies widely by region. Nationally, only about 28% of eligible Black children live in neighborhoods with a Head Start program [15]. In 2019, the children and families served by Head Start were 37% Hispanic/Latino and 30% Black/African American [16].

In 2015, to enhance program quality, Head Start was directed to promote classroom diversity [17]. Head Start programs can enroll over-income families who pay a fee. However, implementing this rule often means programs with long waiting lists must weigh providing slots to paying families against serving their original target communities.

One potential solution to this access problem is increased Congressional funding for Head Start programs. An example of the impact of such increased funding can be seen in the pandemic response, which helped states and local providers stabilize their markets. However, simply increasing funding does not address the fundamental issue – there are too few grantees to meet the demand of all eligible children who could benefit from these programs.

18.3   Child Care Development Fund

Unlike the Head Start grant system which provides funds directly to ECE programs, the CCDF offers subsidies to low-income working families for childcare access. Serving nearly 1.4 million children from low-income families, the CCDF allows families to choose a childcare provider that meets all applicable state and local requirements [18].

The CCDF funding is allocated to states as a block grant to cover childcare costs and enhance the quality of childcare programs. Each state has the flexibility to determine how to administer these subsidy programs. However, state-level restrictions can either broaden access or prevent otherwise eligible communities from receiving care.

For example, while some states recognize English as a Second Language (ESL) courses for program eligibility, others impose minimum weekly work hours for one or both parents, which can disproportionately burden families of color engaged in informal or seasonal jobs [19]. Furthermore, verification of work hours is a requirement, even in states without a minimum weekly hour requirement. Some states request social security numbers and do not explicitly state that their inclusion is optional, potentially deterring undocumented or immigrant families from applying.

States also have the option to align CCDF with Head Start and other early childhood programs and can transfer Temporary Assistance for Needy Families (TANF) funding to supplement the CCDF program [20]. Most states prioritize TANF families when distributing funding. However, given TANF's stricter eligibility and documentation requirements, this could pose additional barriers for families eligible for CCDF but not TANF [21].

Similar to Head Start, CCDF presents several access challenges for low-income families. Families must consistently demonstrate their employment or participation in education or training programs. Moreover, issues such as lack of internet access, transportation difficulties, or language barriers can hinder the application process. For families who receive funding, there are additional obstacles. Most subsidies fall short of covering the full costs of quality providers, whose rates often exceed the state's payment cap. Some providers might even refuse to accept CCDF funds due to increased requirements for caregivers, inherent and external biases, and disparate treatment toward families of color that access public benefits. Finally, while CCDF subsidies assist some low-income parents, they inadvertently create a "coverage gap" for middle-income families who find the costs unmanageable [22].

"The best way to improve the American workforce in the 21st century is to invest in early childhood education, to ensure that even the most disadvantaged children have the opportunity to succeed alongside their more advantaged peers."

James Heckman, Nobel Prize-winning Economist

18.4 Additional Federal Programs

Besides the primary federal programs detailed earlier, most of the federal action for early childhood education revolves around grants and funding packages provided to states, which are more adept at effective money distribution through local agencies and partners. Recent congressional efforts have aimed at boosting ECE funding to empower parents to rejoin the workforce.

In response to COVID-19, the federal government approved $50 billion in new funding for ECE across several relief packages (The Coronavirus Aid, Relief, and Economic Security [CARES] Act, Coronavirus Response and Relief Supplemental Appropriations Act [CRRSAA], American Rescue Plan), including the Children's Funding Project. These funds included $52.5 billion for childcare through Child Care & Development Block Grant (CCDBG) or childcare stabilization efforts, $2 billion for Head Start, and an additional $150 billion for Home Visiting programs [23]. This funding was allocated to enhance existing facilities, expand capacity, and improve both access and quality of care for children.

For instance, Whatcom County, Washington, and other small cities within the county pooled their state-allocated funding to provide nearly $700,000 in grants to licensed childcare providers [24]. Similarly, Saint Louis city and county governments devoted portions of CARES Act funding to support childcare providers in underserved neighborhoods and family and home-based providers [25]. As a result of this pandemic-related funding, state lawmakers enacted twice the usual number of ECE-related bills, with 208 bills enacted related to early childhood [26].

Likewise, the Preschool Development Grant Birth through Five Program, a competitive federal grant worth $250 million, aims to enhance states' early childhood programs by building upon existing federal, state, and local early care and learning investments. Granted to state governments, this funding seeks to promote more efficient coordination of existing early childhood services. While not a comprehensive solution, this program could stimulate states to creatively reallocate their existing funding [27].

18.5 Addressing Structural Issues in Childcare Provision

The crux of childcare reform lies in addressing structural issues, particularly those related to the availability of childcare slots, the compensation and qualifications of early childhood educators, and the hours during which care is available.

One of the significant challenges in the early childhood education market pertains to pricing. There is an inherent ceiling on tuition prices, dictated by governmental subsidies and what families are willing or able to pay. However, families and state governments are also demanding better quality care, which necessitates a better-qualified and thus more expensive staff. This leads to a challenging contradiction. For instance, a 2007 amendment to the Head Start program under President Bush required that half of all Head Start teachers hold a bachelor's degree in early childhood education by 2013 [28]. While successful in enhancing the qualifications of educators, this requirement may have unintentionally compounded other challenges, such as recruitment and retention.

One potential solution could involve adjusting reimbursement rates for providers in low-income areas, helping families and providers offset costs more effectively. Yet, this does not address the underlying financial constraints, such as high startup costs, that might incentivize new providers to establish new childcare centers.

Compounding these problems, the ECE workforce faces significant inequalities. Women of color are disproportionately represented and often earn wages that fall below the poverty line. For example, black female full-time educators serving children aged 0–5 earn just 84 cents for every $1 earned by their white counterparts [29]. Even federal policies devised to aid small businesses during the COVID-19 pandemic have inadvertently perpetuated unequal access for childcare providers and Black Americans.

Lastly, the operation hours of most licensed childcare programs, which tend to be conventional business hours, don't align with the shift-based schedules common in many low-wage jobs. These jobs are often held by Black, Indigenous, Latino, Asian and Pacific Islander, and other parents of color. Childcare providers offering flexible hours are more likely to be home based or family run and may not meet the criteria for state subsidy systems or CCDF requirements [30].

18.6 Conclusion: Enhancing Childcare Policies for Better Outcomes

The analysis of current federal programs offers valuable insights into the dynamic nature of childcare policies and their profound impacts on families and communities. It underscores the pivotal role that different levels of government and private entities play in shaping and implementing these policies.

Historically, the federal government has been instrumental in ensuring access to essential services, including childcare, especially for communities that may be overlooked at the state level.

The COVID-19-related grants have highlighted the government's ability to drive improvements and expansions in childcare services. At this level, policymakers should focus on establishing comprehensive childcare and family leave policies that set a standard for quality and accessibility. These may include grants and subsidies to support high-quality childcare services and incentives for states to develop innovative solutions.

State and local authorities have the flexibility to tailor federal policies to better suit the unique needs of their communities. Policymakers at these levels should work toward ensuring affordability, thereby facilitating a broader reach of these programs. They can also focus on enhancing the quality of childcare services and optimizing the allocation of federal grants. Partnerships with local businesses and communities can also be explored to create supportive ecosystems for parents.

The private sector can play a significant role in complementing government efforts. Businesses can implement family-friendly policies, such as flexible working hours, remote work opportunities, and corporate childcare facilities. By doing so, they contribute not only to employee well-being but also to the broader societal goal of accessible childcare.

Research emphasizes the importance of parental presence during a child's early months. Hence, an optimal childcare system should strive for a balanced approach, offering parents the choice between quality childcare services and the opportunity to stay at home. Policymakers across all levels should consider a combination of strategies, such as expanding access to affordable childcare while concurrently developing robust family leave policies.

Ultimately, adopting a multi-faceted approach that involves federal, state, and local authorities, along with private actors, can lead to significant enhancements in long-term outcomes for families and children. By clarifying the roles, responsibilities, and capacities of each stakeholder, we can ensure a coherent and effective strategy that not only addresses the immediate childcare needs but also lays a foundation for the holistic development of future generations.

Equitable Policies to Address Disparities in Early Childhood

Policy Area	Policy	Details
Healthy Child and Parental Support Policies	Medicaid Expansion	Provides access to services during the perinatal period, reducing birth disparities and medical costs for low-wealth families, especially families of color.
	Supplemental Nutrition Assistance Program (SNAP)	Largest nutrition assistance program in the United States, lifting over 3 million children and families out of poverty, linked to improved birth outcomes and various health outcomes.
	Preconception and Prenatal Care	Group prenatal care (GPNC) offers integrated health assessments, education, skills building, and peer social support, potentially reducing racial disparities in healthy pregnancies and births.
	Home Visiting	Programs support parents, promote positive parent–child relationships, and provide tailored services to meet specific family needs, including cultural competence and communication in the preferred language.

Policy Area	Policy	Details
Accessible and High-Quality Early Care and Education Policies	Child Care Subsidy Expansion	Makes child care more affordable and accessible for low-income families, increasing enrollment in child care and supporting maternal employment.
	Compensation Parity for ECE Workforce	Addresses wage gaps within the ECE workforce, aiming to reduce turnover and develop a diverse, competent workforce, which is crucial for supporting diverse children's needs.
	Elimination of Harsh Discipline and Exclusionary Practices	Ensures proper data collection and addresses the school-to-prison pipeline by eliminating suspension and expulsion practices that disproportionately impact Black children, boys, and children with special needs.
	Support for Dual Language Learners (DLLs)	Guarantees equitable services and learning opportunities for DLLs, supporting their academic achievement, bilingualism, and psychosocial development. Ensures that educators are competent in responding to DLLs' needs.
	Equity-Focused ECE Systems and Services	Ensures ECE programs develop equitable systems and services, including culturally responsive pedagogy, family engagement, and professional development opportunities for educators to support all children effectively.
	Access to Special Education Services	Ensures early identification and access to early intervention and special education services for children with special needs, particularly addressing inequities in service provision for children of color and dual language learners.

References

1 Hahn, R.A. and Truman, B.I. (2015). Education improves public health and promotes health equity. *International Journal of Health Services* 45 (4): 657–678.

2 Desjardins, R., Schuller, T., and Schleicher, A. (2006). Measuring the effects of education on health and civic engagement: proceedings from the Copenhagen symposium. https://escholarship.org/uc/item/6h84705f (accessed 27 August 2024).

3 EdBuild. (2019). 23 billion. http://edbuild.org/content/23-billion (accessed 27 August 2024).

4 Turner, E.O. and Beneke, A.J. (2020). 'Softening' school resource officers: the extension of police presence in schools in an era of Black Lives Matter, school shootings, and rising inequality. *Race Ethnicity and Education* 23 (2): 221–240.

5 Richardson, L.D. and Norris, M. (2010). Access to health and health care: how race and ethnicity matter. *Mount Sinai Journal of Medicine: A Journal of Translational and Personalized Medicine* 77 (2): 166–177.

6 Brown v. Board of Education (1954). 347 U.S. 483.

7 Iruka, I.U. (2022). Delivering on the promise of early childhood education for black children: an equity strategy. *New Directions for Child and Adolescent Development* 2022 (183–184): 27–45.

8 Donoghue, E.A. and Council on Early Childhood (2017). Quality early education and child care from birth to kindergarten. *Pediatrics* 140 (2): e20171488.

9 Ramon, I., Chattopadhyay, S.K., Barnett, W.S. et al. (2018). Early childhood education to promote health equity: a community guide economic review. *Journal of Public Health Management and Practice: JPHMP* 24 (1): e8–e15.

10 Heckman, J.J., Moon, S.H., Pinto, R. et al. (2010). The rate of return to the high/scope Perry Preschool Program. *Journal of Public Economics* 94 (1–2): 114–128.

11 The Center for American Progress (2016). Child care deserts: an analysis of child care centers by zip code in 8 states. https://www.americanprogress.org/article/child-care-deserts/ (accessed 27 August 2024).

12 Marsh, K. (2023). *The Love Jones Cohort: Single and Living Alone in the Black Middle Class*. Cambridge University Press.

13 Zigler, E. and Styfco, S.J. (2010). *The Hidden History of Head Start*. Oxford University Press.

14 Committee on Child Health Financing, Racine, A.D., Long, T.F. et al. (2014). Children's Health Insurance Program (CHIP): accomplishments, challenges, and policy recommendations. *Pediatrics* 133 (3): e784–e793.

15 Brandeis University (2020). Data-for-equity research brief: unequal availability of head start: how neighborhood matters. https://www.diversitydatakids.org/sites/default/files/2020-01/ddk_unequal-availability-of-head-start_2020_4.pdf (accessed 27 August 2024).

16 HeadStart Early Childhood Learning & Knowledge Center (2019). Head start program facts: fiscal year 2019. https://eclkc.ohs.acf.hhs.gov/about-us/article/head-start-program-facts-fiscal-year-2019 (accessed 27 August 2024).

17 Delaney, K.K. and Krepps, K. (2021). Exploring head start teacher and leader perceptions of the pre-K classroom assessment scoring system as a part of the head start designation renewal system. *Early Childhood Research Quarterly* 55: 214–229.

18 Office of Child Care (2016). *Child Care and Development Fund Final Rule Frequently Asked Questions*. U.S. Department of Health and Human Services, Administration for Children and Families. https://www.acf.hhs.gov/occ/faq/child-care-and-development-fund-final-rule-frequently-asked-questions.

19 Hill, Z., Gennetian, L.A., and Mendez, J. (2019). A descriptive profile of state child care and development fund policies in states with high populations of low-income Hispanic children. *Early Childhood Research Quarterly* 47: 111–123.

20 Office of Child Care (2022). OCC fact sheet. https://www.acf.hhs.gov/occ/fact-sheet (accessed 27 August 2024).

21 The National Research Center on Hispanic Children & Families (2019). How state-level child care development fund policies may shape access and utilization among Hispanic families. https://www.hispanicresearchcenter.org/research-resources/how-state-level-child-care-development-fund-policies-may-shape-access-and-utilization-among-hispanic-families/ (accessed 27 August 2024).

22 DC Policy Center (2017). Four principles to guide child care policy in D.C. https://www.dcpolicycenter.org/publications/four-principles-to-guide-child-care-policy-in-d-c/ (accessed 27 August 2024).

23 The Office of Child Care (2023). COVID relief funding for child care. https://childcareta.acf.hhs.gov/covid-relief-funding-child-care (accessed 27 August 2024).

24 Whatcom County, Washington (2023). Healthy children's fund. https://www.whatcomcounty.us/4069/Healthy-Childrens-Fund (accessed 27 August 2024).

25 Adams, G. and Pratt, E. (2021). *Assessing child Care Subsidies Through an Equity Lens*. Washington, DC: Urban Institute.

26 Lovejoy, A. (2024). *States Are Taking Action to Address the Child Care Crisis*. Center for American Progress. https://www.americanprogress.org/article/states-are-taking-action-to-address-the-child-care-crisis/.

27 Office of Elementary & Secondary Education (2023). Awards. https://oese.ed.gov/offices/office-of-discretionary-grants-support-services/innovation-early-learning/preschool-development-grants/awards/ (accessed 27 August 2024).

28 The White House (2007). President Bush signs "Improving Head Start for School Readiness Act of 2007" into law. https://georgewbush-whitehouse.archives.gov/news/releases/2007/12/20071212-3.html (Accessed 27 August 2024).

29 The Center for American Progress (2016). Underpaid and unequal: racial wage disparities in the early childhood workforce. https://www.americanprogress.org/article/underpaid-and-unequal/ (accessed 27 August 2024).

30 Greszler, R. and Burke, L.M. (2020). *Rethinking Early Childhood Education and Childcare in the COVID-19 Era*. Backgrounder. No. 3533. Heritage Foundation.

19

Enacting Paid Family Leave for Health Equity

Abstract

Millions of Americans juggle employment with caring for aging family members or children, yet limited workers have access to paid family leave. This lack of access is particularly acute for low-income employees and women of color, who are the least likely to have meaningful paid family leave. When leave is available, it may not be practical for these workers to take it due to inadequate wage replacement or fear of job loss. Comprehensive paid family leave is crucial for promoting health equity by improving health outcomes, reducing socioeconomic disparities, and supporting women's participation in the workforce. This chapter addresses the intersection of paid family leave and health equity. It begins by providing background on the current state of paid leave in the United States, highlighting the limited access and disparities that exist. Next, it examines the evidence demonstrating how comprehensive paid leave policies can address inequities by improving health outcomes, providing economic stability, and advancing gender and racial equity. The chapter then offers strategies for designing paid leave policies that effectively promote equity and increase uptake among those who need it most. Finally, it concludes by summarizing key principles policymakers should follow to develop and implement effective, equitable paid family leave policies.

Keywords *paid family leave; health equity; economic stability; racial disparities; low-income workers; job protection; wage replacement; caregiving responsibilities*

> *Linda, a single mother and retail worker, faces the daunting task of caring for her elderly father who recently suffered a stroke. With no access to paid family leave, she risks her job and financial stability each time she needs to attend her father's medical appointments. The constant stress of choosing between her family's well-being and her livelihood underscores the urgent need for policies that protect workers like her.*
>
> *Thomas, an African American bus driver in his mid-30s, struggles with the decision to take unpaid leave after the birth of his daughter. The lack of adequate wage replacement makes it financially impossible for him to stay home, depriving him of precious early bonding time with his child. This scenario highlights the disproportionate impact of current paid leave policies on workers of color and the pressing need for inclusive reform.*

Achieving Health Equity: The Role of Law and Policy, First Edition. Y. Tony Yang.
© 2025 John Wiley & Sons Ltd. Published 2025 by John Wiley & Sons Ltd.

19.1 Barriers to Equitable Paid Family Leave in the United States

The United States stands alone among developed nations in its lack of a national paid family leave policy, leaving American workers, particularly those from low-income and marginalized communities, at risk of falling behind their global counterparts. The COVID-19 pandemic has further exposed the glaring inequities in paid leave access and underscored the critical importance of comprehensive paid leave policies.

Access to employer-provided paid family leave is limited, with only 13–14% of workers benefiting from such policies, primarily those in high-paying, professional occupations at large companies [1]. The disparity is even more stark for low-wage workers, with a mere 6% having access to paid family leave [2]. Significant racial inequities also persist, as workers of color are less likely to have paid family leave compared to their white counterparts [3]. While the federal Family and Medical Leave Act (FMLA) offers up to 12 weeks of unpaid job-protected leave, its coverage extends to only about 60% of the workforce, and many eligible workers cannot afford to take unpaid leave [4].

During the pandemic, the absence of comprehensive paid leave policies forced workers to choose between their health, their family's well-being, and their financial stability [5]. Low-income workers, women, and people of color were disproportionately affected, as they were more likely to hold jobs without paid leave benefits [6]. Emergency legislation, such as the Families First Coronavirus Response Act, aimed at expanding paid sick leave during the pandemic inadvertently exacerbated existing disparities, leaving many vulnerable workers ineligible for these temporary measures [7].

As the nation looks to rebuild, policymakers must prioritize the development and implementation of comprehensive paid leave policies that ensure all workers, regardless of socioeconomic status, race, or employment type, have the ability to care for themselves and their families without risking their health or financial security. Addressing these longstanding inequities is crucial for fostering a more resilient and equitable workforce, prepared to weather future crises and support the well-being of all individuals and families. The current landscape of paid family leave in the United States, characterized by limited access, significant disparities, and inadequate protections, necessitates a comprehensive approach that prioritizes accessibility, affordability, and job security for all workers.

> *"Separating a mom from her baby, because she does not have sufficient income to stay home, is NOT a family value, it is the opposite."*
>
> U.S. Senator Bernie Sanders

19.2 The Impact of Paid Leave Policies on Vulnerable Workers and the Far-Reaching Benefits for Health and Equity

Paid leave policies have a disproportionate impact on low-income workers, women, and people of color, who are less likely to have access to flexible hours, paid leave, and the ability to work from home. Women, particularly Black women, find themselves in a precarious position as they are more likely to be both primary caregivers and breadwinners for their families [8]. The lack of paid family leave often forces these women to choose between their caregiving responsibilities and maintaining their employment and income [9].

Black women are especially vulnerable to the effects of inadequate leave policies due to their unique roles, coupled with existing health inequities [10]. They are disproportionately employed in low-paid jobs with few benefits and face higher rates of leave request denials compared to white workers. The financial impact of taking unpaid leave is staggering, with Black women losing an estimated $3.9 billion in wages each year [11]. This financial pressure discourages them from taking leave when needed and creates additional stress when they do.

In addition to the financial burden, Black mothers and their newborns are more likely to experience health problems after childbirth, yet they are less likely to have access to care. Paid family leave plays a crucial role in the health and well-being of those who depend on care, as it offers a wide range of short- and long-term health benefits for workers and their families [12]. Research consistently demonstrates that paid time to care for oneself or a loved one leads to improved health outcomes, reduced healthcare costs, and increased health equity [13].

Paid family leave has particularly significant benefits for new parents and newborns, promoting bonding, breastfeeding, on-time vaccinations, and overall child development [14]. These policies also contribute to better maternal health by allowing mothers to rest and recover after childbirth [15]. Moreover, paid family leave addresses gender and racial disparities in the workplace, fostering a more inclusive workforce without detrimentally impacting employers [16].

The evidence is clear: paid family leave is a powerful tool for promoting public health and health equity. By supporting workers, particularly those from vulnerable populations, in caring for themselves and their loved ones, these policies have the potential to improve health outcomes across the lifespan. Policymakers must recognize the far-reaching benefits of paid family leave and prioritize the implementation of comprehensive policies that ensure all workers, regardless of socioeconomic status or race, have access to this critical support. Only by addressing these inequities can we create a more equitable and inclusive society that values the health and well-being of all its members.

19.3 Designing Effective and Equitable Paid Family Leave Policies: Key Strategies for Inclusivity and Uptake

Paid family leave is a policy that allows employees to take paid time off during pregnancy, after the birth or adoption of a child, or when a young child or other family member needs care [17]. Comprehensive paid family leave policies serve as a powerful tool to address the needs of low-income communities and communities of color, promoting health outcomes and improving economic stability [18]. However, access to paid family leave is far from universal, with disparities in coverage based on factors such as employer size, occupation, and income level.

To develop equitable paid leave programs, it's essential for policymakers to focus on the specific needs of low-income workers and women of color [19]. These programs should aim to increase access to leave without worsening existing economic and health disparities. Effective and inclusive paid family leave policies can be designed by implementing a national coverage that includes all workers, regardless of their employer's size or industry. It's also crucial to enhance oversight through public administration to prevent employers from arbitrarily denying leave requests. The policies should incorporate job protection provisions that allow workers to take necessary leave without the fear of losing their jobs, along with antidiscrimination measures to ensure people of color can access these benefits. Adequate wage replacement rates, especially for low-income workers, are necessary to support the livelihoods of those on leave [20]. Additionally, ensuring that paid leave is portable and covers individuals across multiple jobs can make a significant difference. Broadening the scope of what qualifies for leave – including a generous duration and inclusive definitions of family and gender identities – is key. Finally, dedicated funding for outreach, education, and enforcement will help raise awareness and improve the utilization of paid leave programs.

In addition to these policy elements, policymakers and advocates should focus on strategies for increasing uptake to improve equity. This includes raising awareness of leave policies and job protection provisions, incorporating both short-term and long-term medical leave, expanding allowable leave durations, and increasing wage replacement rates. By adopting comprehensive leave policies that better support the needs of workers, we can promote racial, gender, and economic equality in the workplace and beyond.

Crafting comprehensive paid family leave policies that address the needs of low-income workers, women, and people of color is crucial for promoting health equity [21]. By ensuring that all workers have access to paid leave, regardless of their occupation, company size, or income level, we can create a more level playing field and reduce the health disparities that stem from unequal access to this critical benefit. Policymakers must prioritize the development and implementation of effective paid family leave policies that provide adequate wage replacement, job protection, and coverage for all workers, thereby fostering a healthier, more equitable society.

Creating equitable paid leave programs requires a multifaceted approach that prioritizes the needs of those who have been historically underserved and marginalized. By designing policies that expand access, provide meaningful benefits, and promote uptake, we can ensure that all workers have the opportunity to care for themselves and their loved ones without sacrificing their economic security or well-being.

Various Aspects of Paid Family Leave Policies and Their Impact on Public Health and Equity

Category	Aspect	Impact on Public Health and Equity
Policy Design	Increased leave duration	Facilitates better postpartum recovery for mothers and enhances early childhood development
	Higher benefit amounts	Makes it financially feasible for more workers, especially low income, to take leave, reducing health disparities
	No waiting period	Allows immediate access to benefits, critical for timely support during childbirth or family health issues
Job Security	Job protection	Increases the likelihood that employees will take leave, supporting family stability and employee retention
Inclusivity	Universal coverage	Ensures that all workers, including part-time and gig workers, have access to leave, promoting inclusivity
	Expansion of family definitions	Supports nontraditional families, ensuring that various family structures can benefit from leave policies
Health	Health outcomes	Associated with lower infant mortality rates, increased breastfeeding, and reduced postpartum depression
Economic Impact	Economic security	Provides stability during leave periods, preventing financial crises due to unpaid leave
	Support for childcare	Helps parents provide consistent and quality care, reducing stress and improving long-term child welfare
Equity and Access	Equity among workers	Addresses disparities by ensuring workers of color and lower income have equal access to paid leave benefits

19.4 Conclusion: Paid Leave: A Crucial Step Toward Health and Economic Equity

Paid leave is a vital step toward achieving health and economic equity, particularly for women and people of color. By providing workers with the ability to take time off to receive medical care and care for family members without sacrificing their income or job security, paid leave policies can help keep these populations in the workforce, promoting greater equality and stability.

To ensure that paid leave policies are effective in supporting workers and their families, policymakers must pass laws that guarantee access to these benefits. Crucially, these policies should include appropriate wage replacement rates and job protection provisions to encourage workers who need leave to take it without fear of financial hardship or job loss.

While some states and private employers have already taken steps to promote paid family and medical leave policies, federal action is essential to ensure that all Americans, regardless of where they live or work, have access to these critical benefits. A comprehensive, national paid leave policy would provide a foundation for supporting the health and economic stability of workers and their families across the country.

By prioritizing the development and implementation of robust paid leave policies, policymakers have the opportunity to create a more equitable and inclusive workforce, one that values the well-being of all workers and recognizes the importance of balancing work and family responsibilities. In doing so, we can take a significant step toward building a society that truly promotes health and economic equity for all.

References

1 U.S. Bureau of Labor Statistics (2019). Racial and ethnic disparities in access to and use of paid family and medical leave: evidence from four nationally representative datasets. https://www.bls.gov/opub/mlr/2019/article/racial-and-ethnic-disparities-in-access-to-and-use-of-paid-family-and-medical-leave.htm (accessed 27 August 2024).

2 Bureau of Labor Statistics, U.S. Department of Labor (2022). A look at paid family leave by wage category in 2021. *The Economics Daily.* https://www.bls.gov/opub/ted/2022/a-look-at-paid-family-leave-by-wage-category-in-2021.htm.

3 Goodman, J.M., Williams, C., and Dow, W.H. (2021). Racial/ethnic inequities in paid parental leave access. *Health Equity* 5 (1): 738–749. https://doi.org/10.1089/heq.2021.0001.

4 Shepherd-Banigan, M. and Bell, J.F. (2014). Paid leave benefits among a national sample of working mothers with infants in the United States. *Maternal and Child Health Journal* 18 (1): 286–295. https://doi.org/10.1007/s10995-013-1264-3.

5 Pollack, C.C., Deverakonda, A., Hassan, F. et al. (2023). The impact of state paid sick leave policies on weekday workplace mobility during the COVID-19 pandemic. *Public Health* 215: 118–123. https://doi.org/10.1016/j.puhe.2022.08.019.

6 Goodman, J.M., Elser, H., and Dow, W.H. (2020). Among low-income women in San Francisco, low awareness of paid parental leave benefits inhibits take-up. *Health Affairs (Project Hope)* 39 (7): 1157–1165. https://doi.org/10.1377/hlthaff.2020.00157.

7 Act, E.P.S.L. (2020). Families first coronavirus response act. *Public Law* 116–217.

8 Schneider, D. and Harknett, K. (2019). Consequences of routine work-schedule instability for worker health and well-being. *American Sociological Review* 84 (1): 82–114. https://doi.org/10.1177/0003122418823184.

9 Han, W.J., Ruhn, C., and Waldfogel, J. (2009). Parental leave policies and parents' employment and leave-taking. *Journal of Policy Analysis and Management: [The Journal of the Association for Public Policy Analysis and Management]* 28 (1): 29–54. https://doi.org/10.1002/pam.20398.

10 Goodman, J.M. and Schneider, D. (2023). Racial/ethnic and gender inequities in the sufficiency of paid leave during the COVID-19 pandemic: evidence from the service sector. *American Journal of Industrial Medicine* 66 (11): 928–937. https://doi.org/10.1002/ajim.23533.

11 Tucker, J. and Vogtman, J. (2021). *When Hard Work Is Not Enough: Women in Low-Paid Jobs.* National Women's Law Center.

12 Nandi, A., Jahagirdar, D., Dimitris, M.C. et al. (2018). The impact of parental and medical leave policies on socioeconomic and health outcomes in OECD countries: a systematic review of the empirical literature. *The Milbank Quarterly* 96 (3): 434–471. https://doi.org/10.1111/1468-0009.12340.

13 Yang, Y.T., Wallington, S.F., and Morain, S. (2022). Paid leave for fathers: policy, practice, and reform. *The Milbank Quarterly* 100 (4): 973–990. https://doi.org/10.1111/1468-0009.12590.

14 Arnautovic, T.I. and Dammann, C.E.L. (2023). The neonatal perspective of paid family medical leave (PFML). *Journal of Perinatology: Official Journal of the California Perinatal Association* 43 (8): 1055–1058. https://doi.org/10.1038/s41372-021-01300-6.

15 Hewitt, B., Strazdins, L., and Martin, B. (2017). The benefits of paid maternity leave for mothers' post-partum health and wellbeing: evidence from an Australian evaluation. *Social Science & Medicine* 1982 (182): 97–105. https://doi.org/10.1016/j.socscimed.2017.04.022.

16 Elser, H., Williams, C., Dow, W.H., and Goodman, J.M. (2022). Inequities in paid parental leave across industry and occupational class: drivers and simulated policy remedies. *SSM – Population Health* 18: 101045. https://doi.org/10.1016/j.ssmph.2022.101045.

17 Malamitsi-Puchner, A., Addati, L., Eydal, G.B. et al. (2023). Paid leave to support parenting – a neglected tool to improve societal well-being and prosperity. *Acta Paediatrica (Oslo, Norway: 1992)* 112 (10): 2045–2049. https://doi.org/10.1111/apa.16929.

18 Wething, H. (2022). Paid sick leave policy impacts on health and care utilization in the United States: why policy design matters. *Journal of Public Health Policy* 43 (4): 530–541. https://doi.org/10.1057/s41271-022-00371-9.

19 Haro-Ramos, A.Y. and Bacong, A.M. (2023). Disparities in unmet needed paid leave across race, ethnicity and citizenship status among employed Californians: a cross-sectional study. *Public Health* 221: 97–105. https://doi.org/10.1016/j.puhe.2023.06.013.

20 Davison, H.K. and Blackburn, A.S. (2023). The case for offering paid leave: benefits to the employer, employee, and society. *Compensation and Benefits Review* 55 (1): 3–18. https://doi.org/10.1177/08863687221131728.

21 Montez, K., Thomson, S., and Shabo, V. (2020). An opportunity to promote health equity: national paid family and medical leave. *Pediatrics* 146 (3): e20201122. https://doi.org/10.1542/peds.2020-1122.

20

Enhancing Rural, Remote, and Tribal Health Equity Through Policies

Abstract

This chapter examines the challenges faced by Americans living in rural, remote, and tribal areas in terms of health outcomes and access to quality healthcare services. It highlights the multifaceted policy approach required to advance health equity for these underserved populations, addressing the unique social, economic, environmental, and geographic factors impacting their health. The chapter discusses recent federal frameworks, such as the Centers for Medicare and Medicaid Services (CMS) Framework for Advancing Health Care in Rural, Tribal, and Geographically Isolated Communities, and state legislative trends aimed at improving health and healthcare access in these communities. It also identifies remaining gaps and provides recommendations for federal policymakers to accelerate progress toward equitable rural and tribal health. The chapter emphasizes the urgent need for a sustained, multisectoral effort to address both the medical and nonmedical drivers of health inequity, seizing the opportunities presented by COVID-19 pandemic recovery efforts to catalyze transformative investments in rural health infrastructure, workforce, and community well-being. Ultimately, the chapter argues that achieving rural and tribal health equity is not only a moral imperative but also essential for the nation's overall health and prosperity.

Keywords *rural health equity; tribal health disparities; healthcare access; telehealth expansion; workforce shortages; social determinants of health; federal policies; COVID-19 impact*

> *In a remote Alaskan village, Hunter, a tribal elder with diabetes, struggles to access the specialist care he needs. The nearest endocrinologist is over 200 miles away, and the village's understaffed clinic lacks the resources to provide comprehensive diabetes management. As a result, the elder's condition worsens, leading to avoidable complications and a lower quality of life.*
>
> *A rural hospital in the heart of Appalachia faces imminent closure due to financial instability, exacerbated by the COVID-19 pandemic. The hospital's shutdown would leave thousands of residents without access to emergency care and essential health services, forcing them to travel long distances to seek treatment. The community grapples with the potential loss of not only their primary healthcare provider but also a significant economic driver and source of employment.*

Achieving Health Equity: The Role of Law and Policy, First Edition. Y. Tony Yang.
© 2025 John Wiley & Sons Ltd. Published 2025 by John Wiley & Sons Ltd.

> *Adsila, a young Native American mother living on a reservation struggles to find affordable, nutritious food for her family. The nearest grocery store is an hour's drive away, and the only local food options are high-priced, low-quality processed foods at the gas station. Despite qualifying for SNAP benefits, the limited availability of healthy food options contributes to the family's poor dietary habits and increased risk of obesity and chronic diseases.*

20.1 Challenges Facing Rural, Remote, and Tribal Health

Approximately 61 million people, or around 15% of the US population, live in rural and remote areas [1]. These Americans are more likely to die prematurely from the five leading causes of death – heart disease, cancer, unintentional injury, chronic lower respiratory disease, and stroke. Poverty rates and age-adjusted mortality rates are also higher [2], while health insurance coverage is lower, in rural compared to urban areas [3].

For tribal populations, health disparities are even more stark. American Indians and Alaska Natives, whether living in rural or urban settings, have higher rates of chronic diseases, such as diabetes and hypertension, compared to national averages [4]. The Indian Health Service (IHS), which is responsible for providing federal health services to American Indians and Alaska Natives, has been chronically underfunded, leading to significant gaps in access to care and health outcomes [5].

Several factors drive these poor health outcomes in rural, remote, and tribal communities. Geographic isolation and low population density make it difficult to sustain healthcare services in these areas. Workforce shortages are more acute, with fewer physicians, specialists, and behavioral health providers per capita compared to urban areas [6]. When local hospitals or clinics close due to financial instability, residents must travel longer distances to access care, which can be particularly challenging for those with limited transportation options or mobility issues [7].

High rates of poverty and un-insurance also create significant financial barriers to accessing healthcare services in rural and remote areas. Many residents may forego needed care due to cost concerns or lack of coverage [8]. Additionally, these communities often lack adequate public health infrastructure, such as disease surveillance systems, health promotion programs, and emergency preparedness resources [9].

The COVID-19 pandemic has further exposed and exacerbated these long-standing health inequities. Rural and tribal communities have experienced higher rates of COVID-19 cases, hospitalizations, and deaths compared to urban areas. The pandemic has also strained the already fragile rural healthcare system, with many hospitals and clinics facing financial losses due to suspension of elective procedures and reduced patient volumes [10].

> *"American Indians and Alaska Natives born today have a life expectancy that is 5.5 years less than the U.S. all races population. American Indians and Alaska Natives continue to die at higher rates than other Americans in many categories, including chronic liver disease and cirrhosis, diabetes mellitus, unintentional injuries, assault/homicide, intentional self-harm/suicide, and chronic lower respiratory diseases."*
>
> Indian Health Services, HHS (2019)

20.2 Advancing Rural and Tribal Health Equity Through Federal Policies

Recognizing the urgent need for coordinated cross-agency efforts to address these persistent inequities, the Biden administration and Congress have launched several promising initiatives focused specifically on improving rural, remote, and tribal health.

In November 2022, the CMS released its Framework for Advancing Health Care in Rural, Tribal, and Geographically Isolated Communities. The Framework outlines six key priorities [11]. The first priority is applying a community-informed geographic lens to CMS policies and programs. This involves considering the unique needs and challenges of rural, tribal, and geographically isolated communities when developing and implementing policies and programs. The second priority is increasing the collection and use of standardized data to drive improvements. This includes improving data collection methods and systems to better understand the health needs and disparities facing these communities, and using this data to inform targeted interventions and track progress over time. Strengthening and supporting the rural health workforce is the third priority. This recognizes the critical role that healthcare providers play in ensuring access to care in underserved areas, and the need for targeted efforts to recruit, retain, and support rural healthcare professionals. The fourth priority is optimizing medical and communication technology for these communities. This includes expanding access to telehealth and other digital health tools, as well as improving the interoperability of health information systems to facilitate care coordination and data sharing. Expanding access to comprehensive health coverage, benefits, and services is the fifth priority. This involves working with states, health plans, and providers to ensure that rural and underserved populations have access to the full range of services they need to maintain and improve their health, including preventive care, chronic disease management, and behavioral health services. The sixth and final priority is driving innovation and value-based care models suitable for rural contexts. This recognizes the unique challenges of delivering care in low-volume, geographically dispersed settings, and the need for flexible payment models that incentivize quality and value rather than volume. The Framework aims to support the development and scaling of alternative payment models and delivery system reforms that are tailored to the needs of rural communities.

Importantly, the CMS Framework was developed through extensive engagement with rural and tribal stakeholders, including listening sessions, tribal consultations, and public input. This community-driven approach aims to ensure CMS programs and policies are more responsive to the unique needs, challenges, and strengths of these populations.

The Framework proposes concrete actions CMS will take over the next five years to advance each priority. For example, to enhance data collection and use, CMS will work with partners to address barriers to interoperability and leverage technologies like telehealth to improve care coordination. To expand access to coverage and benefits, CMS will support state Medicaid agencies and health plans in covering a broader array of services, including those that address social determinants of health such as transportation and housing [12].

To drive rural-appropriate value-based care, CMS will examine participation barriers for rural providers and design flexible payment models suitable for facilities with low patient volumes. Across all areas, CMS emphasizes the importance of ongoing engagement and co-creation with rural and tribal communities to ensure policies and programs meet their needs.

The CMS Framework aligns with and supports broader health equity initiatives across the Department of Health and Human Services (HHS), including the HHS Rural Health Action Plan, the CDC SDOH

Accelerator Plans, and IHS Strategic Plan [13]. By leveraging its role as the largest payer of healthcare services, CMS aims to be a catalyst for systemwide transformation toward more equitable rural and tribal health.

In addition to the CMS Framework, the White House launched a Rural Infrastructure Tour to engage local elected officials and community leaders on place-based strategies to advance equity. The 2021 American Rescue Plan and 2022 Inflation Reduction Act also included significant investments in rural healthcare access and affordability, such as enhanced subsidies for ACA Marketplace coverage, Medicaid expansion incentives, and funds for rural health clinic and hospital infrastructure [14].

In September 2022, the Biden Administration released a whole-of-government Federal Plan for Equitable Long-Term Recovery and Resilience (ELTRR). The ELTRR Plan outlines strategies for federal agencies to better align and coordinate efforts related to health equity, community engagement, data collection, and place-based initiatives in under-resourced communities, including those in rural and remote areas. Key recommendations include establishing an interagency data-sharing portal on rural health disparities, expanding eligibility for federal grant programs to include rural nonprofits and community organizations, and developing rural-specific communications campaigns to promote health insurance enrollment and COVID-19 vaccination [15].

For tribal health specifically, the permanent reauthorization of the Indian Health Care Improvement Act in 2010 was a significant milestone in advancing health equity for American Indians and Alaska Natives. The Act authorizes comprehensive health services and programs through IHS, tribal health programs, and urban Indian organizations [16]. More recently, the Consolidated Appropriations Act of 2022 included advance appropriations for IHS for the first time, providing greater funding certainty and reducing the impact of government shutdowns on tribal health services.

However, despite this progress, IHS remains chronically underfunded compared to other federal health programs like Medicare, Medicaid, and the Veterans Health Administration. Per capita spending for IHS is far below that of other federal health programs, limiting the ability of tribal health systems to provide comprehensive, high-quality care [17]. Efforts to elevate the IHS Director position to an HHS Assistant Secretary, which would give greater visibility and influence to tribal health issues, have also stalled in Congress [18].

20.3 State-Level Policy Trends

Key Policies and Equity Initiatives in Advancing Rural, Remote, and Tribal Health Equity

Policy Area	Key Initiatives and Actions	Impact on Health Equity
Regulatory Activities	• Established Rural Emergency Hospital (REH) designation • Finalized Medicaid and CHIP postpartum coverage expansion	• Ensures continued essential health services in rural areas • Expands postpartum care access for new mothers in underserved areas
Payment Policies	• Implemented payment policies for behavioral health and chronic pain management • Introduced supplemental payments for IHS and tribal hospitals	• Enhances financial support for rural and tribal health providers • Addresses needs of underserved communities

Policy Area	Key Initiatives and Actions	Impact on Health Equity
Coverage Expansion	• Supported ACA marketplace coverage and increased issuer participation • Expanded Medicaid eligibility in South Dakota • Extended postpartum coverage	• Reduces uninsured rates and increases access to affordable care • Ensures continuous coverage for vulnerable populations
Health Systems Innovation	• Developed innovative models like Making Care Primary • Supported state initiatives addressing social determinants of health (SDOH)	• Promotes tailored care models for rural areas • Addresses both medical and social factors impacting health
Data Collection and Use	• Increased telehealth data collection • Improved nursing home data transparency • Released health equity data briefs	• Enhances understanding of health disparities • Informs targeted health interventions and policy decisions
Partner Engagement	• Conducted listening sessions and tribal consultations • Engaged with rural and tribal health stakeholders	• Ensures community voices are included in policymaking • Strengthens trust and relationships with underserved communities
Technology and Telehealth	• Extended Medicare telehealth flexibilities • Promoted digital health education and telehealth indicators	• Expands care access via telehealth • Improves digital literacy and telehealth service use
SDOH Initiatives	• Provided guidance for Medicaid-managed care addressing social needs • Released Medicaid Transportation Coverage Guide	• Tackles nonmedical factors like housing and transportation • Supports holistic healthcare approaches for better health outcomes

In addition to federal actions, states are also advancing legislative policies to improve health equity in rural and underserved areas. A review of recent state laws enacted reveals several promising trends.

Expanding loan repayment programs to incentivize healthcare providers to practice in rural and underserved communities is a common strategy. For example, Hawaii enacted a new law providing loan repayment for physicians and other clinicians who commit to working in designated shortage areas, while Iowa expanded eligibility for its existing loan repayment program to include more rural regions. These financial incentives can help address persistent workforce shortages in rural areas [19].

Improving access to behavioral health services is another priority for many states, given the higher rates of substance use disorders and suicide in rural populations. Nevada passed a law allowing rural hospitals to be certified as crisis stabilization centers, enabling them to provide short-term behavioral health services and reduce reliance on scarce inpatient psychiatric beds. Oregon created a new grant program to fund transportation for rural veterans accessing mental health treatment. By integrating behavioral health into primary care settings and leveraging tele-mental health, these policies aim to reduce stigma and increase access to much-needed services [20].

Expanding telehealth flexibilities that were initially enacted during the COVID-19 pandemic is another common theme. Maryland and Vermont, for example, codified requirements for Medicaid and private insurers to cover audio-only telehealth visits at parity with in-person services. West Virginia enacted a new law requiring all health plans to cover telehealth and reimburse at rates negotiated between payers and providers. These policies recognize the vital role of telehealth in delivering care to rural and underserved communities, particularly those with transportation barriers or limited access to specialists [21].

Finally, several states are making significant investments in rural broadband infrastructure to enable greater adoption of telehealth and other digital health technologies. Indiana designated rural health clinics as eligible sites for broadband expansion projects, while Iowa clarified the minimum download/upload speeds required for its broadband grant program targeting rural areas. These efforts are being bolstered by federal funding from the American Rescue Plan and the Infrastructure Investment and Jobs Act, which included billions for broadband deployment in unserved and underserved regions. Closing the digital divide is essential for ensuring rural communities can fully participate in virtual care innovations [22].

20.4 Remaining Gaps and Recommendations

Despite the promising federal and state policy developments outlined above, significant work remains to fully close health equity gaps facing rural, remote, and tribal populations. Key challenges include the lack of granular data on the needs and experiences of rural subpopulations, which limits the ability to target interventions and track progress. While the CMS Framework and ELTRR Plan emphasize the importance of data disaggregation, the technological infrastructure and workforce capacity needed to collect and analyze this data remains limited in many rural areas [23].

Persistent health workforce shortages are another major barrier, with rural communities facing a 19% gap in primary care physicians and 31% gap in specialists compared to urban areas [24]. Expanded loan repayment and scholarships are helpful but insufficient to fully close this gap. More flexible licensure and scope of practice policies, increased rural training opportunities, and innovative care delivery models are also needed to maximize the rural workforce.

Restrictive and outdated payment policies also impede the ability of rural providers to sustainably deliver comprehensive, coordinated care. Medicare and Medicaid regulations often fail to account for the unique challenges of providing care in low-volume, geographically dispersed settings. While the CMS Framework promises to examine rural-appropriate value-based payment models, the details and timelines for these reforms remain unclear [25].

Additionally, the looming expiration of Medicaid continuous coverage requirements tied to the COVID-19 public health emergency could lead to significant coverage losses in rural areas, exacerbating access and affordability challenges [26]. Policies to streamline Medicaid redetermination and facilitate smooth transitions to other coverage sources will be critical to mitigate these risks.

To accelerate progress toward equitable rural and tribal health, federal policymakers should consider the following recommendations:

Enhance rural data collection and use. In addition to supporting data disaggregation as outlined in the CMS Framework, HHS should provide targeted technical assistance and infrastructure funding to help rural providers upgrade electronic health record systems and participate in health information exchanges. The CDC and other agencies should also expand sampling of rural populations in national health surveys to enable more granular analyses of rural subgroups, such as by race/ethnicity, disability status, and sexual orientation/gender identity [27].

Permanently expand access to affordable health coverage. Congress should provide enhanced federal funding for Medicaid expansion in the remaining non-expansion states, which are disproportionately rural. Policymakers should also make the enhanced ACA subsidies permanent and allow individuals to enroll in Marketplace coverage year-round to maximize participation [28]. For uninsured individuals in non-expansion states, the administration should consider extending the COVID-19 Uninsured Program to cover additional services like primary care and behavioral health.

Strengthen rural healthcare delivery infrastructure. Beyond supporting broadband access, federal investments are needed to modernize physical infrastructure of rural hospitals and clinics, many of which are aging and in need of repair. Policymakers should also increase funding for rural residency training programs, rural health clinics, community health centers, and other safety net providers. Regulatory flexibilities around telehealth, facility and physician licensing, and value-based payment should be made permanent where possible [29].

Invest in tribal health systems. To fulfill the federal government's trust responsibility, Congress should enact mandatory, inflation-adjusted funding for IHS rather than relying on discretionary appropriations. Funding levels should be increased to match per capita spending on federal prisoners and Medicaid beneficiaries. All HHS grant programs should have minimum tribal set asides, and reporting requirements should be streamlined to reduce the administrative burden on under-resourced tribal health departments [30].

Address social and economic drivers of rural health inequities. In addition to healthcare access, federal efforts to advance rural health equity must also tackle the underlying social, economic, and environmental determinants. This requires significant investments in affordable housing, transportation infrastructure, nutrition assistance, job creation, and environmental justice initiatives. Grant programs and demonstration projects should incentivize cross-sector collaboration and incorporate health impact assessments to identify unintended consequences.

Strengthen rural community engagement in policymaking. Too often, rural and tribal voices are left out of federal policy decisions that impact their health and well-being. The administration should appoint a Rural Health Equity Advisor in the White House Domestic Policy Council to elevate rural issues across government. Federal agencies should also be required to have rural representation on all relevant advisory committees and conduct rural impact assessments for proposed rules and programs. Ongoing funding should be provided for community-based organizations to facilitate authentic engagement and capacity-building at the local level [31].

20.5 Conclusion: Seizing Opportunities, Achieving Equity

Achieving health equity for the more than 61 million Americans living in rural, remote, and tribal communities is an urgent moral and economic imperative. The persistent disparities in health outcomes, access to care, and social determinants facing these populations are the result of long-standing structural inequities, geographic isolation, and policy failures. Closing these gaps will require a sustained, multisectoral effort that addresses both the medical and nonmedical drivers of health inequity.

The federal frameworks and state policy initiatives outlined in this article provide a promising foundation for this work, but much more remains to be done. The COVID-19 pandemic recovery efforts offer a unique opportunity to catalyze transformative investments in rural health infrastructure, workforce, and community well-being. Federal policymakers should seize this moment to advance a comprehensive rural health equity agenda that includes enhanced data collection, coverage expansions, delivery system reforms, social determinants investments, and authentic community engagement.

Achieving rural and tribal health equity is not only the right thing to do but also essential for the nation's overall health and prosperity. With concerted action and political will, we can ensure that all Americans, regardless of their zip code, have a fair and just opportunity to thrive and reach their full health potential.

References

1 U.S. Health Resources & Services Administration (2024). Defining rural population. https://www.hrsa.gov/rural-health/about-us/what-is-rural (accessed 27 August 2024).

2 Moy, E., Garcia, M.C., Bastian, B. et al. (2017). Leading causes of death in nonmetropolitan and metropolitan areas – United States, 1999–2014. *MMWR Surveillance Summaries* 66 (1): 1–8. https://doi.org/10.15585/mmwr.ss6601a1.

3 Centers for Disease Control and Prevention (2022). About rural health. https://www.cdc.gov/rural-health/php/about/

4 Indian Health Service. (2022). Disparities. https://www.ihs.gov/newsroom/factsheets/disparities/.

5 Warne, D. and Frizzell, L.B. (2014). American Indian health policy: historical trends and contemporary issues. *American Journal of Public Health* 104 (S3): S263–S267. https://doi.org/10.2105/AJPH.2013.301682.

6 Kirch, D.G., Henderson, M.K., and Dill, M.J. (2012). Physician workforce projections in an era of health care reform. *Annual Review of Medicine* 63: 435–445. https://doi.org/10.1146/annurev-med-050310-134634.

7 Douthit, N., Kiv, S., Dwolatzky, T., and Biswas, S. (2015). Exposing some important barriers to health care access in the rural USA. *Public Health* 129 (6): 611–620. https://doi.org/10.1016/j.puhe.2015.04.001.

8 Kaiser Family Foundation. (2021). Health insurance coverage of the total population. https://www.kff.org/other/state-indicator/total-population/ (accessed 27 August 2024).

9 Bolin, J.N., Bellamy, G.R., Ferdinand, A.O. et al. (2015). Rural Healthy People 2020: new decade, same challenges. *The Journal of Rural Health* 31 (3): 326–333. https://doi.org/10.1111/jrh.12116.

10 Kaufman, B.G., Whitaker, R., Pink, G., and Holmes, G.M. (2020). Half of rural residents at high risk of serious illness due to COVID-19, creating stress on rural hospitals. *The Journal of Rural Health* 36 (4): 584–590. https://doi.org/10.1111/jrh.12481.

11 Centers for Medicare and Medicaid Services (2022). CMS framework for advancing health care in rural, tribal, and geographically isolated communities. https://www.cms.gov/files/document/cms-geographic-framework.pdf.

12 Warshaw, R. (2017). Health disparities affect millions in rural U.S. communities. *AAMC News* https://www.aamc.org/news-insights/health-disparities-affect-millions-rural-us-communities.

13 U.S. Department of Health and Human Services (2020). HHS rural health action plan. https://www.hhs.gov/sites/default/files/hhs-rural-action-plan.pdf (accessed 9 September 2024).

14 The White House (2023). The Biden-Harris Administration is taking actions to improve the health of rural communities and help rural health care providers stay open. https://www.hhs.gov/about/news/2023/11/03/department-health-human-services-actions-support-rural-america-rural-health-care-providers.html

15 Office of Disease Prevention and Health Promotion, Office of the Assistant Secretary for Health, Office of the Secretary, U.S. Department of Health and Human Services (2022). Federal plan for equitable long-term recovery and resilience (ELTRR). https://health.gov/news/tag/federal-plan-eltrr.

16 Indian Health Care Improvement Act (2010). 25 U.S.C. §§ 1601-1683.

17 Warne, D., Kaur, J., and Perdue, D. (2012). American Indian/Alaska native cancer policy: systemic approaches to reducing cancer disparities. *Journal of Cancer Education* 27 (1): 18–23. https://doi.org/10.1007/s13187-012-0322-7.

18 National Indian Health Board (2024). 2024 Legislative and Policy Agenda for Indian Health. https://www.nihb.org/resources/2024NIHBLegislativeandPolicyAgenda.pdf

19 Pathman, D.E., Konrad, T.R., King, T.S. et al. (2004). Outcomes of states' scholarship, loan repayment, and related programs for physicians. *Medical Care* 42 (6): 560–568. https://doi.org/10.1097/01.mlr.0000128003.81622.ef.

20 Morales, D.A., Barksdale, C.L., and Beckel-Mitchener, A.C. (2020). A call to action to address rural mental health disparities. *Journal of Clinical and Translational Science* 4 (5): 463–467. https://doi.org/10.1017/cts.2020.42.

21 Marcin, J.P., Shaikh, U., and Steinhorn, R.H. (2016). Addressing health disparities in rural communities using telehealth. *Pediatric Research* 79 (1–2): 169–176. https://doi.org/10.1038/pr.2015.192.

22 Federal Communications Commission (2021). Fourteenth broadband deployment report. https://docs.fcc.gov/public/attachments/FCC-21-18A1.pdf.

23 Melillo, K.D. (2020). Community-based research priorities for rural older adults: a pilot study. *Journal of Gerontological Nursing* 46 (7): 13–20. https://doi.org/10.3928/00989134-20200605-03.

24 Skinner, L., Staiger, D.O., Auerbach, D.I., and Buerhaus, P.I. (2019). Implications of an aging rural physician workforce. *The New England Journal of Medicine* 381 (4): 299–301. https://doi.org/10.1056/NEJMp1900808.

25 Navathe, A.S., Liao, J.M., and Emanuel, E.J. (2020). Aligning payment reform and delivery innovation in Medicare. *JAMA* 323 (5): 409–410. https://doi.org/10.1001/jama.2019.20843.

26 Corallo, B. and Rudowitz, R. (2022). *Analysis of Recent National Trends in Medicaid and CHIP Enrollment.* Kaiser Family Foundation. https://www.kff.org/coronavirus-covid-19/issue-brief/analysis-of-recent-national-trends-in-medicaid-and-chip-enrollment/.

27 Hale, N., Probst, J., and Robertson, A. (2016). Rural area deprivation and hospitalizations among children for ambulatory care sensitive conditions. *Journal of Community Health* 41 (3): 451–460. https://doi.org/10.1007/s10900-015-0113-2.

28 Garfield, R., Orgera, K., and Rudowitz, R. (2021). *Implications of the ACA Medicaid Expansion: A Look at the Data and Evidence.* Kaiser Family Foundation. https://www.kff.org/medicaid/issue-brief/implications-of-the-aca-medicaid-expansion-a-look-at-the-data-and-evidence/.

29 Haque, W., Ahmadzada, M., Neisyif, W. et al. (2021). The impact of telemedicine and telehealth in healthcare systems: a systematic literature review. *Journal of Telemedicine and Telecare* 27 (10): 609–620. https://doi.org/10.1177/1357633X20960639.

30 Warne, D. and Bane, A. (2019). The impact of racism on American Indian health: challenges and responses. In: *The Economics of Racism* (ed. P. Muennig, W. Johnson, and E.N. Reeves), 199–214. Palgrave Macmillan. https://doi.org/10.1007/978-3-030-10950-9_12.

31 Henning-Smith, C., Moscovice, I., and Kozhimannil, K. (2019). Differences in social isolation and its relationship to health by rurality. *The Journal of Rural Health* 35 (4): 540–549. https://doi.org/10.1111/jrh.12344.

21

Addressing Medical Debt on Marginalized Communities: Potential Reforms

Abstract

This chapter explores the pervasive issue of medical debt in the United States, focusing on its disproportionate impact on vulnerable populations and examining the government's role in addressing these disparities. The chapter begins by highlighting the prevalence and far-reaching consequences of medical debt, particularly for communities of color and low-income individuals. It then examines the No Surprises Act, which aims to protect consumers from unexpected medical bills, while also discussing the law's limitations and the importance of effective enforcement. Further, the chapter delves into the potential of Medicaid expansion and enrollment adjustments in reducing medical debt, alongside the role of the Affordable Care Act (ACA) in expanding appeal rights and funding consumer assistance programs. It also showcases how certain state laws surpass federal protections to ensure more affordable care. Legislative and policy initiatives, such as Arizona's ballot initiative to reform medical debt collection practices and the challenges associated with a proposed medical debt cancellation plan, are also discussed. The chapter concludes by presenting a range of policy recommendations from medical organizations and patient advocacy groups, encompassing changes to provider interactions, cost controls, and insurance reforms. Finally, it emphasizes key considerations for policymakers, stressing the importance of patient education and language accessibility in effectively addressing the medical debt crisis. By implementing comprehensive strategies that include patient education, robust consumer protections, and systemic reforms, policymakers can mitigate the burden of medical debt and promote overall well-being for all individuals.

Keywords *medical debt; financial burden; no surprises act; Medicaid expansion; health disparities; debt collecion reform; consumer protections; policy recommendations*

> *James, a Black retiree, faced a daunting pile of medical bills after his unexpected heart surgery. Despite having insurance, the bills were steep, and some were from out-of-network providers he didn't knowingly choose. Overwhelmed and unsure, James didn't know his rights under the No Surprises Act, leaving him vulnerable to aggressive debt collection practices that threatened his financial stability.*

Achieving Health Equity: The Role of Law and Policy, First Edition. Y. Tony Yang.
© 2025 John Wiley & Sons Ltd. Published 2025 by John Wiley & Sons Ltd.

> *Sarah, a single mother in Arizona, juggled multiple jobs to stay afloat but still struggled with medical debt from her daughter's chronic illness. When Arizona introduced a ballot initiative to cap interest rates on medical debt, Sarah saw a glimmer of hope. The proposed changes meant she could potentially protect her home from creditors and reduce her weekly payments, alleviating the constant choice between her daughter's health and their basic needs.*

21.1 The Burden and Disproportionate Impact of Medical Debt

Medical debt, which arises when patients are unable to pay for necessary health treatments, unaffordable deductibles, or surprise bills from out-of-network providers, is a common issue affecting many households. According to the Kaiser Family Foundation (KFF), approximately 25% of adults aged 18–64 struggled with paying medical bills in 2021, with 17.4% of insured households and 27.9% of uninsured households facing medical debt [1]. Notably, nearly 80% of medical debt is held by households with zero or negative net worth [2]. Even with price transparency, patients often have little ability to compare prices prior to seeking treatment, especially in emergency situations.

The consequences of medical debt extend beyond financial strain, exacerbating poor health outcomes and existing health disparities [3]. It can adversely affect economic stability and mobility, increase stress levels, and reduce access to medical care. Furthermore, medical debt collections in credit reports can hinder individuals' ability to secure housing, increase prices for cars or insurance, and make it more challenging to find employment [4]. These difficulties may even prevent people from moving to neighborhoods with health-promoting infrastructure. Additionally, medical debt may be disguised as other forms of debt, such as credit card payments or neglected bills, suggesting that the total amount of debt caused by medical issues is likely much higher than what is reflected on credit reports.

Communities of color and lower-income individuals are disproportionately affected by medical debt, as they are more likely to be un- or underinsured [5]. High medical costs and the resulting debt discourage these populations from seeking necessary care, leading to decreased use of medical services and worsening symptoms and diagnoses. A 2022 study found that 56% of Black adults owe money for medical or dental bills, compared to 37% of white adults [6]. Black patients are less likely to have generational wealth, reducing the chances of having a safety net of savings to face high medical bills [7]. Moreover, the debt collection industry systematically targets Black debtors more aggressively than other races, particularly for smaller debts [8]. The KFF poll revealed that about 60% of Black adults with medical debts under $2500 reported being contacted by a collection agency in the past five years, compared to only 40% of white adults with similar debt.

> *"Nearly one in five Americans have medical debt. Black households are disproportionately affected, carrying higher amounts of debt at higher rates."*
>
> The Commonwealth Fund

21.2 Government's Role in Addressing Medical Debt Disparities

In the face of mounting medical debt that disproportionately affects vulnerable populations, the government has implemented various measures to alleviate this burden and promote equity [9]. Key legislation and policies aim to protect consumers from the financial strain of unexpected medical expenses, improve access to affordable care, and enhance transparency in medical billing. By addressing these disparities, the government seeks to mitigate the impact of medical debt on households across the nation. The following sections delve into specific initiatives such as the No Surprises Act, Medicaid expansion, consumer appeal rights, and state-level protections that collectively contribute to this effort.

21.2.1 The No Surprises Act: Protections, Limitations, and Enforcement

The No Surprises Act, enacted in 2021, aims to shield consumers from unexpected medical bills when receiving care from out-of-network providers in situations beyond their control [10]. The law specifically addresses surprise medical bills in three scenarios: (i) receiving emergency care at an out-of-network facility or from an out-of-network provider; (ii) using air ambulance emergency transport services; and (iii) receiving non-emergency care at an in-network facility but being treated by an out-of-network healthcare provider without knowingly electing that provider or consenting to be billed [11]. Furthermore, providers are prohibited from billing patients more than the applicable in-network cost-sharing amount, with potential penalties of up to $10,000 per violation.

The No Surprises Act was designed to complement state laws, particularly in areas where federal law (such as The Employee Retirement Income Security Act of 1974 [ERISA]) typically preempts state law, and to extend protection for facilities and services that some state laws overlooked [12]. However, the law grants states substantial discretion in determining which payments will be considered, how arbitration will be conducted, and what state payment determination processes will entail. This leaves room for providers to lobby and leverage power at the state level for favorable processes.

Similar to the ACA, the No Surprises Act involves collaboration between states and the federal government for enforcement [10]. Three-quarters of states have chosen to enforce the law, with the majority opting for some form of collaborative enforcement agreement with the federal government [13]. However, the law's enforcement provisions rely heavily on consumer complaints rather than a federal or state monitoring system. Consequently, if the state or federal government fails to properly inform consumers of their rights under the law, patients may be unaware of their protections.

The Act also mandates that providers give uninsured or self-pay patients a good faith estimate of the cost of care [14]. It also calls for various studies on provider networks, health costs, provider concentration, and the role of private equity. While this may provide additional information to help patients avoid being blindsided by their eventual bill, transparency without further reforms may still ultimately leave patients with the difficult choice between accessing unaffordable care (and incurring debt) or forgoing necessary interventions.

21.2.2 Medicaid Expansion and Enrollment Adjustments Reduce Medical Debt

The decision of a state to expand Medicaid under the ACA is associated with lower levels of medical debt [15]. Although individuals with insurance can still accumulate medical debt, health insurance provides financial benefits by reducing the likelihood of higher billing. A recent study estimates that Medicaid expansion directly reduced newly accrued medical debt by 35% [16]. Notably, most states that have chosen not to expand their Medicaid program are located in the South, a region known for higher racial disparities in health and wealth.

Some states have experimented with adjustments to enrollment periods for qualified individuals [17]. For instance, Maryland allows patients 240 days after receiving a hospital bill to qualify for federal financial assistance programs, such as Medicaid, in case the hospital care leads to worsened financial circumstances. Implementing initiatives that connect patient advocates with patients to help them navigate and access government assistance programs could lead to significant cost savings and reduce the burden of medical debt [18].

21.2.3 Expanding Appeal Rights and Funding Consumer Assistance Programs

The ACA mandates that all consumers in non-grandfathered health plans have the right to appeal denials, initially internally to the plan and then to an independent external reviewer. However, under current federal rules, only denials based on medical necessity can be appealed to an independent external reviewer. The No Surprises Act expanded the scope of external review to include coverage disputes related to surprise medical bills and mental health parity [19].

These policy changes are connected to the Consumer Assistance Programs established under the ACA [20]. These programs were designed to educate the public about their rights and protections under private health plans and assist consumers in resolving disputes with their health plans, including filing approvals. The programs help individuals with a range of problems, now encompassing surprise medical bills and denials. However, states received minimal funding for these programs in 2010, and there have been no appropriations since then. Both the Build Back Better Act and the FY 2022 Labor-HHS Appropriations Act included provisions that would appropriate funding for these essential consumer assistance programs.

21.2.4 State Laws Surpassing Federal Protections and Ensuring Affordable Care

Certain state laws provide more comprehensive protections than the No Surprises Act, covering a wider range of services (such as ground ambulances) and facilities (including skilled nursing facilities, dialysis centers, and outpatient settings) [21]. New Mexico and a handful of other states have enacted laws that require hospitals to proactively screen patients to determine their eligibility for free or discounted care, as well as public assistance programs like Medicaid [22]. Likewise, Maryland mandates that hospitals ensure free or discounted care and reimburse patients who pay for medical services that should have been less expensive [23].

21.3 Legislative and Policy Initiatives to Mitigate Medical Debt

In the ongoing effort to address the pervasive issue of medical debt, various legislative and policy initiatives are being proposed and implemented across the United States. These measures aim to reform debt collection practices, provide relief for indebted individuals, and implement systemic changes to reduce the financial burden of healthcare costs. The following sections explore specific initiatives, including Arizona's ballot initiative to reform medical debt collection, challenges surrounding the proposal for medical debt cancellation, policy recommendations for provider interactions and cost controls, and the efforts to remove medical debt from credit reports.

21.3.1 Arizona Ballot Initiative: Reforming Medical Debt Collection Practices

In Arizona, a current ballot initiative aimed to alleviate the impact of medical debt by reforming the procedures used by providers and collection agencies for debt collection [24]. The initiative proposed to reduce the interest rate on medical debt from 10% to 3%. It also sought to increase the value of a debtor's home that is protected from creditors, from $250,000 to $400,000, and to decrease the portion of the debtor's weekly disposable income subject to debt collection from 25% to 10%.

Critics argued that the measure affected all collection remedies rather than specifically targeting medical debt [20]. They also pointed out that the initiative did not address the underlying costs of healthcare, merely softening the blow of collections later. While these concerns are valid, reducing the interest owed on medical debt will free up funds for people to pay off their debt more quickly and decrease the amount they need to pay each month. This should help alleviate situations where people are forced to choose between paying their medical bills and purchasing other necessities.

21.3.2 Challenges of Medical Debt Cancellation Proposal

During his 2020 presidential campaign, Bernie Sanders proposed canceling medical debt [25], which, in theory, would mirror the federal government's efforts to forgive student loans. A recent Brookings study showed that reducing the amount of medical debt held by all households would disproportionately benefit Black people [26]. However, this proposal presents substantially more challenges than student loan forgiveness, as Congress would need to grant authority for the government to purchase the medical debt held by hospitals and collection agencies – a massive undertaking.

21.3.3 Provider Interactions, Cost Controls, and Insurance Reforms

Medical organizations and patient advocacy groups have put forth a range of policy recommendations to address the issue of medical debt [27]. These recommendations encompass changes to how providers interact with patients. For instance, the government could expand comprehensive financial assistance policies to cover hospitals and a broader range of healthcare providers or allocate more funding for public hospitals that serve as safety net providers for people who are unable to pay for services. However, it is crucial to ensure that these providers have sufficient funding to recruit caregivers and provide quality care to their patients. Additionally, the federal or state government could implement cost–control measures or limits on facility fees.

On the insurance side, changes could be made to reduce the financial burden on the underinsured [28]. One approach is to place limits on cost-sharing or out-of-network billing by implementing standards that govern which providers fall within the network. However, it is important to recognize that medical debt is a persistent struggle even among households with health insurance and middle incomes, indicating that expanding insurance coverage alone will not fully resolve the medical debt problem.

21.3.4 Remove Medical Debt from Credit Reports

In September 2023, the Consumer Financial Protection Bureau (CFPB) announced a significant move to initiate a rulemaking process aimed at removing medical bills from Americans' credit reports [29]. This decision is driven by research indicating that medical debt has little predictive value in credit decisions, yet tens of millions of households are burdened with such debt on their credit reports [30]. The CFPB's proposals under consideration would have far-reaching implications. First, consumer reporting companies would be prohibited from including medical debts and collection information on consumer reports used for underwriting decisions by creditors. Second, creditors would be barred from using medical collections information when evaluating borrowers' credit applications. This would effectively narrow the existing exception created in 2005 that allowed creditors to rely on medical data as "financial information." Crucially, the proposed changes would also address coercive debt collection practices. As unpaid medical bills would no longer appear on consumers' credit reports used by creditors, debt collectors would lose the leverage of using the credit reporting system to pressure consumers into paying questionable debts. Overall, the CFPB's proposed changes seek to alleviate the financial strain caused by medical crises, curb coercive debt collection tactics, and ensure that creditors do not rely on data often plagued with inaccuracies and mistakes. This move represents a significant step towards protecting consumers and promoting fairness in the credit reporting system. While this provides relief, it does not eliminate the need to pay outstanding medical bills.

Key Policies and Equity Considerations for Addressing Medical Debt

Area of Focus	Policy	Equity Consideration
Financial Assistance Policies	Require hospitals to provide financial assistance to low-income residents	Ensures low-income patients can access care without incurring insurmountable debt.
Community Benefit Standards	Mandate community benefit spending for nonprofit hospitals	Aims to ensure that nonprofit hospitals give back to the community in meaningful ways, including financial assistance and investments in social determinants of health.
Billing and Collections Practices	Regulate hospital billing and debt collection practices	Prevents aggressive collections and ensures fair treatment of patients. Includes requirements for payment plans, limits on interest rates, and oversight of debt collection agencies.
Interest on Medical Debt	Cap or prohibit interest charges on medical debt	Reduces the financial burden on patients, particularly those from low-income backgrounds, by preventing debt from escalating due to high interest rates.
Lien and Foreclosure Protections	Limit or prohibit liens and foreclosures on patients' homes	Protects homeownership for patients with medical debt, preventing loss of housing due to medical financial burdens.
Wage Garnishment Limits	Restrict wage garnishment for medical debt	Protects patients' income, ensuring they can meet basic needs even while repaying medical debt.
Reporting Requirements	Mandate detailed reporting by hospitals on financial assistance and bad debt	Enhances transparency and accountability, ensuring hospitals adhere to financial assistance policies and highlighting disparities in debt collection practices.

21.4 Conclusion: Key Considerations for Policymakers

To effectively address the pervasive issue of medical debt, policymakers must consider several critical factors [31]. First, the current system often places the onus on patients to identify and report billing discrepancies to insurers or government agencies. This assumes that patients are well-informed consumers, yet many rely on their healthcare providers for accurate information. It is essential that patients have access to the necessary knowledge to recognize inaccuracies in their medical bills and understand the appropriate channels for reporting these issues.

Moreover, the disproportionate impact of medical debt on low-income families highlights the urgent need for accessible and user-friendly appeal options. Information and services must be communicated in clear, straightforward language to ensure that individuals fully understand their medical bills, denial notices, and their rights. This transparency is crucial in empowering patients to navigate their healthcare-related financial obligations effectively.

Furthermore, addressing medical debt requires a multifaceted approach that goes beyond mere financial relief. Policymakers should focus on systemic changes, such as improving the transparency and accuracy of medical billing, enforcing consumer protections like the No Surprises Act, and expanding Medicaid to reduce the incidence of medical debt. Additionally, enhancing funding for consumer assistance programs can provide crucial support for individuals struggling with medical debt, helping them to understand their rights and options.

Ultimately, comprehensive strategies that incorporate patient education, robust consumer protections, and systemic reforms are essential in mitigating the burden of medical debt. By focusing on these key considerations, policymakers can create a more equitable healthcare system that alleviates financial strain and promotes overall well-being for all individuals.

References

1 Lopes, L., Kearney, A., Montero, A. et al. (2022). *Health Care Debt in the U.S.: The Broad Consequences of Medical and Dental Bills*. Kaiser Family Foundation https://www.kff.org/health-costs/report/kff-health-care-debt-survey/.

2 Kluender, R., Mahoney, N., Wong, F., and Yin, W. (2021). Medical Debt in the US, 2009-2020. *JAMA* 326 (3): 250–256.

3 Himmelstein, D.U., Dickman, S.L., McCormick, D. et al. (2022). Prevalence and risk factors for medical debt and subsequent changes in social determinants of health in the US. *JAMA Network Open* 5 (9): –e2231898.

4 Wiltshire, J.C., Enard, K.R., Colato, E.G., and Orban, B.L. (2020). Problems paying medical bills and mental health symptoms post-Affordable Care Act. *AIMS Public Health* 7 (2): 274.

5 Barcellos, S.H. and Jacobson, M. (2015). The effects of Medicare on medical expenditure risk and financial strain. *American Economic Journal: Economic Policy* 7 (4): 41–70.

6 KFF Health News (2022). Diagnosis: debt. *KFF Health News* https://kffhealthnews.org/diagnosis-debt/.

7 Zewde, N. and Wimer, C. (2019). Antipoverty impact of Medicaid growing with state expansions over time. *Health Affairs* 38 (1): 132–138.

8 Charron-Chénier, R. and Seamster, L. (2021). Racialized debts: racial exclusion from credit tools and information networks. *Critical Sociology* 47 (6): 977–992.

9 Haynes, B.L. (2022). *The Racial Health and Wealth Gap: Impact of Medical Debt on Black Families*. National Consumer Law Center.

10 Hoadley, J. and Lucia, K. (2022). The No Surprises Act: a bipartisan achievement to protect consumers from unexpected medical bills. *Journal of Health Politics, Policy and Law* 47 (1): 93–109.

11 Pollitz, K. (2021). *No Surprises Act Implementation: What to Expect in 2022*. Kaiser Family Foundation.

12 Hoadley, J., Lucia, K., Volk, J. et al. (2023). No Surprises Act. https://www.rwjf.org/en/insights/our-research/2023/04/no-surprises-act--perspectives-on-status-of-consumer-protections-against-balance-billing.html.

13 Medicaid and CHIP Payment and Access Commission (MACPAC) (2022). Overview of the affordable care act and Medicaid. https://www.macpac.gov/subtopic/overview-of-the-affordable-care-act-and-medicaid/ (accessed 27 August 2024).

14 Richmond, L.M. (2022). No Surprises Act brings new billing rules, disclosures; doctors sue. *Psychiatric News* 57 (02): https://doi.org/10.1176/appi.pn.2022.2.38.

15 Rudowitz, R. and Antonisse, L. (2018). *Implications of the ACA Medicaid Expansion: A Look at the Data and Evidence*. Henry J Kaiser Family Foundation.

16 Brevoort, K., Grodzicki, D., and Hackmann, M.B. (2020). The credit consequences of unpaid medical bills. *Journal of Public Economics* 187: 104203.

17 Finkelstein, A., Taubman, S., Wright, B. et al. (2012). The Oregon health insurance experiment: evidence from the first year. *The Quarterly Journal of Economics* 127 (3): 1057–1106.

18 Adams, A., Kluender, R., Mahoney, N. et al. (2022). The impact of financial assistance programs on health care utilization: evidence from Kaiser Permanente. *American Economic Review: Insights* 4 (3): 389–407. https://doi.org/10.1257/aeri.20210515.

19 Keith, K., Hoadley, J., and Lucia, K.W. (2021). *Banning Surprise Bills, Part 2: Good Faith Estimates, External Review, and More*. Health Affairs Forefront.

20 Keith, K., Hoadley, J., and Lucia, K.W. (2022). *Recent Guidance to Implement the No Surprises Act*. Health Affairs Forefront.

21 Hoadley, J., Keith, K., and Lucia, K.W. (2020). *Unpacking the No Surprises Act: An Opportunity to Protect Millions*. Health Affairs Forefront.

22 Ollove, M. (2022). *New Safeguards May Help Those Who Are Drowning in Medical Debt*. Stateline. https://stateline.org/2022/08/24/new-safeguards-may-help-those-who-are-drowning-in-medical-debt/.

23 Ollove, M. (2022). *New Safeguards in Maryland and Other States May Help Those Who Are Drowning in Medical Debt*. Maryland Matters. https://marylandmatters.org/2022/08/29/new-safeguards-in-maryland-and-other-states-may-help-those-who-are-drowning-in-medical-debt/.

24 Ballotpedia. (2022). Arizona proposition 209, healthcare debt interest rate limit and debt collection exemptions initiative. https://ballotpedia.org/Arizona_Proposition_209_Healthcare_Debt_Interest_Rate_Limit_and_Debt_Collection_Exemptions_Initiative_(2022)

25 Sanders, B. (2024). *It's OK to be Angry About Capitalism*. Crown.

26 Perry, A.M., Crear-Perry, J., Romer, C., and Adjeiwaa-Manu, N. (2021). *The Racial Implications of Medical Debt: How Moving Toward Universal Health Care and Other Reforms Can Address Them*. Brookings. https://www.brookings.edu/articles/the-racial-implications-of-medical-debt-how-moving-toward-universal-health-care-and-other-reforms-can-address-them/.

27 Rosenbaum, S. (2015). *Additional Requirements for Charitable Hospitals: Final Rules on Community Health Needs Assessments and Financial Assistance.* Health Affairs Forefront.

28 Banthin, J.S. and Bernard, D.M. (2006). Changes in financial burdens for health care: national estimates for the population younger than 65 years, 1996 to 2003. *JAMA* 296 (22): 2712–2719.

29 The Consumer Financial Protection Bureau (2023). CFPB kicks off rulemaking to remove medical bills from credit reports. https://www.consumerfinance.gov/about-us/newsroom/cfpb-kicks-off-rulemaking-to-remove-medical-bills-from-credit-reports/ (accessed 27 August 2024).

30 Brevoort, K.P. and Kambara, M. (2015). Are all collections equal? The case of medical debt. *Journal of Credit Risk* 11 (4): 73–97.

31 Gotberg, B.E. and Sousa, M.D. (2019). Moving beyond medical debt. *American Bankruptcy Institute Law Review* 27: 93.

22

Preserving Diversity: Impact of Affirmative Action Ruling on Healthcare

Abstract

The chapter begins by discussing the Supreme Court's June 2023 ruling that deemed race-conscious college admissions policies unconstitutional. This decision poses a significant challenge to efforts to increase the representation of ethnic minorities in nursing, medical, and health science schools. The chapter then highlights the crucial importance of diversity in healthcare, as it directly impacts health equity. Research shows diversity improves patient-provider relationships, health outcomes, and access to care, especially for underserved communities. However, minoritized groups remain severely underrepresented in the health professions. Next, the chapter explores the potential impacts of the Court overturning affirmative action. Prohibiting race-conscious admissions could substantially decrease diversity and exacerbate disparities, as seen in states that previously enacted bans. The ruling puts schools in a difficult position between accreditation standards and legal compliance. It risks creating a self-perpetuating cycle of declining diversity and rising implicit bias. The chapter then delves into strategies schools can use to maintain diversity post-ruling. This includes rethinking applicant evaluation to look beyond grades and test scores; using race-neutral proxies like socioeconomic status; investing heavily in pipeline programs to engage diverse students from K-12 through college; revamping recruitment and yield activities; and reimagining curriculum and institutional climate with inclusion in mind. Additionally, it emphasizes the need for committed leadership, innovative cross-sector collaborations, and robust accountability systems to keep diversity efforts on track. It concludes with an urgent call to action for healthcare stakeholders to mobilize a multifaceted response to protect diversity. Even without affirmative action, progress is still possible with steadfast commitment from the entire healthcare ecosystem.

Keywords *affirmative action; healthcare diversity; supreme court; health equity; race-conscious admissions; pipeline programs; socioeconomic status; medical education*

> *When Ayana, a Black high school student passionate about science, visited her local hospital, she noticed the lack of healthcare professionals who looked like her. Despite her strong grades and interest in medicine, she wondered if she truly belonged in this field. Ayana's story underscores the importance of representation in inspiring the next generation of diverse healthcare leaders.*

Achieving Health Equity: The Role of Law and Policy, First Edition. Y. Tony Yang.
© 2025 John Wiley & Sons Ltd. Published 2025 by John Wiley & Sons Ltd.

Dr Patel, a renowned surgeon, built a successful career but never forgot his roots. Growing up in a low-income immigrant family, he faced numerous barriers to pursuing medicine. Now, as a member of his hospital's diversity committee, Dr Patel is alarmed by the potential impact of the Supreme Court's affirmative action ruling. He knows firsthand how race-conscious admissions policies opened doors for talented minority students like himself. Without these policies, he fears the progress made in diversifying the medical field could be erased.

As the Dean of Admissions at a top nursing school, Lisa has long been a champion for diversity. However, the recent Supreme Court decision has left her grappling with how to legally maintain a diverse student body. She and her team must now navigate a complex landscape, finding innovative ways to attract and support minority students without the tool of affirmative action. Lisa knows the stakes are high – the diversity of the nursing workforce has a direct impact on health equity for the communities they serve.

22.1 Supreme Court Ruling Threatens Diversity in Healthcare Education

In June 2023, the US Supreme Court issued a groundbreaking ruling in the cases Students for Fair Admissions v. University of North Carolina and Students for Fair Admissions Inc. v. President and Fellows of Harvard College [1]. The court determined that affirmative action policies considering race and ethnicity as key criteria for college admissions are unconstitutional, as they breach the equal protection clause of the US Constitution. This landmark decision marks a turning point in efforts to bolster the representation of people from ethnic minorities in higher education. It also places a formidable hurdle on the path to diversity in US nursing, medical, and broader healthcare science schools, with substantial implications for health equity [2].

Affirmative action has played a crucial role in increasing diversity in medical education and the healthcare workforce over the past 50 years. Its loss threatens to undermine decades of progress and exacerbate existing disparities. Medical and health professional schools must now pioneer innovative strategies within the boundaries of the law to sustain diversity.

22.2 The Importance of Diversity in Healthcare

Diversity in the healthcare workforce is crucial not only for representation but also for directly impacting health equity among the populations served. A diverse and culturally competent healthcare workforce is essential for promoting positive health outcomes and enhancing the quality of care for all, especially for minority groups. Research consistently demonstrates the benefits of diversity in healthcare. For example, a 2023 study found that for every 10% increase in Black primary care physicians, the life expectancy of Black individuals rose by one month [3]. Diversity also significantly improves communication, comfort levels, and trust in patient-practitioner relationships [4]. Racial and language concordance between patients and providers correlates with better patient satisfaction and health outcomes [5]. Additionally, professionals from disadvantaged backgrounds often serve in communities with limited healthcare access [6].

Despite these benefits, there is a significant disparity in the representation of minority groups in the healthcare workforce. Although Black people make up 13% of the US population, they represent only 5% of physicians – a percentage that has remained unchanged for 50 years. It is estimated that there is a deficit of about 114,000 Black doctors and 81,000 Hispanic doctors compared to population proportions [7]. Similar to medical and health professional schools, nursing, dental, and other health professional schools face comparable challenges in achieving diversity. Affirmative action has been a critical tool in addressing systemic inequities that hinder minorities' paths to medical and other health professional schools [8]. The loss of affirmative action threatens to exacerbate this already challenging situation, further limiting diversity in healthcare and potentially worsening health disparities for minoritized groups.

"While our country grows more diverse, historically marginalized communities have been left behind on nearly every health indicator. A physician workforce that reflects the diversity of the nation is key to eliminating racial inequities. There is convincing evidence that racially diverse care teams produce measurably positive health outcomes for patients in historically marginalized populations."
Jesse M. Ehrenfeld, M.D., President, American Medical Association

22.3 Impact of Overturning Affirmative Action

The Supreme Court cases, brought by the organization Students for Fair Admissions, allege the universities' race-conscious admissions policies amount to racial discrimination in violation of the Equal Protection Clause and Title VI of the Civil Rights Act [9]. This prohibition extends beyond admissions to any educational programs like scholarships, financial aid, and leadership positions. It impacts the education of the next generation of physicians, nurses, and other healthcare providers. More broadly, it becomes challenging to seek diversity in hospital administration without violating nondiscrimination laws – an ironic outcome for civil rights laws originally meant to protect minorities.

The natural experiment of several states banning affirmative action already provides insight into the potential impacts. A 2022 study found states with bans saw a 4.8 percentage point decline in underrepresented minority students in public medical and health professional schools, while control states saw a 0.7-point increase [10]. This forecasts what could happen nationally as the Supreme Court bans race-conscious admissions.

Medical and health professional schools are in a difficult position, torn between accreditation standards requiring effective policies to achieve racial and ethnic inclusion, and a Supreme Court prohibition on considering race. Accreditation standards need to change to reflect the new legal reality.

The ruling's impact would likely be self-perpetuating. Racial and ethnic diversity helps make spaces more inclusive to people from differing backgrounds. African American physicians have been shown to have far less implicit bias than white physicians [11]. A less diverse medical profession could bring heightened bias, leading to a downward spiral where medical spaces become increasingly homogenous.

Crucially, losing minority physicians would negatively impact health equity. Racial concordance between providers and patients is associated with improved communication, lower ED use, and better health outcomes [12]. Although this doesn't necessarily mean assigning physicians by race, it raises serious concerns about worsening disparities if the medical workforce becomes less representative of the diverse US population. Unique health issues affecting certain racial/ethnic groups may go unnoticed or unaddressed without diverse providers attuned to them.

22.4 Maintaining and Improving Diversity Post-ruling

Due to the Supreme Court decision, medical and health professional institutions should strategize now on how to preserve diversity without running afoul of the law. While the loss of race-conscious admissions poses a significant challenge, a multifaceted approach drawing on race-neutral strategies can still promote diversity and inclusion. Key areas of focus should include the following.

22.4.1 Rethinking Merit and Applicant Evaluation

The Court's decision seems to endorse a narrow, numbers-driven view of merit-based mainly on GPAs and standardized test (such as MCAT) scores. But these metrics are incomplete predictors of success as a physician. Medical and health professional schools can push back by doubling down on holistic applicant review, considering a wide range of attributes like socioeconomic background, lived experience, cultural competence, commitment to serving the underserved, and distance traveled [13].

Evaluation should also interrogate how conventional metrics and admissions processes may disadvantage minority applicants. For example, research shows the MCAT has significant racial and ethnic score disparities, reflecting systemic inequities in access to test prep [8]. Overemphasis on MCAT performance will likely decrease diversity.

Medical and health professional schools can consider de-emphasizing or eliminating the standardized test (such as MCAT) requirement, as a growing number have done in recent years. One study found students with scores well below the national mean can succeed in medical school with proper support; MCAT was not a linear predictor of key outcomes [14]. Waiving standardized tests for disadvantaged students and providing free prep courses are other promising approaches.

Schools should also consider ending admissions preferences that favor the privileged, such as legacy admissions or connections to donors and VIPs. Some have already moved in this direction: Amid the affirmative action cases, Johns Hopkins and Icahn School of Medicine at Mount Sinai dropped legacy admissions to increase fairness.

22.4.2 Proxies and Race-Neutral Alternatives

With the prohibition on considering race directly, many medical and health professional schools will need to rely on proxies and race-neutral alternatives to maintain a diverse class. Socioeconomic status is one of the most promising options – a strategy of giving admissions preferences based on family income, wealth, education level, and neighborhood. This approach targets the intersection of racial and socioeconomic disadvantage. While it won't fully replicate the diversity achieved through affirmative action, it's likely the closest legal proxy.

Other potential race-neutral metrics include geography, language skills, and experience with prejudice/discrimination (although the latter can be thorny as privileged applicants may claim it too).

Some law schools have found success with new essay questions and application materials designed to surface diversity of background and perspective in race-neutral ways [15].

However, any proxy approach requires careful design, as the Court may look askance at policies it sees as mere pretexts for considering race. Medical and health professional schools will need to consult legal counsel to thread this needle. Defenders of proxy strategies argue they are not aimed at race alone, but at capturing disadvantage and difference more broadly.

22.4.3   Invest in Pipeline Programs and Partnerships

One of the most impactful strategies medical and health professional schools can adopt is investing in pipeline programs that engage and prepare minoritized students well before the admissions stage [16]. This approach includes several key initiatives aimed at building a robust and diverse applicant pool.

K-12 outreach programs are crucial for exposing children in underserved communities to healthcare careers early and often. These programs provide mentoring, field trips, and hands-on science experiences, sparking interest in healthcare professions from a young age. Establishing partnerships with community colleges is essential for recruiting talented students [17]. These partnerships should offer clear pathways and transfer agreements to four-year universities and medical and health professional schools, ensuring that prerequisites align and credits transfer seamlessly.

Postbaccalaureate and master's programs are vital for students needing to strengthen their academic records before applying to medical and health professional schools. These programs should include standardized test preparation, research experience, and comprehensive guidance on the medical school application process. Providing robust premed advising and mentoring is critical for supporting college students from underrepresented backgrounds [18]. Connecting these students with physicians and other health professional mentors who share similar life experiences can offer invaluable support and insight.

Offering paid summer research opportunities and enrichment programs for promising undergraduates can significantly enhance their readiness and competitiveness for medical school [19]. These efforts require substantial investments in funding and personnel but are essential for building a pipeline of competitive, diverse applicants. Importantly, these programs are legal because they target students based on disadvantage, not explicitly on race. By focusing on these initiatives, medical and health professional schools can make significant strides in promoting diversity and equity in healthcare.

22.4.4   Revamp Recruitment and Yield Activities

Medical and health professional schools must overhaul their recruitment and applicant yield activities to sustain diversity. Several key strategies are essential for achieving this goal.

Expanding recruitment targets is crucial. Schools should actively recruit at more Historically Black Colleges and Universities (HBCUs), Hispanic-Serving Institutions (HSIs), and Tribal Colleges. Additionally, reaching out to Black and Hispanic student groups at predominantly White institutions and using geo-demographic data to target high schools and zip codes with large underrepresented minority (URM) populations can broaden the pool of potential applicants.

Mobilizing diverse alumni networks can significantly enhance recruitment efforts [20]. Alumni of color can assist with recruitment, interviewing, and second-look visits, offering prospective students the chance to see people who look like them and hear authentic accounts of the medical and health professional school experience. This connection can be powerful in making prospective students feel welcomed and understood.

Eliminating application barriers is vital. Schools should reduce or waive application fees for disadvantaged students based on race-neutral income criteria and offer application workshops and mock interviews to support these students through the application process [21]. This can help level the playing field for students who might otherwise be deterred by the cost and complexity of the application process.

Revamping the interview approach can help assess a broader range of backgrounds and perspectives [22]. Interviews should be structured to evaluate diversity and inclusion competencies, and interviewers should receive training on bias and cultural competence. This ensures that the interview process is fair and inclusive.

Enhancing second-look programming for admitted minoritized students can make a significant impact. These visits should be high-touch and high-impact, connecting students with affinity groups, diversity, equity, and inclusion (DEI) offices, diverse faculty, and alumni to showcase the supportive community they would join. This helps admitted students envision themselves thriving in the school's environment.

Providing scholarships and financial support is essential. Schools should raise scholarship funds for disadvantaged students using race-neutral criteria such as family income and first-generation status, making world-class financial aid a key component of their recruitment strategy [23]. Financial support can be a decisive factor in a student's decision to enroll.

A strong, multifaceted diversity recruitment strategy demonstrates to underrepresented students that they are valued and wanted. In the post-affirmative action landscape, making these students feel welcome and supported will be more important than ever.

22.4.5   Reimagine Curriculum, Climate, and Inclusion

Medical and health professional schools must extend their diversity efforts beyond admissions to foster equity, diversity, and inclusion throughout the entire educational experience. To achieve this, schools should implement several key strategies.

Reforming the curriculum is essential. Health equity, social determinants of health, and anti-racism should be integrated throughout the curriculum rather than confined to standalone electives [24]. Teaching culturally responsive care is also critical. Diversifying faculty is a priority. Schools should focus on hiring and promoting diverse faculty members, especially in leadership roles, as representation is crucial for students [25]. Offering department incentives for making progress in diversity can help achieve this goal.

Robust training on DEI competencies should be mandatory for all faculty, staff, and students [26]. This training should cover implicit bias, microaggressions, allyship, and upstander skills, making DEI a central component of professional development. Supporting affinity groups is vital. Schools should fully fund student affinity groups, particularly those for underrepresented minorities, and compensate diverse student leaders who support their peers [27].

Making it easy to report bias is crucial. Schools should establish clear, easy, and confidential systems for reporting bias incidents and microaggressions. Conducting annual climate surveys and acting on the data is also important. Involving the community is key [28]. Schools should partner with local communities of color on education and research initiatives, making community members feel welcome on campus and recruiting them to advisory boards.

Transforming medical and health professional schools into truly inclusive environments is a long-term commitment, not a quick fix. When students of color feel valued and supported, they are more likely to persist and thrive.

22.4.6 Leadership, Accountability, and Collaboration

Preserving diversity in the post-affirmative action era will require visionary leadership, novel collaborations, and robust accountability systems.

At the leadership level, deans and administrators must champion diversity as a core commitment, not a nice-to-have. This means allocating meaningful funding and staff to DEI initiatives, and tying leadership performance evaluations and promotions to diversity progress. Leaders should also use their platforms to publicly advocate for diversity, countering the divisive narratives that often follow affirmative action decisions.

New cross-sector and cross-institutional partnerships can maximize collective impact on diversity. For example, medical and health professional schools, teaching hospitals, and public health departments could launch citywide or regional diversity initiatives, pooling resources for pipeline programs. Schools could also partner with minority-serving K-12 districts to build early interest in healthcare careers. Statewide and national medical and health professional school associations, as well as groups like the AAMC, should help coordinate and disseminate best practices.

Accountability systems must also be strengthened [29]. Schools should set ambitious diversity goals and transparently report progress against benchmarks. Some may consider tying performance on diversity metrics to administrator compensation. Outside actors like accreditors and rankings organizations should elevate diversity as a key measure of med school quality. And as the NIH has recently done, major research funders could consider diversity of research teams in grant decisions [30].

In the face of adversity, leaders must bring stakeholders together around a shared vision of an equitable, anti-racist healthcare system. Progress is still possible if the medical education community works as one to prioritize diversity, inclusion, and belonging [31].

22.5 Conclusion: Urgent Strategies Needed to Protect Diversity in Healthcare Education

The Supreme Court decision prohibiting race-conscious admissions poses an existential threat to diversity in healthcare. Healthcare leaders, educators, and stakeholders must mobilize urgently to implement a range of strategies to protect diversity to the greatest extent possible. From rethinking applicant evaluation and developing race-neutral alternatives, to strengthening pipeline programs and making inclusion a strategic priority, institutions cannot afford to wait.

While the loss of affirmative action is a devastating blow, it must catalyze a redoubling of efforts and creative solutions. With a tireless commitment to health equity from all corners of the healthcare ecosystem, diversity and inclusion can still advance in the face of this new challenge. The health of the nation depends on it.

Key Policy Strategies for Increasing Health Workforce Diversity

Category	Policy Strategies	Details
Admission Policies	Alternative admission criteria	• Consider socioeconomic status, wealth, underserved community background, or being first-generation college students
Pipeline Programs	Pathway programs	• Provide academic resources, health career information, and encouragement for primary and secondary students interested in health careers
Experiential Learning	Summer work experience/shadowing	• Promote interest in health professions through shadowing and working experiences
Post-Graduate Support	Postbaccalaureate programs	• Support college graduates with pre-health professions education to strengthen their applications
Educational Partnerships	Partnerships with HBCUs and community colleges	• Partner with HBCUs and community colleges to recruit more Black and URM students
	Partnerships with minority student organizations	• Collaborate with minority student organizations to aid in recruitment and create better applicant experiences
Mentorship and Support	Mentorship	• Engage mentors and mentees from underrepresented backgrounds to promote diversity in health professions education
	Supportive environment	• Create supportive environments with student organizations, academic support, and wraparound services
Financial Support	Scholarships	• Provide financial support to attract low-income students to higher education
Bias Mitigation	Anti-bias training in admissions	• Mitigate implicit biases in the admissions process through training
Faculty Diversity	Diverse faculty	• Increase racial diversity among faculty to attract and retain students of color

References

1 Students for Fair Admissions v. Harvard, 600 U.S. 181 (2023). https://www.supremecourt.gov/opinions/22pdf/20-1199_hgdj.pdf (accessed 26 August 2024).

2 Association of American Medical Colleges (2023). AAMC Deeply Disappointed by SCOTUS Decision on Race-ConsciousAdmissions.https://www.aamc.org/news/press-releases/aamc-deeply-disappointed-scotus-decision-race-conscious-admissions

3 Snyder, J.E., Upton, R.D., Hassett, T.C. et al. (2023). Black representation in the primary care physician workforce and its association with population life expectancy and mortality rates in the US. *JAMA Network Open* 6 (4): e236687. https://doi.org/10.1001/jamanetworkopen.2023.6687.

4 Shen, M.J., Peterson, E.B., Costas-Muñiz, R. et al. (2018). The effects of race and racial concordance on patient-physician communication: a systematic review of the literature. *Journal of Racial and Ethnic Health Disparities* 5 (1): 117–140. https://doi.org/10.1007/s40615-017-0350-4.

5 Jetty, A., Jabbarpour, Y., Pollack, J. et al. (2022). Patient-physician racial concordance associated with improved healthcare use and lower healthcare expenditures in minority populations. *Journal of Racial and Ethnic Health Disparities* 9 (1): 68–81. https://doi.org/10.1007/s40615-020-00930-4.

6 Saha, S. and Shipman, S.A. (2008). Race-neutral versus race-conscious workforce policy to improve access to care. *Health Affairs* 27 (1): 234–245. https://doi.org/10.1377/hlthaff.27.1.234.

7 Mora, H., Obayemi, A., Holcomb, K., and Hinson, M. (2022). The national deficit of Black and Hispanic physicians in the US and projected estimates of time to correction. *JAMA Network Open* 5 (8): e2215485. https://doi.org/10.1001/jamanetworkopen.2022.15485.

8 Lucey, C.R. and Saguil, A. (2020). The consequences of structural racism on MCAT scores and medical school admissions: the past is prologue. *Academic Medicine* 95 (3): 351–356. https://doi.org/10.1097/ACM.0000000000002939.

9 Feingold, J.P. (2019). SFFA v. Harvard: how affirmative action myths mask White bonus. *California Law Review* 107 (2): 707–736. https://doi.org/10.15779/Z38BG31Z0V.

10 Ly, D.P., Essien, U.R., Olenski, A.R., and Jena, A.B. (2022). Affirmative action bans and enrollment of students from underrepresented racial and ethnic groups in US public medical schools. *Annals of Internal Medicine* 175 (6): 873–878. https://doi.org/10.7326/M21-4312.

11 Sabin, J.A., Nosek, B.A., Greenwald, A.G., and Rivara, F.P. (2009). Physicians' implicit and explicit attitudes about race by MD race, ethnicity, and gender. *Journal of Health Care for the Poor and Underserved* 20 (3): 896–913. https://doi.org/10.1353/hpu.0.0185.

12 Greenwood, B.N., Hardeman, R.R., Huang, L., and Sojourner, A. (2020). Physician-patient racial concordance and disparities in birthing mortality for newborns. *Proceedings of the National Academy of Sciences* 117 (35): 21194–21200. https://doi.org/10.1073/pnas.1913405117.

13 Witzburg, R.A. and Sondheimer, H.M. (2013). Holistic review – shaping the medical profession one applicant at a time. *New England Journal of Medicine* 368 (17): 1565–1567. https://doi.org/10.1056/NEJMp1300411.

14 Elks, M.L., Herbert-Carter, J., Smith, M. et al. (2018). Shifting the curve: fostering academic success in a diverse student body. *Academic Medicine* 93 (1): 66–70. https://doi.org/10.1097/ACM.0000000000001783.

15 Coleman, C., Keith, J.L., and Webb, E. (n.d.). *Engaging Campus Stakeholders on Enrollment Issues Associated with Student Diversity: A Communication Primer*. College Board, Education Counsel, American Council on Education. https://professionals.collegeboard.org/pdf/engaging-campus-stakeholders-enrolmment-diversity.pdf.

16 Smith, S.G., Nsiah-Kumi, P.A., Jones, P.R., and Pamies, R.J. (2009). Pipeline programs in the health professions, part 1: preserving diversity and reducing health disparities. *Journal of the National Medical Association* 101 (9): 836–851. https://doi.org/10.1016/S0027-9684(15)31030-0.

17 Saha, S., Guiton, G., Wimmers, P.F., and Wilkerson, L. (2008). Student body racial and ethnic composition and diversity-related outcomes in US medical schools. *JAMA* 300 (10): 1135–1145. https://doi.org/10.1001/jama.300.10.1135.

18 Larson, J.S., Orehek, E., and Sandstrom, G.M. (2015). Insights from the underserved: how minority student experiences can inform undergraduate education in psychology. *Scholarship of Teaching and Learning in Psychology* 1 (3): 229–242. https://doi.org/10.1037/stl0000035.

19 Barr, D.A., Gonzalez, M.E., and Wanat, S.F. (2008). The leaky pipeline: factors associated with early decline in interest in premedical studies among underrepresented minority undergraduate students. *Academic Medicine* 83 (5): 503–511. https://doi.org/10.1097/ACM.0b013e31816bda16.

20 Smedley, B.D., Butler, A.S., and Bristow, L.R. (ed.) (2001). *In the Nation's Compelling Interest: Ensuring Diversity in the Health-care Workforce.* National Academies Press. https://doi.org/10.17226/10885.

21 Millo, L., Ho, N., and Ubel, P.A. (2019). The cost of applying to medical school – a barrier to diversifying the profession. *New England Journal of Medicine* 381 (16): 1505–1508. https://doi.org/10.1056/NEJMp1906704.

22 Capers, Q. 4th, Clinchot, D., McDougle, L., and Greenwald, A.G. (2018). Implicit racial bias in medical school admissions. *Academic Medicine* 93 (3): 365–369. https://doi.org/10.1097/ACM.0000000000001388.

23 Aibana, O., Swails, J.L., Flores, R.J., and Love, L. (2019). Bridging the gap: holistic review to increase diversity in graduate medical education. *Academic Medicine* 94 (8): 1137–1141. https://doi.org/10.1097/ACM.0000000000002779.

24 Nolen, L. (2021). How medical education is missing the bull's-eye. *New England Journal of Medicine* 384 (24): 2233–2235. https://doi.org/10.1056/NEJMp2101767.

25 Karani, R., Varpio, L., May, W. et al. (2017). Commentary: racism and bias in health professions education: how educators, faculty developers, and researchers can make a difference. *Academic Medicine* 92 (11S): S1–S6. https://doi.org/10.1097/ACM.0000000000001928.

26 Sukhera, J., Milne, A., Teunissen, P.W. et al. (2020). Adaptive reinventing: implicit bias and the co-construction of social change. *Advances in Health Sciences Education* 25 (2): 297–314. https://doi.org/10.1007/s10459-018-9869-3.

27 Campbell, K.M., Brownstein, N.C., Livingston, H., and Rodríguez, J.E. (2019). Improving underrepresented minority in medicine representation in medical school. *Southern Medical Journal* 112 (4): 203–206. https://doi.org/10.14423/SMJ.0000000000000960.

28 Pradhan, A., Arnott, E., Scott, N., and Shee, A.W. (2020). Pursuing diversity in medical education. *Medical Journal of Australia* 212 (4): 152–153. https://doi.org/10.5694/mja2.50492.

29 Warren, N., Bronder, D., and Williams, M. (2019). Applying an organizational framework to examine diversity and inclusion in the workplace. *Journal of Psychosocial Nursing and Mental Health Services* 57 (6): 16–22. https://doi.org/10.3928/02793695-20190404-04.

30 National Institutes of Health (n.d.). Fiscal years 2023–2027 NIH-wide strategic plan for diversity, equity, inclusion, and accessibility. https://www.nih.gov/sites/default/files/about-nih/nih-wide-strategic-plan-deia-fy23-27.pdf (accessed 26 August 2024).

31 Nivet, M.A. (2015). A diversity 3.0 update: are we moving the needle enough? *Academic Medicine* 90 (12): 1591–1593. https://doi.org/10.1097/ACM.0000000000000950.

23

Reforming the Public Charge Rule for Immigrant Health Equity

Abstract

The chapter explores the challenges faced by immigrants in accessing public services and healthcare, particularly in the context of the Trump administration's 2019 public charge rule and its subsequent rollback by the Biden administration. The chapter begins by highlighting the disparity in healthcare access between immigrants and citizens, which has been exacerbated by the Trump administration's policies and the COVID-19 pandemic. It then delves into the concept of "public charge," tracing its origins in immigration law and its evolution over time. The chapter compares the key differences between the Trump and Biden administrations' public charge rules. Despite the Biden administration's efforts to reverse the Trump-era rule, the chapter emphasizes the persistent chilling effect on immigrants' use of public benefits due to misinformation, fear, and distrust. This hesitancy has negative consequences for immigrants' health and quality of life, as well as implications for healthcare providers and the broader healthcare system. The chapter then explores the limited policy solutions currently available to address immigrant distrust and expand access to benefits, highlighting the need for legislation to send a strong message to immigrant communities. It proposes strategies to rebuild trust and increase immigrant access to public benefits, such as targeted communications, in-language resources, and policies that extend eligibility or remove barriers to enrollment. Finally, the chapter underscores the need for legislative action to provide certainty and stability for immigrants regarding the public charge rule. It argues that congressional action, either rescinding the statute and encouraging the use of public benefits or clearly defining the term "public charge" and its associated public benefit programs, would offer immigrant communities the necessary clarity and assurance regarding their access to federal programs.

Keywords *public charge rule; immigrant health equity; healthcare access; Medicaid enrollment; misinformation; social determinants of health; legislative action*

> *Raquel, a lawful permanent resident, hesitates to enroll in Medicaid despite her eligibility, fearing that accepting public benefits could jeopardize her chances of becoming a US citizen. She forgoes preventive care and struggles to manage her chronic health conditions, ultimately leading to a costly emergency room visit.*

> *Sarina, a pregnant woman from Bhutan, is unsure if enrolling in the Women, Infants, and Children (WIC) program could negatively impact her immigration status. Despite the nutritional risks to her unborn child, she decides not to apply for WIC benefits due to the lack of clear information and lingering fears surrounding the public charge rule.*
>
> *The Nguyen family, Vietnamese refugees, face a difficult decision when their elderly father requires long-term care. They are uncertain whether his use of Medicaid-funded nursing home services could affect their own immigration prospects, leading to increased stress and financial strain as they explore limited alternatives for his care.*

23.1   Barriers to Immigrant Healthcare Access: The Public Charge Rule's Impact

Immigrants face significant obstacles in accessing public services and utilizing crucial health services, such as preventive care, at lower rates compared to citizens [1]. This disparity has been exacerbated by the Trump administration's policies and the COVID-19 pandemic. The 2019 public charge rule, which allows the Department of Homeland Security (DHS) to penalize immigrants who use certain types of federal government benefits, had a particularly profound impact on immigrants' access to public services [2]. Despite federal courts staying the use of the 2019 public charge rule in 2020 and the Biden administration reversing it in a final rule that took effect in December 2023, the erosion of trust within immigrant communities persists, leading to hesitancy in enrolling themselves and their families in government assistance programs.

Generally, unauthorized immigrants are ineligible for federal health care coverage programs unless they are classified as "qualified immigrants" [3]. Qualified immigrants may have access to various federal public benefits, including Supplemental Security Income (SSI), Supplemental Nutrition Assistance Program (SNAP), Temporary Assistance for Needy Families (TANF), Emergency Medicaid, Medicare Part A (subject to work history requirements), Medicare Part D, Department of Housing and Urban Development (HUD) public housing and Section 8 Programs, and Social Security.

The concept of "public charge" originated in the 1882 Immigration Act, which denied entry to immigrants deemed "unable to take care of themselves and likely to become a public charge" [4]. In 1890, Congress introduced a provision allowing for the deportation of immigrants who became public charges after arrival. Currently, being classified as a public charge or potential public charge can result in the denial of admission for certain immigrants or the inability to obtain lawful permanent resident status. The Trump administration's modifications to the public charge rule eliminated the exemption for health-related benefits and permitted sanctions on immigrants who received assistance through Medicaid, Medicare Part D, SNAP, and housing subsidies [5]. From 1999 to 2019, both the DHS and the Department of State defined public charge as an individual who is or is likely to become primarily reliant on public cash assistance or government-funded institutionalization for long-term care.

> *"Migration is an expression of the human aspiration for dignity, safety and a better future. It is part of the social fabric, part of our very make-up as a human family."*
> Former Secretary-General of the United Nations, Ban Ki-moon

23.2 Comparing Trump and Biden Public Charge Rules

The Trump and Biden administrations' public charge rules diverge in two key aspects [6]: the definition of public charge, which encompasses the federal and state programs that may be considered in public charge determination, and the manner in which factors are weighed by adjudicators when assessing an individual's risk of becoming a public charge. This section will examine each of these differences in detail.

23.2.1 Defining Public Charge

Before 1991, the definition of public charge was narrow, focusing on the probability of requiring cash assistance for income maintenance or long-term institutionalization. In 2019, the Trump administration's rule expanded the list of public benefits to include nine additional categories of public assistance, such as receiving "Medicaid, food stamps, or housing benefits for an aggregate of 12 months out of 36" within any time period prior to the determination.

In September 2022, the DHS published a final rule that redefined the phrase "likely to become a public charge" to align with the pre-2019 guidance [7]. This definition is considerably more limited than the Trump-era rule and concentrates on the receipt of two types of public benefits: (i) cash assistance for income maintenance and (ii) long-term institutionalization. Cash assistance for income maintenance encompasses Social Security Income, TANF cash assistance, and state and local cash assistance programs designed to support the resident's daily living expenses. Long-term institutionalization includes institutionalization in a nursing home or mental health facility. However, Home and Community-Based Services are not considered in a public charge determination, and these restrictions cannot be applied in a manner that discriminates against people with disabilities. If the individual is or has been institutionalized, the adjudicator must consider evidence that institutionalization violated the Americans with Disabilities Act (ADA) or other federal laws.

23.2.2 Difference in Application

The Trump administration's public charge rule not only expanded the range of public assistance programs considered in public charge determinations but also made it easier for individuals to meet the "public charge" threshold due to the way adjudicators were instructed to weigh the factors [2]. Instead of weighing the factors equally, the Trump administration rule assigned some factors as "heavily weigh negative" and others as "heavily weigh positive" for or against a public charge determination. For example, the rule considered the presence of a medical condition likely to require extensive medical treatment, combined with the absence of health insurance, as a factor heavily weighted towards finding the individual to be a public charge. Conversely, having private, nonsubsidized health insurance was heavily weighted in the individual's favor. This analysis led to substantially more people being designated as public charges. Between October 1, 2018, and July 2019, the State Department denied 5343 immigrant visa applications for Mexican nationals on the grounds that the applicants were so poor or infirm that they risked becoming a "public charge" [8]. During the same period, 12,179 visas were rejected on public charge grounds.

In contrast, under the 2022 Rule, DHS instructs adjudicators to consider the totality of an individual's current circumstances to determine if they are likely to become a public charge in the future [7].

The adjudicator should consider the individual's age, health, family status, assets, education, and skills. Under the Biden administration's rule, denials based on the likelihood that a person will become a public charge must be accompanied by an articulation of the reasons for the decision to denial.

Policy and Equity in Immigration and Immigrant Healthcare

Policy Area	Trump Administration	Biden Administration	Equity Considerations
Public Charge Rule	Expanded definition of public charge to include noncash benefits like Medicaid, SNAP, and housing assistance.	Reverted to pre-2019 definition focusing on cash assistance and long-term institutionalization.	Trump's rule increased fear and reduced benefit enrollment among immigrants. Biden's rule aims to reduce fear but distrust remains.
Healthcare Access	Barriers increased through expanded public charge rule, making many immigrants reluctant to use health services.	Rollback of expanded public charge rule, with efforts to reassure immigrant communities of safe benefit use.	Despite policy changes, misinformation and fear persist, limiting healthcare access for immigrants.
Economic Stability	Increased denial of visas based on potential future public charge status, affecting economic stability of immigrants.	Reduction in visa denials by focusing on the totality of circumstances rather than heavily weighted negative factors.	Economic stability of immigrants improved but trust needs rebuilding to encourage benefit use.
Legal Status Impact	Stricter enforcement and expanded criteria for public charge determinations.	More lenient approach with a focus on the individual's current circumstances.	Equitable access to public benefits is still hindered by lingering fears of future policy changes.
Social Determinants	Worsened by targeting housing and food assistance programs under public charge rule.	Efforts to clarify nonimpact on housing and food assistance, encouraging benefit use.	Persistent distrust and misinformation continue to affect immigrants' access to essential services.

23.3 The Chilling Effect: Immigrant Hesitancy to Access Public Benefits Despite Policy Changes

Despite the Biden administration's rollback of the Trump-era public charge rule and the inclusion of clarifying language in the final rule regarding the individuals subject to public charge determinations, the specific federal programs considered, and the way factors are weighed, immigrant communities have not returned to public assistance programs [9]. This hesitancy is likely due to misinformation, fear, and distrust.

Navigating immigration policy is complex and frustrating, and many communities lack access to in-language resources that effectively communicate the new rule and its applicability [10]. To avoid potential immigration challenges, many individuals may simply choose to forgo federal programs rather than risk being wrong. Additionally, due to inadequate resources explaining the Biden administration's rule, immigrants may erroneously fear that they could be impacted if they choose to sign up for public benefits.

They might also wrongly believe that their families or children cannot receive benefits if they are a member of a limited group that could be affected by a public charge determination. Moreover, even if an individual knows they may not be subject to a public charge designation currently, they might believe that signing up for benefits could harm their case if future administrations continue to change the rule. This uncertainty exacerbates existing distrust in the system and may lead people to forgo benefits entirely.

However, immigrants forgoing public benefits will have negative consequences for their health and quality of life [11]. Uninsured immigrants may choose to delay seeking healthcare until they face an emergency, requiring expensive treatment in an emergency department. Consequently, hospitals and providers may continue to bear the costs of uncompensated care in these situations. Furthermore, because the Trump rule also targeted housing and food instability programs, which are other social determinants of health, immigrants' poor health may be further exacerbated by their living conditions.

The most significant impact of the Trump-era public charge rule, apart from the increased determinations that individuals were public charges leading to visa denials, was the substantial chilling effect on immigrants' use of public benefits [12]. Migration Policy Institute analysis showed that from 2016 to 2019, participation in TANF, SNAP, and Medicaid declined more rapidly for noncitizens than US citizens, with the drop accelerating when the Trump policy change was announced [13]. A 2021 survey found that "1 in 4 potentially undocumented Hispanic adults and over 1 in 10 lawful permanent resident Hispanic adults reported that they or a family member did not participate in a government assistance program in the past three years due to immigration-related fears" [14]. Similarly, 50% of surveyed Asian Community Health Center patients reported not having enough information about how recent immigration policy changes, including the public charge rule, impact them and their families [15]. One in four reported that they or a family member in their household avoided participating in a publicly funded health, nutrition, or housing program in the prior year due to immigration-related fears. Nearly half of the families that needed assistance during the pandemic abstained from applying due to concerns over how doing so could impact their immigration status.

Under the Trump administration rule, even groups exempt from public charge assessments used fewer benefits, and in many situations, "chilled" populations were not targets of the public charge rule [16]. Some immigrant populations were avoiding other food and assistance programs that were not included in either of the public charge rules [17]. For instance, some data suggests that immigrant pregnant women refused Women, Infants, and Children (WIC) services, immigrant parents declined to enroll in state food assistance and free lunch programs, and a New York City health center found that patients with HIV or AIDS were hesitating to enroll in, or were disenrolling from the city-run HIV/AIDS services administration program out of fear that the program's services fell under the public charge rule [18]. A study found that compared to citizen children with US-born parents, SNAP participation among children from families with a noncitizen parent began decreasing from 2015 to 2016 and dropped substantially from 2017 to 2019 [19].

23.4 Limited Policy Solutions to Address Immigrant Distrust and Expand Access to Benefits

At present, there are limited related policies that effectively address the communication and distrust issues that arise when connecting immigrant communities with public benefits [20]. Although the Biden administration recently increased funding for navigator programs that assist individuals in enrolling for public benefits, legislation, rather than rulemaking, would send the strongest message to immigrants that these services are safe and beneficial to use [21]. While legislation has been proposed at the federal level to expand health coverage eligibility for immigrants, there is no clear path to passage in Congress [22]. However, at the state level, a small but increasing number of states have extended fully state-funded coverage to certain low-income individuals, regardless of their immigration status [23].

23.5 Strategies to Rebuild Trust and Increase Immigrant Access to Public Benefits

Moving forward, the current executive branch's primary focus should be on consistently emphasizing that the 2019 Rule is no longer in effect and that immigrants can and should access public benefits [24]. Communications should target families with children who could significantly benefit from additional food or housing assistance [25]. Public payers must ensure that their application materials clearly state in multiple languages that the public charge rule does not impact access to coverage through Medicaid, the Children's Health Insurance Program (CHIP), or the Affordable Care Act (ACA) marketplace [26].

As communications are disseminated, the administration and local health departments should prioritize providing in-language resources to community hubs, such as churches or childcare centers [27]. The administration should also consider implementing policies that extend eligibility or remove barriers to enrollment [28]. For example, qualified adult immigrants are currently subject to a five-year waiting period before becoming eligible for SNAP benefits [29]. Eliminating this waiting period for adults could facilitate participation for the children in their households [30].

23.6 The Need for Legislative Action to Provide Certainty and Stability for Immigrants

Despite the Biden administration's rollback of the Trump administration's public charge rule, its impact on immigrants' lives has been far-reaching and persistent [31]. The Biden administration must take further steps to communicate that the rule has been reversed; however, immigrants may continue to distrust a rule that can be altered whenever there is a change in the governing party. While no viable legislation has been introduced yet to address this issue, congressional action that either rescinds the statute and encourages the use of public benefits or, alternatively, clearly defines the term "public charge" and its associated public benefit programs would provide stability in this policy area and offer immigrant communities certainty regarding the federal programs they can and cannot access.

References

1 Artiga, S., Garfield, R., and Damico, A. (2019). *Estimated Impacts of Final Public Charge Inadmissibility Rule on Immigrants and Medicaid Coverage*. Kaiser Family Foundation.

2 Capps, R., Gelatt, J., and Greenberg, M. (2020). *The Public-Charge Rule: Broad Impacts, But Few Will Be Denied Green Cards Based on Actual Benefits Use*. Migration Policy Institute.

3 Fortuny, K. and Chaudry, A. (2011). *A Comprehensive Review of Immigrant Access to Health and Human Services*. Washington, DC: Urban Institute.

4 Vialet, J.C. and Education and Public Welfare Division (1991). *A Brief History of US Immigration Policy*. Congressional Research Service, Library of Congress.

5 Daval, J. (2020). The problem with public charge. *Yale Law Journal* 130: 998.

6 Konisky, D.M. and Nolette, P. (2021). The state of American Federalism, 2020–2021: deepening partisanship amid tumultuous times. *Publius: The Journal of Federalism* 51 (3): 327–364.

7 Department of Homeland Security (2022). Public charge ground of inadmissibility. *Federal Register* 87 (186): 55472–55590.

8 Hesson, T. (2019). *Exclusive: Visa Denials to Poor Mexicans Skyrocket Under Trump's State Department*. Politico. https://www.politico.com/story/2019/08/06/visa-denials-poor-mexicans-trump-1637094.

9 Bernstein, H., McTarnaghan, S., and Gonzalez, D. (2019). *Safety Net Access in the Context of the Public Charge Rule*. Urban Institute. https://www.urban.org/research/publication/safety-net-access-context-public-charge-rule.

10 Pereira, K.M., Crosnoe, R., Fortuny, K. et al. (2012). *Barriers to Immigrants' Access to Health and Human Services Programs*. Office of the Assistant Secretary for Planning and Evaluation.

11 Artiga, S. and Diaz, M. (2019). *Health Coverage and Care of Undocumented Immigrants*. Kaiser Family Foundation. https://www.kff.org/racial-equity-and-health-policy/issue-brief/health-coverage-and-care-of-undocumented-immigrants/.

12 Bernstein, H., Gonzalez, D., Karpman, M., and Zuckerman, S. (2019). *One in Seven Adults in Immigrant Families Reported Avoiding Public Benefit Programs in 2018*. Urban Institute. https://www.urban.org/research/publication/one-seven-adults-immigrant-families-reported-avoiding-public-benefit-programs-2018.

13 Capps, R., Fix, M., and Batalova, J. (2020). *Anticipated "Chilling Effects" of the Public-Charge Rule Are Real: Census Data Reflect Steep Decline in Benefits Use by Immigrant Families*. Migration Policy Institute. https://www.migrationpolicy.org/news/anticipated-chilling-effects-public-charge-rule-are-real.

14 Bernstein, H., Gonzalez, D., and Karpman, M. (2021). *Adults in Low-Income Immigrant Families Were Deeply Affected by the COVID-19 Crisis Yet Avoided Safety Net Programs in 2020*. Urban Institute. https://www.urban.org/research/publication/adults-low-income-immigrant-families-were-deeply-affected-covid-19-crisis-yet-avoided-safety-net-programs-2020.

15 Pillai, D. and Artiga, S. (2022). *Changes to the Public Charge Inadmissibility Rule and the Implications for Health Care*. Kaiser Family Foundation Retrieved 24 April 2023.

16 Batalova, J., Fix, M., and Greenberg, M. (2018). *Chilling Effects: The Expected Public Charge Rule and Its Impact on Legal Immigrant Families' Public Benefits Use*. Migration Policy Institute. https://www.migrationpolicy.org/research/chilling-effects-expected-public-charge-rule-impact-legal-immigrant-families.

17 Protecting Immigrant Families (2020). Changes to "public charge" immigration rules: implications for health and health care. https://protectingimmigrantfamilies.org/wp-content/uploads/2020/02/Public-Charge-Fact-Sheet-Updated-February-2020.pdf (accessed 26 August 2024).

18 Maru, S., Glenn, L., Belfon, K. et al. (2021). Utilization of maternal health care among immigrant mothers in New York City, 2016-2018. *Journal of Urban Health: Bulletin of the New York Academy of Medicine* 98 (6): 711–726. https://doi.org/10.1007/s11524-021-00584-5.

19 Bovell-Ammon, A., Ettinger de Cuba, S., Coleman, S. et al. (2019). Trends in food insecurity and SNAP participation among immigrant families of US-born young children. *Children* 6 (4): 55.

20 Tolbert, J., Artiga, S., and Pham, O. (2019). *Impact of Shifting Immigration Policy on Medicaid Enrollment and Utilization of Care Among Health Center Patients*. Kaiser Family Foundation. https://www.kff.org/medicaid/issue-brief/impact-of-shifting-immigration-policy-on-medicaid-enrollment-and-utilization-of-care-among-health-center-patients/.

21 Zallman, L., Finnegan, K.E., Himmelstein, D.U. et al. (2019). Implications of changing public charge immigration rules for children who need medical care. *JAMA Pediatrics* 173 (9): 901–902.

22 National Immigration Law Center (2021). Immigrants and the affordable care act (ACA). https://www.nilc.org/issues/health-care/immigrantshcr/ (accessed 26 August 2023).

23 Brooks, T., Roygardner, L., Artiga, S. et al. (2020). *Medicaid and CHIP Eligibility, Enrollment, and Cost-Sharing Policies as of January 2020: Findings from a 50-State Survey*. Kaiser Family Foundation. https://www.kff.org/medicaid/report/medicaid-and-chip-eligibility-enrollment-and-cost-sharing-policies-as-of-january-2020-findings-from-a-50-state-survey/.

24 Parmet, W.E. (2019). *The Trump Administration's New Public Charge Rule: Implications for Health Care & Public Health*. Health Affairs Blog. https://www.healthaffairs.org/content/forefront/trump-administration-s-new-public-charge-rule-implications-health-care-public-health.

25 Artiga, S. and Pham, O. (2019). *Recent Medicaid/CHIP Enrollment Declines and Barriers to Maintaining Coverage*. Kaiser Family Foundation. https://www.kff.org/medicaid/issue-brief/recent-medicaid-chip-enrollment-declines-and-barriers-to-maintaining-coverage/.

26 Kaiser Family Foundation (2019). Proposed changes to "public charge" policies for immigrants: implications for health coverage. https://www.kff.org/racial-equity-and-health-policy/fact-sheet/proposed-changes-to-public-charge-policies-for-immigrants-implications-for-health-coverage/ (accessed 26 August 2024).

27 Perreira, K.M. and Pedroza, J.M. (2019). Policies of exclusion: implications for the health of immigrants and their children. *Annual Review of Public Health* 40: 147–166.

28 Perreira, K.M., Yoshikawa, H., and Oberlander, J. (2018). A new threat to immigrants' health – the public-charge rule. *The New England Journal of Medicine* 379 (10): 901–903.

29 National Immigration Law Center (2020). Overview of immigrant eligibility for federal programs. https://www.nilc.org/issues/economic-support/overview-immeligfedprograms/ (accessed 26 August 2024).

30 Chilton, M., Black, M.M., Berkowitz, C. et al. (2009). Food insecurity and risk of poor health among US-born children of immigrants. *American Journal of Public Health* 99 (3): 556–562.

31 Haley, J. M., Kenney, G. M., Bernstein, H., & Gonzalez, D. (2020). One in Five Adults in Immigrant Families with Children Reported Chilling Effects on Public Benefit Receipt in 2019. Urban Institute. https://www.urban.org/research/publication/one-five-adults-immigrant-families-children-reported-chilling-effects-public-benefit-receipt-2019 (accessed 26 August 2024).

24

Promoting Health in All Policies (HiAP) Approach

Abstract

The chapter explores the integration of health considerations into all aspects of policymaking to achieve health equity, discussing the foundational principles and broad applications of HiAP. It begins with an introduction to the concept, highlighting the necessity of addressing socioeconomic, racial, gender, and educational disparities in health as endorsed by the World Health Organization. The discussion then transitions to how legal frameworks can facilitate multi-sector collaboration across areas like transportation, housing, and education. The chapter details the creation, operational goals, successes, and challenges of California's HiAP Task Force as a case study. It offers practical advice on overcoming implementation challenges, securing funding, managing stakeholder engagement, and ensuring the longevity of HiAP initiatives. Additionally, the chapter examines the specific challenges HiAP faced during the COVID-19 pandemic, reflecting on lessons learned and how these insights can inform future strategies. The chapter concludes by summarizing the overall lessons from HiAP implementations, emphasizing the importance of policymaking research to effectively integrate health equity into public policy across various governmental and societal contexts.

Keywords *Health in All Policies (HiAP); health equity; multi-sector collaboration; social determinants of health; legal frameworks; policy integration; COVID-19 pandemic; public health governance,*

Aliyah, a single mother living in a low-income neighborhood, struggles to provide healthy meals for her children due to the lack of affordable, fresh produce in her area. The city council, unaware of the health implications of their zoning decisions, continues to approve fast-food restaurants and convenience stores in Aliyah's community, exacerbating the problem of food deserts and contributing to higher rates of obesity and diet-related illnesses.

Ethan, a bright high school student from an underserved community, dreams of attending college but finds himself falling behind his peers from more affluent neighborhoods. His school, underfunded and understaffed, lacks the resources to provide the quality education he needs to succeed. Policymakers, focused solely on short-term budget concerns, fail to recognize the long-term health and economic consequences of neglecting education in disadvantaged communities.

> *Liam, a construction worker, suffers from chronic respiratory issues due to years of exposure to air pollution at his job sites. Despite his declining health, Liam cannot afford to miss work or seek medical care, as his employer does not provide adequate health insurance. The lack of collaboration between labor, healthcare, and environmental agencies leaves workers like Liam vulnerable to the health consequences of poor working conditions.*

24.1 Integrating HiAP: A Strategic Approach to Achieving Health Equity

Health equity aims to provide everyone the opportunity to achieve their full health potential without being disadvantaged by their social position or other socially determined circumstances. Despite significant medical advancements, health equity remains elusive. Experts now understand that government policies significantly influence the structural determinants of health inequities, such as socioeconomic status, race, gender, and education. In response, governments at various levels are adopting an approach termed "Health in All Policies" (HiAP). Championed by the World Health Organization (WHO), HiAP seeks to avoid harmful health impacts and enhance population health and equity. The WHO also asserts that HiAP bolsters policymakers' accountability and stresses the repercussions of public policies on health systems and overall well-being [1].

HiAP lacks a universally accepted definition; however, it is generally described as a strategy that guides leaders and policymakers to consider health, well-being, and equity during the policy and service development, implementation, and evaluation stages. This collaborative approach mandates that health considerations be integrated into the decision-making processes of diverse government sectors. Several US cities have implemented HiAP initiatives [2]. For example, in 2014, Seattle/King County established a multiagency task force to evaluate the health equity impact of county activities, achieving milestones such as creating trails in low-income areas for physical activity and fostering collaboration between criminal justice and education departments to reduce school expulsions.

> *"Health is a state of complete physical, mental and social well-being, and not merely the absence of disease or infirmity. The enjoyment of the highest attainable standard of health is one of the fundamental rights of every human being without distinction of race, religion, political belief, economic or social condition."*
>
> Constitution of the World Health Organization

Addressing the social determinants of health, which the WHO defines as conditions that encompass complete physical, mental, and social well-being, is a crucial function of HiAP. Many of these determinants fall outside traditional public health agency control, making it essential for all policymakers to consider health impacts in their decisions. While clinical care is vital, it accounts for only 15–20% of a population's overall health and longevity [3]. Social determinants, by contrast, have a significantly larger effect on longevity and quality of life. Studies have shown that addressing factors such as inadequate education could enhance population health more substantially than new medical treatments [4]. Moreover, environmental sustainability directly influences health and equity. Recognizing these factors, HiAP requires officials from sectors like education and treasury to assess the health implications of their policies, ensuring a broader and more effective approach to public health.

24.2 Legal Frameworks Facilitating Multi-sector Collaboration for HiAP

Implementing HiAP requires multi-sector collaboration across transportation, agriculture, housing, employment, planning, business, education, and energy. The National Academy of Medicine (formerly Institute of Medicine) advises governments to consider HiAP in major legislative, regulatory, and policy decisions that could significantly impact public health [5]. To effectively foster this collaboration, the law can serve as a powerful tool in various ways.

The law can mandate interdepartmental collaboration to enhance health outcomes. For example, in California, former Governor Schwarzenegger established a HiAP Task Force and mandated cooperation among all executive agencies and the state's public health department [6]. These agencies, which include those overseeing business, transportation, housing, natural resources, and the environment, are tasked with improving health collectively. Similarly, in Knox County, Tennessee, the local health department must collaborate with other county departments to address public health concerns [7].

Where the law does not explicitly require collaboration, it can still authorize or imply it. In Vermont, a state statute permits the state health commissioner to collaborate with the motor vehicle department on health aspects of motor vehicle licensing [7]. In Baltimore, the City Charter empowers the health commissioner to establish policies for treating and preventing illness, enabling collaboration across government departments [7]. Idaho's law broadly authorizes its district boards of health to protect public health, supporting interagency cooperation, particularly when courts interpret such authority expansively [7]. Additionally, in New York City, a multidisciplinary Child Fatality Review Team operates through regular meetings and annual recommendations to city leaders, illustrating how laws can formalize collaborative processes [8].

Laws can also establish formal mechanisms for collaboration, such as task forces or advisory boards. In Ohio, the Ex-Offender Reentry Coalition, formed by various state departments, works together to reduce recidivism, providing findings and recommendations to the state legislature [9]. Post-mass shootings, an executive order in New Jersey led to the formation of a task force focused on the root causes of mass violence, culminating in a permanent multidisciplinary team for prevention efforts [10].

An essential element of enabling such collaborative initiatives through law is funding. The establishment of new agencies or task forces often requires significant financial resources. The law can facilitate this through appropriations, grants, or social impact bonds. For instance, in Washington, DC, the Mayor's Council on Physical Fitness, Health, and Nutrition not only brings together leaders from health, education, and parks departments but also supports its initiatives through a dedicated fitness fund sourced from appropriations, gifts, and donations [11]. Similarly, in Texas, an executive order established the Governor's Advisory Council on Physical Fitness, with the legislature allocating $800,000 for grants to various cities.

In summary, the legal framework can effectively support HiAP by mandating, authorizing, or encouraging collaboration across various government sectors and ensuring the necessary funding to sustain these efforts.

24.3 Establishment and Impact of California's HiAP Task Force

As outlined earlier, in February 2010, former California Governor Schwarzenegger launched the HiAP Task Force at the "Summit on Health, Nutrition and Obesity: Actions for Healthy Living" [12]. This initiative was established through an executive order under the auspices of California's Strategic Growth

Council (SGC), with the California Department of Public Health (CDPH) acting as the facilitator. The executive order tasked the Task Force with identifying key programs and strategies to enhance Californian health, submitting a report with these recommendations to the SGC, outlining the potential health benefits of these recommendations, examining the opportunities for and barriers to interagency collaboration, and holding regular workshops to gather and incorporate stakeholder feedback.

Convened in March 2010, the HiAP Task Force comprised 19 state agencies, departments, and offices, including those focused on education, agriculture, social services, the attorney general, and health and human services [6]. In its initial meetings, the Task Force set several "aspirational goals" aimed at promoting active transportation, healthy housing, accessible parks and green spaces, community safety through violence prevention, access to healthy foods, and informed public policymaking.

The Task Force established criteria such as population health impact, evidentiary support, equity impact, measurability, and feasibility to guide its recommendations [13]. By December 2010, it had approved 34 recommendations, organized into 6 thematic areas reflecting its goals. By June 2011, it identified eleven priority recommendations.

By 2012, the Task Force shifted toward implementing these recommendations [12]. A significant role was to reconcile diverse policy goals across departments, such as integrating transportation, air quality, and land use planning, which occasionally conflicted, for example, the siting of affordable housing near busy roadways. To address these issues, it established a multiagency Housing Siting and Air Quality Workgroup to foster understanding and strategies for inter-agency harmonization, focusing on improving indoor air quality in polluted areas.

An evaluation two years later underscored the Task Force's achievements [6]. Key success factors included actionable recommendations, broad sectoral participation, and a directive from high-level leadership. Many Task Force members reported increased trust in other state agencies, and noted enhanced collaboration with non-governmental and community organizations. Members also indicated that their involvement had spurred broader intersectoral collaboration, with the HiAP policy serving as a governance model.

24.4 Strategies for Enhancing and Sustaining HiAP Initiatives

Understanding the challenges faced by California's HiAP Task Force is crucial for refining and effectively implementing similar measures elsewhere [12]. Initially, the Task Force relied heavily on external funding from nonprofit organizations. As its successes grew, so did the demands for its services at local and federal levels, which strained its resources. To avoid similar challenges, future HiAP implementations should ensure robust funding and prepare for potential expansions [14].

California was a pioneer in establishing a state-level HiAP Task Force, which initially faced difficulties in enacting its recommendations. However, as more states and localities have adopted HiAP measures, opportunities for collaboration and learning from each other's experiences have increased, enhancing localized efforts and the overall effectiveness of HiAP initiatives.

Members of the California HiAP Task Force have highlighted the ongoing challenge of balancing specific, actionable policies with broader health and equity goals. The effort to manage immediate tasks alongside long-term strategic planning is complicated further by the implementation consuming resources that could contribute to broader objectives. Moreover, frequent turnover among leadership and partners complicates continuity, as new stakeholders often require time to align with established priorities.

To address these issues, experts recommend several strategies. First, securing active, high-level political support is crucial for ensuring HiAP's legitimacy and sustainability [15]. Intergovernmental collaboration across various sectors should be fostered, beginning with high-priority areas, even if not all agencies are immediately involved. Engaging with non-governmental organizations and philanthropic entities early and continuously leverages their expertise, support, and funding. Involving members of the populations most affected by HiAP initiatives is key to effective health promotion.

Learning from HiAP models in similar settings can help identify effective strategies for breaking down silos, such as shared staffing, data, and professional development opportunities. The HiAP framework should be used to address and resolve inter-agency conflicts, such as differing priorities between urban development and environmental health. Regular feedback from participating agencies is essential to refine the HiAP process, favoring smaller, issue-based collaborative groups over large meetings.

Setting realistic expectations for outcomes by combining short-term projects with visible impacts and long-term initiatives for broader change is also vital. Exploring how legal frameworks, academic research, and professional legal advice can support HiAP initiatives can further enhance its effectiveness. Starting with modest efforts to build cross-sector relationships can evolve into significant, long-term successes.

These recommendations aim to enhance collaboration, ensure sustainability, and effectively integrate health and equity into government decision-making across sectors.

Policy and Equity in Health in All Policies

Aspect	Key Points
What is Health in All Policies	• A collaborative approach to improving health by incorporating health considerations into decision-making across sectors and policy areas • Promotes health, equity, and sustainability
Why Health in All Policies is needed	• Addresses social determinants of health which are key drivers of health outcomes and health inequities • Engages other sectors that influence social determinants to promote health and equity
Looking Through a Health and Equity Lens	• A systematic way to find opportunities to improve health and equity and embed them in decision-making • Can range from informal discussions to formal health impact assessments • Considers distribution of health impacts across a population
Choosing Policies to Work on	• Consider potential for improving health, equity, sustainability • Look for co-benefits and win-wins across agencies' goals • Engage stakeholders to ensure policies address community needs
Structural Changes to Embed Equity	• Incorporate health and equity into government processes like strategic planning, budgeting, grant-making • Provide health and equity training for non-health agency staff • Establish shared goals and metrics related to health equity
Stakeholder Engagement	• Enables Health in All Policies to be responsive to community needs, especially those facing inequities • Requires building relationships with community organizations representing disadvantaged groups
Data and Evidence	• Use data disaggregated by race, income, neighborhood to reveal health inequities • Evidence-based and evidence-informed strategies, with community input, to address inequities

24.5 Challenges and Strategic Insights for Implementing HiAP Amidst a Pandemic

As discussed earlier, HiAP programs aim to mitigate health inequities, a need underscored by the COVID-19 pandemic, which vividly demonstrated how structural determinants like income and social/environmental conditions can exacerbate health disparities [16]. The pandemic particularly impacted those with underlying health conditions and those unable to work safely, highlighting the potential role of HiAP in addressing such crises. However, the response to the pandemic revealed significant shortcomings in the existing HiAP frameworks.

Instead of deploying new public health strategies, many health departments were forced to delay these initiatives and divert resources, reflecting the complex challenges HiAP programs face in reshaping public healthcare. While the logic behind HiAP is compelling to its advocates, the transition from a government's public commitment to the actual implementation of a comprehensive HiAP model is not guaranteed [17]. The advice often given to those developing HiAP programs – such as increasing governmental awareness and support, adopting standardized HiAP models and toolkits, and seeking partnerships – proved to be a plausible but ultimately incomplete strategy. Furthermore, the effectiveness of HiAP implementation is often compromised by the commitment to existing healthcare policies and fiscal retrenchment.

Most research on HiAP combines rational planning, hopeful anticipation, and programmatic logic. Yet, this approach has not led to effective implementation. Researchers argue for a shift toward policy-making research, which more directly addresses the "implementation gap" by exploring the complexities of policy enactment [18]. This type of research can provide HiAP advocates with the insights necessary to bridge this gap effectively. During the COVID-19 pandemic, this approach suggested several strategies for HiAP advocates, including treating HiAP as a political project rather than a mere technical solution, re-evaluating the effectiveness of intersectoral action and collaboration in light of power imbalances and the tendency toward policy specialization, rethinking taken-for-granted concepts like co-production and policy learning, navigating trade-offs between the desire for uniform outcomes and the reality of significant variations in HiAP application, and avoiding the temptation to reinvent strategies in the face of challenges to health improvement.

These insights highlight the need for a more nuanced understanding of HiAP as a tool for public health governance, capable of addressing complex health challenges in a politically and socially stratified landscape.

24.6 Conclusion: Lessons and Challenges in Implementing HiAP

It's difficult to dispute the potential benefits of fully functional HiAP measures for community health. Research clearly demonstrates the impact of structural determinants such as socioeconomic status and race on individual health, and HiAP is specifically designed to address these factors in all areas of decision-making. As HiAP measures become more common among state and local governments, it is crucial that these entities understand how to effectively utilize legal frameworks to promote and facilitate collaboration among policymakers. California, the first state to implement HiAP, experienced many successes but also encountered significant challenges. These challenges provide valuable lessons for other governments implementing HiAP measures.

The COVID-19 pandemic highlighted a critical opportunity for the successful deployment of HiAP measures, particularly as the virus disproportionately affected those most vulnerable to health inequities. However, obstacles such as state retrenchment impeded the effective application of HiAP strategies during the pandemic. Researchers now suggest that HiAP advocates should refocus on policymaking research [19]. This shift will better equip them to advocate effectively for HiAP implementation by understanding the complexities of policy development and the systemic changes required to integrate health equity into public policy effectively.

References

1 (2014). Health in all policies (HiAP) framework for country action. *Health Promotion International* 29 (Suppl 1): i19–i28. https://doi.org/10.1093/heapro/dau035.

2 Wernham, A. and Teutsch, S.M. (2015). Health in all policies for big cities. *Journal of Public Health Management and Practice: JPHMP* 21 (Suppl 1): S56–S65. https://doi.org/10.1097/PHH.0000000000000130.

3 McGinnis, J.M., Williams-Russo, P., and Knickman, J.R. (2002). The case for more active policy attention to health promotion. *Health Affairs (Project Hope)* 21 (2): 78–93. https://doi.org/10.1377/hlthaff.21.2.78.

4 Woolf, S.H., Johnson, R.E., Phillips, R.L. Jr., and Philipsen, M. (2007). Giving everyone the health of the educated: an examination of whether social change would save more lives than medical advances. *American Journal of Public Health* 97 (4): 679–683. https://doi.org/10.2105/AJPH.2005.084848.

5 Institute of Medicine (US) Committee on Public Health Strategies to Improve Health (2011). *For the Public's Health: The Role of Measurement in Action and Accountability*. National Academies Press (US).

6 Rudolph, L., Caplan, J., Mitchell, C. et al. 2013. Health in all policies: improving health through intersectoral collaboration. NAM Perspectives. Discussion Paper, National Academy of Medicine, Washington, DC. https://doi.org/10.31478/201309a.

7 Gakh, M. (2015). Law, the health in all policies approach, and cross-sector collaboration. *Public Health Reports (Washington, D.C.: 1974)* 130 (1): 96–100. https://doi.org/10.1177/003335491513000112.

8 Batra, E.K., Quinlan, K., Palusci, V.J. et al. (2024). Child fatality review. *Pediatrics* 153 (3): e2023065481. https://doi.org/10.1542/peds.2023-065481.

9 Pogorzelski, W., Wolff, N., Pan, K.Y., and Blitz, C.L. (2005). Behavioral health problems, ex-offender reentry policies, and the "Second Chance Act". *American Journal of Public Health* 95 (10): 1718–1724. https://doi.org/10.2105/AJPH.2005.065805.

10 Cooper, M.C. and Siegel, B. (1994). Violence: changing the paradigm in New Jersey. *New Jersey Medicine: The Journal of the Medical Society of New Jersey* 91 (12): 836–839.

11 DC Office of the Deputy Mayor for Health and Human Services (2019). Mayor's council on physical fitness, health, and nutrition. https://dmhhs.dc.gov/physicalfitness (accessed 26 August 2024).

12 Pepin, D., Winig, B.D., Carr, D., and Jacobson, P.D. (2017). Collaborating for health: health in all policies and the law. *The Journal of Law, Medicine & Ethics: A Journal of the American Society of Law, Medicine & Ethics* 45 (1_suppl): 60–64. https://doi.org/10.1177/1073110517703327.

13 Gase, L.N., Schooley, T., Lee, M. et al. (2017). A practice-grounded approach for evaluating health in all policies initiatives in the United States. *Journal of Public Health Management and Practice: JPHMP* 23 (4): 339–347. https://doi.org/10.1097/PHH.0000000000000427.

14 Guglielmin, M., Muntaner, C., O'Campo, P., and Shankardass, K. (2018). A scoping review of the implementation of health in all policies at the local level. *Health Policy* 122 (3): 284–292.

15 Shankardass, K., Muntaner, C., Kokkinen, L. et al. (2018). The implementation of health in all policies initiatives: a systems framework for government action. *Health Research Policy and Systems* 16 (1): 26. https://doi.org/10.1186/s12961-018-0295-z.

16 Abrams, E.M. and Szefler, S.J. (2020). COVID-19 and the impact of social determinants of health. *The Lancet. Respiratory Medicine* 8 (7): 659–661. https://doi.org/10.1016/S2213-2600(20)30234-4.

17 Baum, F., Delany-Crowe, T., MacDougall, C. et al. (2019). To what extent can the activities of the South Australian health in all policies initiative be linked to population health outcomes using a program theory-based evaluation? *BMC Public Health* 19 (1): 88. https://doi.org/10.1186/s12889-019-6408-y.

18 Warwick-Booth, L. and Rowlands, S. (2020). Policies for health in the 21st century. In: *Health Promotion: Global Principles and Practice*, 75. CABI Books. https://www.cabidigitallibrary.org/doi/10.1079/9781789245332.0003.

19 Exworthy, M. (2008). Policy to tackle the social determinants of health: using conceptual models to understand the policy process. *Health Policy and Planning* 23 (5): 318–327. https://doi.org/10.1093/heapol/czn022.

25

Rethinking Preemption for Health Equity

Abstract

Preemption is a legal doctrine that enables a higher level of government to restrict or abolish the authority of a lower level of government to regulate a particular issue. While preemption is not inherently positive or negative, it can serve as an obstacle to public health measures and exacerbate inequities. Historically, preemption has been used to the detriment of vulnerable populations, and the COVID-19 pandemic highlighted the potential negative public health consequences of limiting local governments' powers. State and local governments are typically more attuned to the specific needs of their communities and serve as "laboratories" for experimenting with innovative public health policies that may not be part of federal policy. When preemption restricts the authority of local governments, it can hinder grassroots movements and stifle public health innovation, ultimately impeding the implementation of effective public health measures. Moreover, local governments are often better positioned to address the unique needs of vulnerable and disadvantaged populations within their communities. When state laws restrict local authority to regulate certain areas, it can disproportionately harm racial minorities and lower socioeconomic groups. This chapter begins by examining the relationship between preemption and health disparities. It then provides an overview of preemption and discusses its impact during the COVID-19 pandemic. The chapter also explores the disproportionate effects of preemption on racial minorities, low-income groups, and other pre-existing inequities. Finally, it concludes with recommendations for improving the preemption framework to better address inequities.

Keywords   *preemption; health equity; local authority; public health regulation; COVID-19 impact; socioeconomic disparities; state versus local governance; legislative frameworks*

> *Linda, a public health official in a small rural town, faces the challenge of implementing crucial health measures tailored to her community's unique needs. However, state laws consistently override her efforts, preventing initiatives like increased minimum sick days, which are vital for the town's many low-income workers. The frustration mounts as she watches preventable health disparities widen, illustrating the stifling impact of preemption on local public health innovation.*

Achieving Health Equity: The Role of Law and Policy, First Edition. Y. Tony Yang.
© 2025 John Wiley & Sons Ltd. Published 2025 by John Wiley & Sons Ltd.

Tom, the mayor of a diverse city, struggles to enact housing reforms to protect his constituents from rising rents and evictions during the COVID-19 pandemic. Despite his efforts, state preemption laws block these critical measures, leaving vulnerable populations at risk. His experience underscores the argument that preemption often disproportionately harms racial minorities and low-income groups, exacerbating existing inequities.

25.1 The Double-Edged Sword of Preemption in Public Health Regulation

Preemption in public health regulation is a complex issue with both potential benefits and drawbacks [1]. While patchwork responses across different jurisdictions may be insufficient to address public health matters, and varying policies at different levels of government can create confusion or tension, preemption can ensure uniform regulation, prevent conflicts between different levels of government, and advance well-being and equity. However, preemption can also be misused to disadvantage certain groups of people or hinder efforts to address specific problems.

In some cases, preemptive laws can prevent state and local governments from acting to protect their citizens by restricting local action, rather than utilizing lower-level governments as incubators for innovative policies with the potential to improve health and reduce health inequities. Preemptive interference can have direct and indirect effects on public health and a chilling effect on local communities' power to benefit their residents [2].

Preemption affects local regulation of various areas of life that have significant impacts on public health, such as housing, economic interests, and discrimination. Many states preempt housing regulations, including zoning, rent, and antidiscrimination policies, which can restrict the housing security and rights of vulnerable people [3]. Additionally, states may preempt the ability of local jurisdictions to mandate earned sick days or other employee benefits, limiting workers' access to medical care. Some states also limit local government authority to regulate restaurants, preventing local innovation to promote healthy diets and nutritional awareness [4], while others limit civil rights protections for groups such as sexual minorities, preventing local governments from protecting these individuals from discrimination [5].

Moreover, preemptive restrictions limiting local and fiscal authority to raise and spend revenue can prevent local governments from taking prompt action to address their unique needs, such as improving broadband internet access, which affects access to telemedicine, education, and remote work.

Preemption can also create tension between different levels of government, with preempted governments potentially pushing back on preemptive laws, attempting to regulate restricted areas, or refusing to enforce preemptive orders [6]. This tension can lead to confusion and distrust, undermining the cooperation, local innovation, and unified messaging that would benefit public health.

However, preemption is not always detrimental to public health. It can be used to further objectives that require nationwide uniformity, and it may be prompted by state or local inaction. Although federal or state mandates may not always reflect the needs of a local community, they can set a uniform baseline for localities to build upon and tailor to their unique needs [1]. In some cases, federal preemption can even be used to combat state misuse of preemption.

25.2   Preemption During the COVID-19 Pandemic: Challenges and Consequences

During interstate and international public health emergencies like COVID-19, preemptive actions may be taken to ensure a uniform response across federal, state, and local jurisdictions [6]. However, it was more common for state orders to preempt local authorities, preventing local governments from taking actions they deemed necessary to protect public health.

Preemption can take three forms: floor, ceiling, and vacuum. Federal preemption typically establishes a regulatory floor, setting baseline standards while allowing local governments to implement additional restrictions based on local conditions. During COVID-19, states often established regulatory ceilings, preventing local governments from imposing stricter requirements than the state. For example, if a state set a ceiling on social gathering restrictions by limiting gatherings to no more than 50 people, a local government could not impose a stricter limit of 10 people. In rare instances, states created a regulatory vacuum by not issuing state laws but restricting the authority of local officials to regulate certain areas.

States used their preemptive power to limit local governments' authority to respond to the pandemic in various ways, such as restricting local governments from imposing social distancing regulations, business shutdowns, masking, and curfew orders [6]. Housing became a critical issue during COVID-19, and state housing preemption laws prevented local governments from addressing local housing inequities.

States blocking local efforts to respond to the pandemic created friction between different levels of government [7]. Pre-existing preemption policies concerning broadband access, discrimination, and business regulation created new challenges for local governments trying to respond to their communities' needs. This had a chilling effect on local authorities and hindered the development of innovative solutions at the local level during a time when innovation and creative problem-solving were needed to promote public health.

While preemption is not inherently bad and can sometimes provide relief through uniform policies across jurisdictions, such as the Public Readiness and Emergency Preparedness Act enacted by Congress, most pandemic-era examples of preemption did not promote public health. Instead, they reduced the health and safety protections that state and local governments could impose, often leaving already vulnerable populations worse off when their local governments could not enact policies or provide aid.

> *"...if you believe that as much power as possible ought to be devolved from the federal to state governments, it follows that as much power as possible ought to be devolved to local governments. As a general rule, political power ought always to rest closest to those whom it will affect."*
>
> John Phelan, Center of the American Experiment

25.3   Preemption's Disproportionate Impact on Vulnerable Populations and Inequities

The COVID-19 pandemic exacerbated existing inequalities along racial lines, and preemption played a significant role in this outcome [7]. By restricting the local authority to mitigate the public health and economic fallout of the pandemic, preemption effectively reinforced inequalities during the crisis.

Setting restrictions on the actions localities could take to address community needs worsened inequality among vulnerable groups. Scholars suggest that preemption could have been used to promote health and economic equality by advancing public health goals and ensuring that local governments were better equipped to deal with the pandemic [6]. However, most pandemic-era examples of preemption did not promote public health, instead reducing the health and safety protections that state and local governments could impose, often leaving already vulnerable populations worse off when their local governments could not enact policies or provide aid.

Preemption can have a discriminatory effect on racial, socioeconomic, and other minority or disadvantaged groups, impacting public health, economic opportunity, voting rights, civil rights, and racial equality [7]. State preemption of local measures to prevent the spread of COVID-19 may worsen health inequities by excluding racial minorities and low-income people from opportunities and health benefits that local laws could provide. For example, if local governments are preempted from implementing mask mandates, improving broadband access, or offering sick leave policies, racial minorities and lower socioeconomic groups are most affected (because they were more likely to work in person and be at risk of illness during the pandemic). This is particularly concerning given that the pandemic has deepened existing inequalities along racial lines.

Preemption can be imposed to favor certain groups over others. In the South, preemption has a long history of reinforcing racism and favoring white property owners, with Southern state governments using preemption to create barriers for people of color [8]. Preemption may also favor the interests of corporations or certain industries with economic interests in deregulation, restricting the power of local governments to address the needs of their vulnerable constituents and perpetuating disparities among racial and socioeconomic groups.

The structure and framework of state and local laws, such as "home rule" and "Dillon's Rule," also influence how preemption can be used to disadvantage particular groups of people [9]. Dillon's Rule states create substantial barriers to local action by restricting local authority to powers expressly granted by the state, creating a presumption of state preemption. The preemptive authority of Dillon's Rule states strips local power and disproportionately harms black and brown workers, low-income workers, and women.

Preemption can be used to stymie local power to regulate labor standards, civil rights, public health and safety, technology, environmental protection, land use, and taxes [10]. All of these issue areas directly and indirectly impact health, safety, and economic opportunities, particularly for racial minorities and low-income groups. For instance, preempting local governments from improving broadband internet access affects how people connect to the world, including their access to telemedicine, education, and remote work. While technology has increased healthcare accessibility during the pandemic, policies that restrict a government's ability to ensure equitable internet access only widen gaps in health disparity.

Moreover, preemptive restrictions limiting local and fiscal authority to raise and spend revenue prohibit localities from using such revenue to reinvest in local services and the local economy, which can have a greater impact on public health [7]. Other preemptive policies have been used to restrict housing regulations, including zoning, rent, and anti-discrimination policies, limiting the housing security and rights of vulnerable people. States may also preempt the ability of local jurisdictions to mandate earned sick days or other employee benefits, limiting workers' ability to obtain medical care. Some preemptive laws also limit civil rights protections for groups such as sexual minorities, preventing local governments from protecting these individuals from discrimination.

To address these disparities, local governments should be given the authority to act in the interests of the most vulnerable members of their communities. Local governments have the advantage of a more intimate level of governance, with officials often having firsthand experience with community challenges, allowing them to develop more directed and specific policies tailored to the unique needs of their constituents. Preemption that restricts this local authority can exacerbate inequities and limit the ability of local governments to effectively address public health crises like the COVID-19 pandemic.

25.4 Conclusion: Toward an Equity-First Preemption Framework

Preemption is not inherently adverse to positive public health outcomes [11]. When used strategically, preemptive policies can serve as a powerful tool to ensure uniform regulation, protect against conflicts between different levels of government, and advance well-being and equity. However, because preemption is being used as a tool to perpetuate inequities and reduce innovation, federal and state legislators should avoid framing preemptive legislation in a way that hinders public health action [12]. As we move forward through the COVID-19 pandemic and beyond, policymakers should consider how preemption can be adapted to better serve the interests of all people, promote public health, and reduce inequities [13, 14].

There is a need for fresh approaches to preemption that elevate social, economic, and health interests while limiting inequity and discrimination. Experts recommend several steps that federal, state, and local governments can take to improve preemption as it relates to public health and equity. These include investing in research to gather empirical data on the public health effects of preemption, developing a robust evidence base to inform preemption policy considerations, emphasizing that preemptive clauses should draw on this evidence base, and ensuring that consideration of disproportionately impacted populations is core to all policies. Other recommendations include involving representation of disproportionately impacted communities in all phases of policy drafting, obtaining input from the public health science community on preemption's potential benefits and harms, including savings clauses to protect future public health legislation, enacting preemptive legislation that serves as a regulatory floor rather than a regulatory ceiling, considering waiver provisions, removing existing preemption of more protective local COVID-19 laws, strengthening home rule, considering federal preemptive intervention to combat state misuse, and disallowing regulatory vacuums.

An equity-first preemption framework could improve the effects of preemption on public health, equity, and good governance [15]. Some scholars characterize preemption as both a cause of and a means to alleviate inequities, and an equity-first approach reconciles preemption's potential to advance and hinder health equity. The equity-first preemption framework would assess when preemption will enhance or inhibit equity and ensure that local governments are not preempted from improving public health and equity.

Laws and policies play significant roles in perpetuating health inequities. Local governments are sometimes preempted from addressing the needs of their communities when preemption restricts their ability to regulate in certain areas. Local action is often tailored to the unique challenges of individual communities, and state preemption bars the pursuit of healthier, more equitable futures. This inhibits responsiveness and impedes efforts to remedy existing laws that may have discriminatory effects.

Under existing frameworks, preemption laws are classified primarily on the basis of their mechanical operation – that is, whether the law establishes a regulatory floor, a regulatory ceiling, or a regulatory vacuum. In contrast, equity-first would support local governments' ability to innovate and respond to the needs and values of people they represent while also acknowledging the need for states and the federal government to block local actions that are likely to create or perpetuate inequities. An equity-first framework would shift the analysis from the mechanics of the law to the anticipated impact on health and health equity.

An equity-first preemption framework would harness the power of preemption to counter harmful policies and promote fairness. To ensure policies developed under this framework promote health equity, policymakers can utilize the Racial Equity and Policy (REAP) framework to examine the anticipated effects of drafted guidelines [16]. The REAP framework prompts policymakers to evaluate a policy according to key assessments centered on three considerations: disproportionality, decentralization, and voice. This assessment examines the actors and institutions responsible for drafting the policy, the biases that may exist, and the context through which the policy will be constructed and implemented. By identifying the components and context of a law that may enable inequities, lawmakers can reconstruct the policy to mitigate these implications.

Advocates for equity-first frameworks say that while this approach is promising, more research needs to be done in this area to establish an effective framework based on empirical evidence. If equity-first is pursued as a reform to the current mechanical preemption framework, research would be essential to developing an effective model.

State Preemption on Local Health Equity Policies

Policy Area	Equity Implications of Preemption
General	• "New preemption" trend increasingly aims to prevent any local regulation, often propelled by corporate interests • Fails to consider health equity implications and impedes local efforts to remedy historical harms, undermining democracy • Can threaten public health innovations that start locally to reduce inequities
Affordable and Fair Housing	• Preempts local laws protecting against housing discrimination based on source of income, which disproportionately harms people of color • Preempts local inclusionary zoning, rent control, and other policies aimed at increasing affordable housing
Food and Beverages	• Some states preempt nearly all local nutrition-related policies, prohibiting efforts to reduce "food-based health disparities" • Preemption of sugary drink taxes limits local ability to reduce consumption and raise revenue to address health issues in underserved communities
Tobacco, Alcohol, and Guns	• Preemption of local smokefree air laws, e-cigarette regulations, and tobacco control policies obstruct campaigns to advance equitable health outcomes • Most states preempt local gun safety laws despite high rates of gun deaths
Economic Well-Being	• Many states preempt local paid sick leave, minimum wage, fair scheduling, and prevailing wage laws aimed at promoting equitable labor practices, leaving workers without protections

References

1 Pomeranz, J.L. and Pertschuk, M. (2017). State preemption: a significant and quiet threat to public health in the United States. *American Journal of Public Health* 107 (6): 900–902. https://doi.org/10.2105/AJPH. 2017.303756.

2 Melton-Fant, C., Carr, D., and Montez, J.K. (2021). *Addressing Health Equity in the New Preemption Era.* Health Affairs Forefront.

3 Michener, J. (2023). Entrenching inequity, eroding democracy: state preemption of local housing policy. *Journal of Health Politics, Policy and Law* 48 (2): 157–185. https://doi.org/10.1215/03616878-10234156.

4 Barbour, L., Lindberg, R., Woods, J. et al. (2022). Local urban government policies to facilitate healthy and environmentally sustainable diet-related practices: a scoping review. *Public Health Nutrition* 25 (2): 471–487. https://doi.org/10.1017/S1368980021004432.

5 Pomeranz, J.L. (2018). Challenging and preventing policies that prohibit local civil rights protections for lesbian, gay, bisexual, transgender, and queer people. *American Journal of Public Health* 108 (1): 67–72. https://doi.org/10.2105/AJPH.2017.304116.

6 Carr, D., Adler, S., Winig, B.D., and Montez, J.K. (2020). Equity first: conceptualizing a normative framework to assess the role of preemption in public health. *The Milbank Quarterly* 98 (1): 131–149. https://doi.org/10.1111/1468-0009.12444.

7 Yang, Y.T. and Berg, C.J. (2022). How preemption can lead to inequity. *International Journal of Environmental Research and Public Health* 19 (17): 10476. https://doi.org/10.3390/ijerph191710476.

8 Blair, H., Cooper, D., and Worker, J. (2020). *Preempting Progress: State Interference in Local Policymaking Prevents People of Color, Women, and Low-Income Workers from Making Ends Meet in the South.* Economic Policy Institute. https://www.epi.org/publication/preemption-in-the-south/.

9 Latham, J.R. (2016). Dillon's rule versus home rule: a comprehensive, comparative review of the impacts. Honors theses. University of Mississippi.

10 Phillips, L.E. (2017). Impeding innovation: state preemption of progressive local regulations. *Columbia Law Review* 117: 2225.

11 Gardbaum, S.A. (1993). Nature of preemption. *Cornell Law Review* 79: 767.

12 Melton-Fant, C. (2022). New preemption as a tool of structural racism: implications for racial health inequities. *The Journal of Law, Medicine & Ethics* 50 (1): 15–22.

13 Mello, M.M. and Gostin, L.O. (2023). Public health law modernization 2.0: rebalancing public health powers and individual liberty in the age of COVID-19: analysis examines the need to rebalance public health powers and individual liberty in the COVID-19 era. *Health Affairs* 42 (3): 318–327.

14 Wu, X., Ma, L., Low, D. et al. (2024). Beyond precautionary principle: policy-making under uncertainty and complexity. *Policy Design and Practice* 7 (1): 1–16.

15 Haddow, K., Carr, D., Winig, B.D., and Adler, S. (2020). Preemption, public health, and equity in the time of COVID-19. In: *Assessing Legal Responses to COVID-19* (July 31, 2020) (ed. S. Burris, S. de Guia, L. Gable, et al.). Boston: Public Health Law Watch.

16 The Commonwealth Fund (2022). A racial equity framework for assessing health policy. https://www. commonwealthfund.org/publications/issue-briefs/2022/jan/racial-equity-framework-assessing-health-policy (accessed 26 August 2024).

26

Achieving Health and Economic Equity Through Broadband Access and Policy

Abstract

This chapter explores the critical role of broadband access in achieving health and economic equity in the United States. It begins by defining broadband and highlighting its increasing importance in daily life, especially since the pandemic, when many activities and services shifted online. The chapter then discusses the digital divide, which disproportionately affects rural and minority communities, perpetuating systemic inequities. It emphasizes the importance of lawmakers at all levels of government in spearheading efforts to achieve equitable internet access. The chapter goes on to examine federal efforts to support broadband access and digital equity, including funding, data collection, and policy initiatives. It then delves into state-level strategies for promoting digital equity, showcasing promising practices identified by the Pew Charitable Trusts, such as stakeholder outreach and engagement, policy frameworks, planning and capacity building, funding and operations, and program evaluation and evolution. The chapter also highlights the effectiveness of local broadband initiatives in addressing community-specific digital needs, providing examples from Delta County, Colorado, and Wimauma Village, Florida. Finally, the chapter concludes by emphasizing the emergence of broadband access as a critical factor in achieving health and economic equity. It calls for policymakers to capitalize on the growing interest and momentum surrounding digital equity by establishing high-speed internet access as an essential component of the public values guaranteed and safeguarded by the government. The chapter underscores that addressing the digital divide is not only a matter of fairness but also a crucial step in promoting overall health and economic well-being for the entire nation.

Keywords *broadband access; digital divide; health equity; telehealth services; rural connectivity; federal and state policies; economic equity; digital infrastructure*

> *Evelyn, an elderly woman in a remote Alaskan village, needed regular check-ups for her chronic condition. The nearest hospital was hours away, making frequent visits nearly impossible. With the introduction of telehealth services, Evelyn could consult her doctor virtually, saving time and reducing health risks associated with long travel distances. However, without stable internet access, she often missed critical appointments, jeopardizing her health.*

> *In a remote Native American reservation, the tribal health center struggles to provide adequate care for its patients. Without reliable broadband connectivity, the center cannot implement telemedicine services or access online medical resources, leaving the community vulnerable to preventable health issues. The lack of internet access also hinders the tribe's ability to apply for grants and funding opportunities that could improve their healthcare infrastructure and overall well-being.*

26.1 Broadband: A Crucial Determinant of Health Equity

Broadband, defined as high-speed and reliable internet, has become increasingly crucial to daily life, especially since the pandemic when many activities and services shifted online, including schools, workplaces, and medical visits [1]. Consequently, data use on home internet networks surged by 47% between March 2019 and March 2020 [2]. This digital revolution has introduced numerous new online services associated with positive health and economic outcomes, such as distance education, telemedicine, streamlined job search and application processes, grocery delivery, and online social services [3]. Moreover, remote work, school, and healthcare are not constrained by the same geographic limitations as their traditional counterparts, thus enhancing flexibility and accessibility. However, the millions of Americans without reliable high-speed internet face growing disadvantages related to education, healthcare, and employment, as these new services require broadband access.

As researchers continue to investigate the relationship between broadband and education, employment, and health outcomes, policymakers at all levels of government can leverage their influence to advocate for policies that establish internet access as an essential public utility. Although many of broadband's impacts remain unknown, public acceptance is growing that high-speed internet access extends beyond mere entertainment and communication opportunities. Broadband has emerged as a critical factor in health and economic success in the United States, and many of those without access already face disadvantages related to other social determinants of health [4]. This supports the conclusion that digital equity is inextricably linked to health equity, and ensuring internet access facilitates better social and health outcomes.

Even before the pandemic, national organizations began referring to broadband access as a "super-determinant" of health due to its connection to various known social determinants of health, such as education and employment [5]. It is well-established that improved education and employment prospects contribute to better health outcomes. Studies also demonstrate that a lack of broadband access can negatively impact education and employment opportunities, including by eliminating the possibility of participating in online classrooms and remote work [6]. For instance, an individual who could not attend online school during the pandemic may have fallen behind by one grade or more, delaying their entry into the workforce and their ability to earn an income and secure health insurance. Thus, broadband access can have a disproportionate, indirect impact on an individual's health solely through its influence on other socioeconomic factors.

More recently, broadband access has begun to play a direct role in health equity. Post-pandemic, healthcare services are increasingly moving online, which, in some respects, helps counter health disparities, particularly for those living in rural areas. Telehealth provides these and other disconnected communities with unprecedented access to specialized, chronic, and follow-up care by eliminating geographic barriers. Some local health departments monitor patients and conduct family home visits remotely, in addition to offering other social services. Like schools, public health authorities can use the internet to provide educational resources remotely. Recent studies have quantified the impact of online health services and education by linking broadband access to specific improved health outcomes, such as reduced prevalence of diabetes and smoking and increased consumption of fruit and vegetables [7]. While this research is ongoing, it has prompted examinations of broadband access, affordability, and utilization across socioeconomic groups.

> *"Counties in any quintile of broadband access have on average 9.6% lower diabetes prevalence than those counties in the next lower quintile of access. This change in diabetes prevalence remains when we control for education and income separately or together with age."*
>
> Federal Communications Commission, C2H Research Monograph (2019)

26.2 The Digital Divide: Perpetuating Systemic Inequities

Unfortunately, some communities that could benefit the most from online health and social services lack reliable broadband access, leaving them unable to take advantage of these innovations. Experts refer to this phenomenon as the "digital divide." In America, this issue affects a significant number of people: as of March 2023, the Federal Communications Commission (FCC) estimates that 19 million people in the US lack broadband access. Most of those impacted by the digital divide either live in rural areas or are members of minority groups – such as Blacks, Native Americans, Latinos, and Alaska Natives – living in segregated communities, including Tribal land [8]. The existing inequities experienced by these groups make them particularly vulnerable to the negative consequences of remaining disconnected.

The reasons why the digital divide disproportionately affects rural and minority communities involve both economic incentives and interconnected systemic inequities. Rural communities, in particular, are more expensive and challenging to service [9]. In the United States, broadband access providers have largely completed the "easy" work of connecting densely populated and centralized communities but have not committed to the complex and costly task of building the infrastructure required to make high-speed internet ubiquitous. Minorities living in urban areas, by contrast, may have the option of getting broadband but cannot afford it. Some studies show that minority households are less likely than white households to afford broadband subscriptions, given that they have lower incomes on average [10]. However, lacking broadband access itself can make it more difficult to secure a stable, high-paying job. Inequity can also begin at the student level: children need the internet to succeed in school and to develop the digital skills necessary to be competitive in the job market. Consequently, lacking broadband access perpetuates systemic inequities.

26.3 Lawmakers' Role in Achieving Equitable Broadband Access

Recognizing that broadband access is a crucial social determinant of health, lawmakers must spearhead efforts to achieve equitable internet access in the United States. Progress has been made at the local, state, and federal levels. Some experts have called for studies on the health impacts of broadband and telehealth laws to better inform future decisions by lawmakers, particularly with respect to underserved communities [11]. By prioritizing research and evidence-based policymaking, legislators can work toward bridging the digital divide and ensuring that all Americans have access to the benefits of high-speed internet, ultimately promoting health equity and improved social outcomes.

26.3.1 Federal Efforts to Support Broadband Access and Digital Equity

To date, the federal government has primarily supported broadband access through funding, data collection, and dissemination. In 2021, Congress passed a bipartisan infrastructure law that allocated over $42 billion to states and territories to build internet access. The Department of Commerce's National Telecommunications and Information Administration (NTIA) leads three programs responsible for distributing funding and overseeing broadband projects. The FCC created the National Broadband Map, which provides information about broadband availability in different locations [12]. Users can file challenges with the FCC to add or correct information on the map, while local and state policymakers can use it to identify disconnected communities. Additionally, the FCC runs the Rural Health Care Program, which provides funding for broadband services to expand telehealth access [13]. The Affordable Connectivity Program, created under the Infrastructure Investment and Jobs Act of 2022, directly reduces the cost of broadband services and electronic devices for eligible households [14].

The federal government can also influence broadband access through policy. In 2023, President Biden appointed Anna Gomez as an FCC commissioner; many are hopeful that her confirmation, which gives Democrats a majority on the commission and ended a multi-year deadlock, will lead to greater FCC involvement in digital equity initiatives. The FCC has also argued that the Telecommunications Act of 1996 preempts state laws blocking broadband expansion into rural areas [15]. Although a federal court ruled against this interpretation, Congress could choose to amend the Telecommunications Act or pass another federal law that clearly preempts state laws standing in the way of digital equity. By leveraging both funding and policy, the federal government has the power to drive significant progress in ensuring equitable access to broadband services across the nation.

26.3.2 State-Level Strategies for Promoting Digital Equity

States play a crucial role in digital equity as the primary recipients of federal funding for broadband infrastructure projects. As of 2023, over half of the states have authorities that oversee broadband development. However, states can also hinder digital equity by passing laws that preempt local broadband expansion or impose procedural barriers on such projects. In 2020, the Pew Charitable Trusts (Pew) studied state broadband programs and identified five "promising practices" worthy of replication: stakeholder outreach and engagement; policy framework; planning and capacity building; funding and operations; and program evaluation and evolution [16]. Overall, states tend to find the greatest success when they coordinate with local governments and private parties and commit the time and resources to fostering well-planned broadband projects.

Pew highlighted California's efforts related to stakeholder outreach and engagement [17]. In 2010, the state's legislators created the Broadband Council as a forum for state agency representatives to collaborate on broadband access solutions. The Council is notable for its range of involved stakeholders and task forces, which allow it to provide comprehensive guidance related to broadband access across the state. Participating agencies include the California Emerging Technology Fund, a nonprofit founded in 2005 with $60 million in initial funding dedicated to improving broadband access and affordability. Pew observed that the Fund's existence ensures that underserved people's interests are represented before California lawmakers.

Pew noted that desirable state policy frameworks set goals, define responsibilities, and address the intersection between broadband access and other policy areas [18]. The organization highlighted West Virginia's success in expanding broadband availability through various initiatives, including legislation (e.g. a bill allowing broadband cooperatives, creating a loan guarantee program, and permitting ISPs to use microtrenching technology to install infrastructure) and the state's Broadband Enhancement Council. This board, composed of state legislators, government and agency officials, private citizens, and business representatives, makes policy recommendations and helps communities secure federal and other funding. Crucially, the Council has centered broadband as "critical to the economic future of West Virginia communities," which has unlocked access to various types of federal funding earmarked for economic and community development.

Regarding planning and capacity building, Pew reported on significant regional investments made by Colorado [19]. Importantly, in 2023, Colorado repealed a law requiring local governments to hold referendum votes on proposed broadband provisions. The state's Department of Local Affairs distributes broadband planning grants in two phases. The first phase requires grantees to complete strategic plans for broadband deployment, with mandated participation by providers. This gives regions the opportunity to articulate their goals and assets, aggregate demand, and examine potential solutions. Second, communities interested in additional funding can apply to create more detailed plans. Colorado officials agreed that the strategic plan requirement has resulted in stronger, tailored projects and created opportunities for educating local leaders and involving broadband providers.

For best practices related to funding and operations, Pew highlighted Minnesota's Border-to-Border Broadband Development Grant Program, established in 2014 [20]. As of 2020, 91% of Minnesota households had broadband access at speeds of 25 Mbps/3 Mbps; importantly, Border-to-Border requires that all projects be scalable to provide symmetrical speeds of at least 100 Mbps, building in the potential for future upgrades and avoiding wasting funding on soon-to-be outdated infrastructure. By state statute, Minnesota's Office of Broadband Development (OBD) can provide up to $5 million for as much as half the cost of a broadband infrastructure project. The statute also requires priority for unserved and underserved areas. OBD also gives priority status to projects with strong community support; as a result, grant initiatives often originate with local governments or community groups that partner with local broadband providers.

Finally, Pew stressed the importance of measuring the success of broadband programs against pre-set goals [21]. In addition to helping states calibrate their programs, these determinations can also inform the next steps or lead to a program's expansion into other applications. To illustrate, Pew detailed Tennessee's Economic and Community Development Department, which collects data throughout a grant cycle. Tennessee requires grantees to submit quarterly progress reports, invoices for reimbursement of costs incurred, and project closeout reports and providers to describe digital literacy activities available for customers in the grant area. Tennessee's State Library and Archives also collects data on digital literacy training, including surveys from class attendees. Legislators review annual reports prepared by the Department and use them to evaluate program effectiveness and gaps.

26.3.3 Local Initiatives Addressing Community-Specific Digital Needs

Local broadband initiatives, although narrower in scope compared to state or federal programs, can effectively address acute problems within communities. A prime example is Delta County, Colorado, which experienced economic devastation in the mid-2010s when two coal mining companies that employed nearly 1000 locals closed [22]. At the time, Delta County lacked high-speed internet, making it unattractive to businesses and pushing some employers out. In 2015, Region 10, a local economic development agency, received a state grant to prepare a broadband implementation plan for Delta County. Lightworks Fiber & Consulting, a local family-run business, won the contract to build the broadband network and hired former coal miners to lay fiber-optic cable for the project, demonstrating how local initiatives can not only improve digital infrastructure but also create employment opportunities.

Another example of a community-based initiative is Wimauma Connects, a free internet community initiative in Florida that brings internet access to highly populated but low-income residential communities in Wimauma Village [23]. By focusing on specific local needs, such initiatives can help bridge the digital divide in areas that may be overlooked by larger-scale programs. These targeted efforts showcase the importance of local involvement in addressing the unique challenges faced by individual communities in achieving digital equity [24].

26.4 Conclusion: A Public Value Essential for Health and Economic Equity

Broadband access has emerged as a critical factor in achieving health and economic equity [25]. Recognizing this, many policymakers have taken action through community, state, and federal initiatives, creating funding and programs aimed at making broadband available and affordable for everyone living in America. However, despite these efforts, broadband infrastructure projects are still in progress, and the digital divide remains a serious problem for many rural, low-income, and minority populations [26]. Compounding this issue, some states still have laws that hinder broadband expansion, further exacerbating the inequities faced by these communities [27].

As the importance of digital equity becomes increasingly apparent, now is the time for policymakers to capitalize on the growing interest and momentum surrounding this issue [28]. By establishing high-speed internet access as an essential component of the public values guaranteed and safeguarded by the government, policymakers can ensure that all Americans, regardless of their socioeconomic background or geographic location, have the opportunity to benefit from the vast array of services and resources available online [29]. Addressing the digital divide is not only a matter of fairness but also a crucial step in promoting overall health and economic well-being for the entire nation [30].

Policy and Equity in Broadband Access and Digital Health

Aspect	Details
Broadband as Essential Infrastructure	Broadband is considered essential infrastructure, requiring affordable prices, universal access, and digital skills for a healthy community.
Equity Challenges	Disparities in broadband access persist across states, rural and urban areas, and among different demographic groups, particularly affecting low-income and nonwhite households.
Systemic Barriers	High costs, limited competition among ISPs, and digital skill gaps are major barriers to universal broadband adoption.
Policy Recommendations	Incentivize private investment in underserved areas. Support public broadband networks. Implement direct subsidy programs for affordability. Promote digital literacy through schools, libraries, and nonprofits.
Regulatory Actions	Implement pro-competition policies, enforce ISP service obligations, and support digital inclusion programs through mechanisms like the Community Reinvestment Act.
Community Interventions	Build coalitions with diverse stakeholders. Target institutions that rely on broadband for service delivery. Communicate the importance of broadband in terms policymakers understand. Use measurable impacts to demonstrate broadband's benefits.
Health and Equity Outcomes	Broadband impacts economic stability, education, social supports, and health outcomes by enabling remote healthcare and access to vital information and services.

References

1 Federal Communications Commission (2021). 2021 broadband deployment report. https://docs.fcc.gov/public/attachments/FCC-21-18A1.pdf (accessed 26 August 2024).

2 OpenVault (2020). Broadband insights report (OVBI) 2020. https://openvault.com/ovbi/ (accessed 26 August 2024).

3 Vogels, E.A., Perrin, A., Rainie, L., and Anderson, M. (2020). *53% of Americans Say the Internet Has Been Essential During the COVID-19 Outbreak*. Pew Research Center. https://www.pewresearch.org/internet/2020/04/30/53-of-americans-say-the-internet-has-been-essential-during-the-covid-19-outbreak/.

4 Benda, N.C., Veinot, T.C., Sieck, C.J., and Ancker, J.S. (2020). Broadband internet access is a social determinant of health! *American Journal of Public Health* 110 (8): 1123–1125. https://doi.org/10.2105/AJPH.2020.305784.

5 Bauerly, B.C., McCord, R.F., Hulkower, R., and Pepin, D. (2019). Broadband access as a public health issue: the role of law in expanding broadband access and connecting underserved communities for better health outcomes. *The Journal of Law, Medicine & Ethics* 47 (2_suppl): 39–42. https://doi.org/10.1177/1073110519857314.

6 Hampton, K.N., Fernandez, L., Robertson, C.T., and Bauer, J.M. (2020). Broadband and student performance gaps. James H. and Mary B. Quello Center, Michigan State University. https://quello.msu.edu/wp-content/uploads/2020/03/Broadband_Gap_Quello_Report_MSU.pdf.

7 Reddick, C.G., Enriquez, R., Harris, R.J., and Sharma, B. (2020). Determinants of broadband access and affordability: an analysis of a community survey on the digital divide. *Cities* 106: 102904. https://doi.org/10.1016/j.cities.2020.102904.

8 Tomer, A., Fishbane, L., Siefer, A., and Callahan, B. (2020). *Digital Prosperity: How Broadband Can Deliver Health and Equity to All Communities*. Brookings Institution. https://www.brookings.edu/research/digital-prosperity-how-broadband-can-deliver-health-and-equity-to-all-communities/.

9 Perrin, A. (2019). *Digital Gap Between Rural and Nonrural America Persists*. Pew Research Center. https://www.pewresearch.org/fact-tank/2019/05/31/digital-gap-between-rural-and-nonrural-america-persists/.

10 Dolan, J.E. (2016). Splicing the divide: a review of research on the evolving digital divide among K–12 students. *Journal of Research on Technology in Education* 48 (1): 16–37. https://doi.org/10.1080/15391523.2015.1103147.

11 Frist, B. (2020). COVID-19 and the importance of a national broadband policy. *The Journal of Law, Medicine & Ethics* 48 (2): 206–207. https://doi.org/10.1177/1073110520935333.

12 Federal Communications Commission (2022). National broadband map. https://broadbandmap.fcc.gov/ (accessed 26 August 2024).

13 Federal Communications Commission (2021). Rural health care program. https://www.fcc.gov/general/rural-health-care-program (accessed 26 August 2024).

14 Federal Communications Commission (2022). Affordable connectivity program. https://www.fcc.gov/acp (accessed 26 August 2024).

15 Atkinson, R.D. (2021). *How State and Local Governments Can Use Federal Funds to Spur Equitable Broadband Deployment*. Information Technology and Innovation Foundation. https://itif.org/publications/2021/06/23/how-state-and-local-governments-can-use-federal-funds-spur-equitable.

16 Pew Charitable Trusts (2020). How states are expanding broadband access. https://www.pewtrusts.org/en/research-and-analysis/reports/2020/02/how-states-are-expanding-broadband-access (accessed 26 August 2024).

17 California Broadband Council (2020). Broadband action plan 2020. https://broadbandcouncil.ca.gov/wp-content/uploads/sites/68/2020/12/BB4All-Action-Plan-Final-Draft-v26.pdf

18 West Virginia Broadband Enhancement Council (2020). West Virginia state broadband plan 2020-2025. https://broadband.wv.gov/wp-content/uploads/2020/01/West_Virginia_State_Broadband_Plan_2020-2025.pdf.

19 Colorado Broadband Office (2024). History. https://broadband.colorado.gov/about-the-cbo

20 Minnesota Office of Broadband Development (2021). Border-to-border broadband development grant program. https://mn.gov/deed/programs-services/broadband/grant-program/ (accessed 26 August 2024).

21 Tennessee Department of Economic and Community Development (2020). Tennessee broadband accessibility grant program: program guidelines. https://www.tn.gov/ecd/rural-development/tennessee-broadband-grant-initiative/tnecd-broadband-accessibility-grant.html

22 Region 10 League for Economic Assistance and Planning (2017). Region 10 Broadband. https://region10.net/broadband-partnerships/.

23 Muñoz, M., Pangelinan, J., and Blackmon, H. (2021). Wimauma connects: a case study of a rural broadband initiative. *The Journal of Community Informatics* 17: 1–19. https://doi.org/10.15353/joci.v17i.3701.

24 Ali, C. (2020). The politics of good enough: rural broadband and policy failure in the United States. *International Journal of Communication* 14: 5982–6004. https://ijoc.org/index.php/ijoc/article/view/14799.

25 Khullar, D. and Chokshi, D.A. (2018). *Health, Income, & Poverty: Where We Are & What Could Help.* Health Affairs Health Policy Brief. https://doi.org/10.1377/hpb20180817.901935.

26 Rodriguez-Lonebear, D., Barceló, N.E., Akee, R., and Carroll, S.R. (2020). American Indian Reservations and COVID-19: correlates of early infection rates in the pandemic. *Journal of Public Health Management and Practice* 26 (4): 371–377. https://doi.org/10.1097/PHH.0000000000001206.

27 Strover, S. (2020). Reaching rural America with broadband internet service. *The Conversation.* https://theconversation.com/reaching-rural-america-with-broadband-internet-service-82488.

28 Horrigan, J. B. (2019). Reaching the Unconnected: Benefits for Kids and Schoolwork Drive Broadband Subscriptions, But Digital Skills Training Opens Doors to Household Internet Use for Jobs and Learning. Technology Policy Institute. https://techpolicyinstitute.org/wp-content/uploads/2019/08/Horrigan_Reaching-the-Unconnected.pdf.

29 Prieger, J.E. (2013). The broadband digital divide and the economic benefits of mobile broadband for rural areas. *Telecommunications Policy* 37 (6–7): 483–502.

30 LaRose, R., Gregg, J.L., Strover, S. et al. (2007). Closing the rural broadband gap: promoting adoption of the Internet in rural America. *Telecommunications Policy* 31 (6–7): 359–373. https://doi.org/10.1016/j.telpol.2007.04.004.

27

Expanding Vaccine Equity: Policy Strategies

Abstract

This chapter explores the complex issue of vaccine inequity, examining its root causes, disproportionate impact on vulnerable populations, and government efforts to address these disparities. It delves into the factors contributing to inequitable vaccine access, including socioeconomic disparities, systemic racism, healthcare gaps, and historical mistrust. The chapter discusses how these inequities lead to lower vaccination rates and worse health outcomes among disadvantaged communities. The chapter examines the government's response to vaccine inequity, highlighting the successes and challenges of existing policies and the need for more targeted measures. It explores proposed solutions and global efforts, such as increasing investments in underserved communities, improving vaccine rollout strategies, enhancing data collection, and fostering global cooperation. The role of federalism in vaccine inequity is analyzed, focusing on how the decentralized US public health system can hinder equitable responses across states. The chapter also addresses the importance of data in understanding health disparities and the challenges posed by data gaps. Finally, the chapter concludes with a call to action, emphasizing the federal government's critical role in reducing vaccine inequities and ensuring equal access to vaccines. By learning from the COVID-19 pandemic and adopting a holistic approach to health equity, significant progress can be made in protecting the health and well-being of all Americans.

Keywords   *vaccine equity; COVID-19 vaccine; health disparities; systemic racism; federal policies; socioeconomic barriers; access to healthcare; data collection gaps*

> *Kendra, a single mother from a low-income neighborhood, anxiously refreshed her web browser, trying to secure a COVID-19 vaccine appointment for her elderly father. Despite her best efforts, the complex online registration system and limited access to reliable internet made it nearly impossible to find an available slot. Kendra worried that her father, who faced a higher risk of severe illness due to his age and underlying health conditions, might contract the virus before he could get vaccinated.*

> *James, a rural farm worker, received conflicting information about the safety and effectiveness of the COVID-19 vaccine from his co-workers and social media. With limited access to healthcare providers and trusted sources of information, James was unsure whether to get vaccinated. His hesitancy stemmed from a long history of medical mistreatment and experimentation on communities of color, which had eroded trust in the healthcare system.*

27.1 Vaccine Inequity: Disparities in Access and Health Outcomes

Vaccine inequity is a significant issue that disproportionately affects communities of color and other disadvantaged groups. Scholars argue that vaccines, like other health innovations, can initially widen the gap between the rich and the poor, even though inequality tends to subside as access increases over time [1]. Inequitable access to vaccines is exacerbated by various factors, including education, income, and wealth disparities; job access and working conditions; systemic racism and discrimination; gaps in healthcare access; transportation and neighborhood conditions; and a lack of trust stemming from historical medical racism and experimentation [2].

These factors not only contribute to lower vaccination rates among certain groups but also make racial and ethnic minorities more susceptible to severe illness and death from COVID-19. Surveillance data from the early months of COVID-19 vaccination has consistently shown lower vaccination rates in communities of color, while these same communities have been more likely to experience COVID-19-related hospitalization, morbidity, and mortality, highlighting the inequitable access to vaccines [3].

Various definitions are used to identify populations who may have inequitable access to vaccines, including protected classes under the Civil Rights Act of 1964, individuals with disabilities, those experiencing health disparities, individuals with access and functional needs, and communities identified by the CDC/ATSDR Social Vulnerability Index (SVI) [4]. During the COVID-19 pandemic, the CDC recommended that states use the SVI to identify communities at greater risk of unequal access to COVID-19 vaccination. The SVI takes into account variables such as socioeconomic status, household composition and disability, minority status and language, and housing type and transportation to measure the risk of inequity.

Researchers studying the "inverse equity hypothesis" argue that healthcare innovations, such as vaccines, can amplify inequality [5]. New health technologies are often limited in supply and only accessible to the wealthy initially. As supply increases and exceeds the demand of the wealthy and middle-income individuals, poor people begin to gain access to the technology. This delayed access creates health status gaps between the rich and the poor, which often align with racial disparities in wealth and healthcare. Consequently, racial and ethnic minorities are the most disadvantaged by vaccine inequity [6].

Vaccine inequity among racial and ethnic minorities was evident during the COVID-19 vaccine rollout. The government managed the limited vaccine availability by conducting vaccine distribution in phases, targeting populations at higher risk of contracting COVID-19 or facing serious health outcomes. This phased approach disproportionately limited access to the vaccine for certain racial and ethnic groups. As the vaccine became more widely available, disparities narrowed, but disadvantaged communities still had lower vaccination rates and remained at higher risk during the early phases of the rollout [7]. Data shows that white people accessed COVID-19 vaccinations at rates exceeding their share of cases, while Black and Hispanic people were vaccinated at lower rates [8].

COVID-19 vaccine inequity was not limited to the priorities set in the vaccine rollout; the method of accessing vaccines once they were available also disadvantaged certain groups. Some researchers suggest that voluntary opt-in approaches can increase inequality, as the COVID-19 vaccine requires individuals to seek out the vaccine rather than bringing vaccines to them [9]. Personal barriers, such as financial constraints or lack of information, may prevent people from seeking out the vaccine. Financial constraints could include the inability to afford losing paid work to get the vaccine or rest due to its side effects.

Physical access is also an issue, as some people may not have a car and would face difficulties getting to vaccine centers if they are not accessible by public transportation. Other factors that can create barriers include a lack of internet access, preventing online appointment scheduling, as well as age or language barriers that may make scheduling appointments more challenging. Beyond the limitations to access discussed above, other factors not unique to COVID-19 can also prevent access. For example, a report documented access problems for childhood vaccines among children covered by Medicaid or living in rural areas [10].

While the discussion above primarily focuses on vaccine inequity in the United States, another important area of inequity is that among countries. During the COVID-19 pandemic, some scholars described the policies around COVID-19 vaccines as "vaccine apartheid" [11]. The recommendations discussed in this text aim to address both types of inequities.

> *Vaccine equity was "not rocket science, nor charity. It is smart public health and in everyone's best interest."*
> Former Dr. Tedros Adhanom Ghebreyesus, the Director-General of the World Health Organization

27.2 Government Efforts to Address Vaccine Inequity: Successes and Challenges

The government employs various laws, policies, and regulatory tools to address vaccine-related inequities. Prior to the COVID-19 pandemic, policies were already in place to protect certain groups from discrimination during public health emergencies. Throughout the COVID-19 crisis, the government utilized funding, communication, and educational resources to tackle vaccine inequity and raise awareness and confidence in vaccines. However, despite these efforts, some populations continue to be disproportionately harmed, prompting experts to recommend additional actions.

The government has several tools at its disposal to track data on vulnerable communities and reduce disparities in access to resources like vaccines during public health emergencies. The CDC utilizes the SVI to assess the potential negative effects on communities caused by external stresses on human health [12]. In addition to data tracking, federal laws such as the Civil Rights Act, Rehabilitation Act, Homeland Security Act, Patient Protection and Affordable Care Act, and Stafford Act include provisions prohibiting discrimination or restricting funding of state and local government programs to those that ensure the protection of certain populations. During the COVID-19 pandemic, the federal government provided specific funding for organizations that target and improve vaccine equity efforts for racial and ethnic minority groups.

Furthermore, the federal government established dedicated offices and policies to address inequity. For example, the Health and Human Services (HHS) Office of Minority Health develops health policies and programs to eliminate health disparities among racial and ethnic minority communities [13]. Several pandemic-specific authorities, entities, and policies were created to address vaccine inequities during COVID-19. Notably, the COVID-19 Health Equity Task Force provides specific recommendations to the President regarding resource allocation, distribution of relief funding, communications, and other mitigation strategies to help protect access to vaccines for at-risk and minority communities [14].

Federal Anti-discrimination Guidelines for COVID-19 Vaccination Programs[a]

Category	Policy Area	Details
Legal and Regulatory Framework	Legal Framework	Title VI of the Civil Rights Act of 1964 and Section 1557 of the Affordable Care Act ensure nondiscriminatory practices in federally assisted healthcare, promoting equitable vaccine access regardless of race, color, or national origin
	Presidential Directives	Executive Order 13995 mandates federal agencies to ensure equitable allocation of pandemic resources, including vaccines, and to enforce anti-discrimination laws vigorously
Disparities and Equity	Disparities in COVID-19 Impact	Recognizes that people of color experience disproportionately higher COVID-19 infection and mortality rates and encounter more significant barriers to accessing healthcare and vaccinations
	Contributing Factors to Disparities	Identifies factors causing health disparities such as socioeconomic challenges, overrepresentation in essential jobs, and dependence on public transportation, which increase exposure risks and hinder healthcare access
Enforcement and Compliance	Enforcement of Nondiscrimination	The Office for Civil Rights (OCR) enforces nondiscrimination within healthcare, ensuring fair vaccine distribution and preventing policies that disproportionately affect specific racial or ethnic groups
Operational Guidance	Guidance for Equitable Access	Offers guidelines to prevent discrimination in vaccine distribution, advising on the accessibility of vaccination sites and the availability of multilingual registration information
	Best Practices for Vaccine Access	Suggests collaborating with community organizations to enhance trust and outreach, ensuring language inclusivity in vaccine communications, and overcoming technological barriers to online access

[a] Adapted from Office for Civil Rights, U.S. Department of Health and Human Services (2021, December 20).

While the focus here is on the United States, it is essential to discuss a few crucial issues. There have been several global initiatives aimed at providing vaccine access across the globe, but more could be done. Providing access to vaccines in other countries is not always motivated by a desire to address equity or even for humane reasons; in a globalized world, infectious diseases can travel. Therefore, more contagious diseases that can spread to rich countries encourage an interest in achieving global coverage. The smallpox eradication program was a global collaboration aimed at combating a highly dangerous airborne virus that could travel, and the World Health Organization (WHO) and member states worked together to address it [15]. In 1988, the WHO adopted a polio eradication initiative that had substantial, albeit incomplete, success [16]. In 2012, the WHO endorsed a goal of eliminating measles and rubella across five world regions. Similarly, for COVID-19, collaboration efforts have been made, but they, too, have encountered obstacles.

27.3 Addressing Persistent Vaccine Inequities: Proposed Solutions and Global Efforts

Despite the advances made in addressing vaccine inequity, significant gaps persist in vaccine access both within the United States and globally. The current efforts, while commendable, are insufficient to fully resolve the equity problem. A substantial body of literature examines potential solutions to bridge these gaps and ensure equitable access to vaccines for all [17].

One proposed approach is to increase investments aimed at expanding equitable vaccine access [18]. For instance, a state health administrator emphasized the importance of making "disproportionate investments" in communities of color, describing it as critical in trying to get equitable outcomes through vaccine allocation [19]. By dedicating more resources to underserved communities, the disparities in vaccine distribution can be addressed more effectively.

Another suggested solution focuses on improving vaccine rollout strategies. Scholars have identified several categories of federal regulatory options that could enhance equity from the outset of vaccine rollout [20]. These include providing specific guidance regarding equity goals and obligations, offering default equity plans for state adoption, collecting equity outcome data, publicly disseminating and ranking state equity outcomes, and facilitating information sharing among states. Equity directives should explicitly address race, ethnicity, and social vulnerability in their guidance. Default equity plans would require states to submit a plan to the CDC for evaluation of its equity-enhancing factors, or the federal government could propose a default plan that states can opt into or modify. Compliance could be enforced by tying federal funding to the implementation of these equity plans, which would be designed to encourage transparency and accountability.

To further enhance equity, data collection efforts could be strengthened by having the federal government increase and refine data collection on race and ethnicity. Once the federal government improves data on equity-related outcomes, the CDC should report the data on a state-by-state basis to encourage transparency through the comparison and ranking of states. This would not only hold states accountable for their performance but also motivate them to improve their equity outcomes. Additionally, establishing a platform for states and localities to share strategies and best practices for improving equity would facilitate the flow of information and enable the development of evidence-based approaches to promote equitable vaccine distribution [21].

On a global scale, Médecins Sans Frontières (Doctors Without Borders) has called for a comprehensive response to promote vaccine equity worldwide [22]. Their proposal emphasizes the need to raise funds to support the rollout of vaccines, facilitate global vaccine distribution, avoid vaccine nationalism, share COVID-19 health technology-related knowledge and data, and ensure full transparency around the distribution and development of COVID-19 vaccines. By adopting a coordinated and collaborative approach, the international community can work together to ensure that vaccines are accessible to all, regardless of their country of residence or socioeconomic status.

27.4 Federalism and Vaccine Inequity: Challenges, Criticisms, and Federal Efforts

Vaccine-related disparities impact various demographic groups, including those based on geographic location. Federalism contributes to the complications arising from vaccine disparities across the country, as nonuniform approaches to public health emergencies hinder equitable responses across state lines. For instance, requiring countermeasures in some states but not others leads to a fragmented response.

Federalism places states and territories in the lead for most exercises of public health authority, meaning that control over public health measures is historically a state police power, and the federal government does not typically impose nationwide policies [23]. In the context of COVID-19 vaccinations, the federal government made recommendations (not requirements) for vaccine priority groups, but ultimately, state and local governments designated vaccine priority groups in their respective jurisdictions. This led to different priority groups being recognized in different places, which may have contributed to appearances of inequity. To avoid this type of inequity in future public health emergencies, we can use incentives to ensure equity across states.

However, priorities were not the only issue. State and local governments sought to distribute the vaccine rapidly and, in doing so, relied on information and technology infrastructures that failed to mitigate inequities. The government used systems that depended on the internet for sign-ups and based vaccine allocation on demand. Communities of color, low-income communities, and rural communities are less likely to have access to the internet and may not have the knowledge or time to complete the vaccine appointment sign-up process [24]. Access to vaccination sites was also a potential barrier for at-risk communities. Language barriers, transportation, and physical access are all factors that should have been considered as part of the pandemic response and vaccine rollout [25]. Additionally, while some states offered paid leave for workers taking time off to get vaccinated and those suffering from vaccine side effects, many did not, which would be a serious barrier for workers who cannot afford to lose paid work time.

Some states specifically designed the later phases of their vaccination rollout plans to reach communities that had lower vaccination rates relative to the general population [26]. While some scholars argue that this approach likely helped address inequities, it also highlights the disadvantage these populations faced in the early vaccine rollout phases. While acknowledging systemic injustice and the history that led to it is important, the government is right when it acts to prioritize access for previously underserved groups. However, the government needs to work with community leaders to do so effectively.

Another recommended strategy for the federal government is to partner with neighborhood and nonprofit groups, community providers, and faith-based organizations to encourage outreach and access for disadvantaged groups [27]. Because federal systems have a comparative advantage in collecting and rapidly analyzing data, publicizing information with credibility, disseminating expertise through guidance, enforcing civil rights violations, and supporting information networks, partnerships are an effective way to funnel resources to groups that can facilitate outreach efforts to vulnerable communities.

Scholars criticized the federal government for not utilizing its existing authority and influence to address vaccine inequity during the COVID-19 vaccine rollout. Although states control most public health policy, the federal government purchases the vaccines available in the United States, giving it more authority in directing the use of vaccines, including requiring providers to agree to vaccinate according to priority groups. Some argue that the federal government could have been more active early on in the COVID-19 vaccine rollout to improve equity by providing different incentives or giving more specific guidance to take equity into account when creating priority groups. However, it is important to note that direct race-based distribution would run afoul of our constitutional equal protections as they stand, but allocation based on proxies, such as neighborhoods with high rates of COVID-19 infection, likely would not.

Despite criticisms of the patchwork vaccine rollout at the state level, the federal government did take some steps to address vaccine inequity. The Federal Emergency Management Agency established the Civil Rights Advisory Group to help ensure equity in the allocation of scarce resources, including ensuring that Community Vaccine Centers in the Federal pilot program are located in areas that help serve historically disenfranchised and vulnerable populations [28]. Additionally, the CDC has targeted $3.5 billion in funding to address inequities in vaccine administration [29]. Recipients of this grant money must tailor their vaccination programs to accommodate various groups to enhance accessibility and inclusivity. These groups include racial and ethnic minority groups, specifically non-Hispanic American Indians, Alaska Natives, non-Hispanic Blacks, and Hispanics. Additionally, the programs should focus on those living in communities with a high SVI, as well as those residing in rural areas. Other target groups include individuals with disabilities, those who are homebound or isolated, the underinsured or uninsured, immigrants and/or refugees, and individuals facing transportation limitations.

27.5 Data Gaps: Hindering Efforts to Address Vaccine Inequities

While the federal system may have posed a disadvantage for unifying response efforts to reduce vaccine inequity across the country, it was not the sole barrier contributing to this problem. Another significant challenge that hinders the government's ability to understand and address healthcare inequities is the presence of data gaps.

The COVID-19 Health Equity Task Force specifically addressed the need for better information about health disparities, noting that data gaps impede efforts to help at-risk and underserved communities [30]. Data on certain groups may be incomplete or obscured, making it more challenging to identify and address healthcare inequities affecting these populations. This lack of comprehensive data can lead to an underestimation of the true extent of the disparities and, consequently, an inadequate response to mitigate them.

Despite its efforts, the Department of HHS faces difficulties in collecting data on characteristics that demonstrate disparities. One of the primary reasons for this challenge is that individuals are not required to self-report information, and they often choose not to provide the information on a voluntary basis. This reluctance to share personal data may be even more pronounced among people who have good historical reasons to mistrust the government, further exacerbating the data gaps.

Moreover, privacy laws and infrastructure gaps that impede data sharing create additional barriers to accessing information on disparities. While there are various proposals to improve data collection to better serve communities, until these initiatives become effective, the data gaps remain a significant challenge during public health emergencies [31]. Without better data, proposals to improve equity and access to vaccines may fall short of their intended goals, as they may not accurately identify or target the communities most in need of assistance.

To address these data gaps, the government must work to build trust with communities that have historically been marginalized or mistreated, encouraging them to participate in data collection efforts by ensuring their privacy and demonstrating how the information will be used to improve their health outcomes. Additionally, investing in infrastructure and technology that facilitates secure data sharing between agencies and organizations can help bridge the gaps in information and provide a more comprehensive picture of health disparities.

Furthermore, collaboration between the federal government, state and local authorities, and community organizations is crucial in identifying and reaching out to underserved populations. By leveraging the knowledge and trust that community organizations have built with their constituents, the government can gather more accurate and complete data on health disparities, even in the absence of self-reported information.

27.6 Conclusion: Addressing Vaccine Inequity: Lessons, Strategies, and a Call to Action

Vaccine inequity poses a grave threat to vulnerable groups, putting them at higher risk of severe illness or death from vaccine-preventable diseases. Despite federal regulatory tools aimed at broadening access, the problem persists, indicating the need for more comprehensive and targeted measures.

The COVID-19 pandemic has highlighted stark inequities in vaccine distribution and the disproportionate impact on vulnerable populations. The federal government must learn from this experience and improve data collection, programs, and policies to better serve these communities and promote vaccine equity nationwide.

Prioritizing granular data collection and analysis will help identify disparities and inform targeted interventions. Strengthening partnerships with community-based organizations and local leaders can help overcome barriers and develop culturally sensitive strategies to increase vaccine uptake.

Addressing vaccine inequity requires a holistic approach that recognizes the broader context of health disparities, structural racism, and socioeconomic disadvantage. Investing in policies and programs that promote health equity is crucial.

In conclusion, the federal government plays a critical role in reducing vaccine inequities and ensuring equal access to life-saving vaccines. By learning from the COVID-19 pandemic, improving data collection, strengthening local partnerships, and adopting a holistic approach to health equity, the government can make significant strides in protecting the health and well-being of all Americans.

References

1 Wouters, O.J., Shadlen, K.C., Salcher-Konrad, M. et al. (2021). Challenges in ensuring global access to COVID-19 vaccines: production, affordability, allocation, and deployment. *Lancet (London, England)* 397 (10278): 1023–1034. https://doi.org/10.1016/S0140-6736(21)00306-8.

2 Privor-Dumm, L., Excler, J.L., Gilbert, S. et al. (2023). Vaccine access, equity and justice: COVID-19 vaccines and vaccination. *BMJ Global Health* 8 (6): e011881. https://doi.org/10.1136/bmjgh-2023-011881.

3 Nguyen, L.H., Joshi, A.D., Drew, D.A. et al. (2021). Racial and ethnic differences in COVID-19 vaccine hesitancy and uptake. medRxiv.

4 Song, J., South, E., Solomon, S., and Wiebe, D. (2021). Injustices in pandemic vulnerability: a spatial-statistical analysis of the CDC Social Vulnerability Index and COVID-19 outcomes in the US. medRxiv, 2021-05.

5 Todd, A. and Bambra, C. (2021). Learning from past mistakes? The COVID-19 vaccine and the inverse equity hypothesis. *European Journal of Public Health* 31 (1): 2.

6 Wrigley-Field, E., Kiang, M.V., Riley, A.R. et al. (2021). Geographically targeted COVID-19 vaccination is more equitable and averts more deaths than age-based thresholds alone. *Science Advances* 7 (40): eabj2099. https://doi.org/10.1126/sciadv.abj2099.

7 Choi, K.H., Denice, P.A., and Ramaj, S. (2021). Vaccine and COVID-19 trajectories. *Socius* 7: 23780231211052946.

8 Siegel, M., Critchfield-Jain, I., Boykin, M. et al. (2022). Racial/ethnic disparities in state-level COVID-19 vaccination rates and their association with structural racism. *Journal of Racial and Ethnic Health Disparities* 9 (6): 2361–2374.

9 Weintraub, R.L., Subramanian, L., Karlage, A. et al. (2021). COVID-19 vaccine to vaccination: why leaders must invest in delivery strategies now: analysis describe lessons learned from past pandemics and vaccine campaigns about the path to successful vaccine delivery for COVID-19. *Health Affairs* 40 (1): 33–41.

10 Blewett, L.A., Davidson, G., Bramlett, M.D. et al. (2008). The impact of gaps in health insurance coverage on immunization status for young children. *Health Services Research* 43 (5 Pt 1): 1619–1636. https://doi.org/10.1111/j.1475-6773.2008.00864.x.

11 Figueroa, J.P., Hotez, P.J., Batista, C. et al. (2021). Achieving global equity for COVID-19 vaccines: Stronger international partnerships and greater advocacy and solidarity are needed. *PLoS Medicine* 18 (9): e1003772. https://doi.org/10.1371/journal.pmed.1003772.

12 Nayak, A., Islam, S.J., Mehta, A. et al. (2020). Impact of social vulnerability on COVID-19 incidence and outcomes in the United States. medRxiv, 2020-04.

13 Koh, H.K., Graham, G., and Glied, S.A. (2011). Reducing racial and ethnic disparities: the action plan from the department of health and human services. *Health Affairs* 30 (10): 1822–1829.

14 Kahn, B., Brown, L., Foege, W., and Gayle, H. (ed.) (2020). *Framework for Equitable Allocation of COVID-19 Vaccine*. National Academies Press.

15 Bhattacharya, S. and Campani, C.E.D.A.P. (2020). Re-assessing the foundations: worldwide smallpox eradication, 1957–67. *Medical History* 64 (1): 71–93.

16 Closser, S., Neel, A.H., Gerber, S., and Alonge, O. (2024). From legacy to integration in the global polio eradication initiative: looking back to look forward. *BMJ Global Health* 9 (5): e014758.

17 Singh, B. and Chattu, V.K. (2021). Prioritizing 'equity' in COVID-19 vaccine distribution through global health diplomacy. *Health Promotion Perspective* 11 (3): 281–287. https://doi.org/10.34172/hpp.2021.36.

18 Dzau, V.J., Balatbat, C.A., and Offodile, A.C. (2022). Closing the global vaccine equity gap: equitably distributed manufacturing. *The Lancet* 399 (10339): 1924–1926.

19 Saha, M. (2022). *Designing Interactive Data-Driven Tools for Understanding Urban Accessibility at Scale.* University of Washington.

20 Schmidt, H., Weintraub, R., Williams, M.A. et al. (2020). Equitable allocation of COVID-19 vaccines: an analysis of the initial allocation plans of CDC's jurisdictions with implications for disparate impact monitoring. https://scholarship.law.georgetown.edu/facpub/2333/

21 Dada, D., Djiometio, J.N., McFadden, S.M. et al. (2022). Strategies that promote equity in COVID-19 vaccine uptake for black communities: a review. *Journal of Urban Health* 99 (1): 15–27.

22 Pilkington, V., Keestra, S.M., and Hill, A. (2022). Global COVID-19 vaccine inequity: failures in the first year of distribution and potential solutions for the future. *Frontiers in Public Health* 10: 821117.

23 Hodge, J.G. Jr. (1997). The role of new federalism and public health law. *JL Healthcare* 12: 309.

24 Njoku, A., Joseph, M., and Felix, R. (2021). Changing the narrative: structural barriers and racial and ethnic inequities in COVID-19 vaccination. *International Journal of Environmental Research and Public Health* 18 (18): 9904.

25 Knights, F., Carter, J., Deal, A. et al. (2021). Impact of COVID-19 on migrants' access to primary care and implications for vaccine roll-out: a national qualitative study. *British Journal of General Practice* 71 (709): e583–e595.

26 Jean-Jacques, M. and Bauchner, H. (2021). Vaccine distribution – equity left behind? *JAMA* 325 (9): 829–830.

27 Heinrichs, A., Megibow, E., Taylor, A. et al. (2023). Advancing Vaccine Equity Through Community-Based Organizations. https://www.urban.org/sites/default/files/2023-07/Advancing%20Vaccine%20Equity%20 through%20Community-Based%20Organizations.pdf

28 Hick, J.L., Hanfling, D., Wynia, M.K., and Toner, E. (2021). Crisis standards of care and COVID-19: what did we learn? How do we ensure equity? What should we do? *NAM Perspectives* 2021.

29 Fiebelkorn, A.P., Adelsberg, S., Anthony, R. et al. (2024). The role of funded partnerships in working towards decreasing COVID-19 vaccination disparities, United States, March 2021–December 2022. *Vaccine.*

30 Lin, J.S., Webber, E.M., Bean, S.I., and Evans, C.V. (2024). Development of a health equity framework for the US preventive services task force. *JAMA Network Open* 7 (3): –e241875.

31 Zhang, H. and Shaw, R. (2020). Identifying research trends and gaps in the context of COVID-19. *International Journal of Environmental Research and Public Health* 17 (10): 3370.

28

Disaggregating Data: Unveiling the Diversity and Disparities Within the AAPI Population

Abstract

This chapter explores the complexity and importance of disaggregating data for Asian Americans and Pacific Islanders (AAPI) in the United States. It begins by discussing the historical context of the term "Asian American" and the diversity within the AAPI population, which encompasses over 20 million people from various countries and regions, speaking more than 100 languages. The chapter then delves into the problems associated with data aggregation, which can obscure significant differences among AAPI subgroups, particularly in terms of economic status and health outcomes. This aggregation of data contributes to the perpetuation of the Model Minority Myth, masking the disparities and challenges faced by different AAPI communities. The chapter then examines the inconsistent approach to data disaggregation at the federal level, contrasting it with state-led initiatives in California, New York, Massachusetts, Rhode Island, and Washington. These states have taken steps to mandate the collection and reporting of disaggregated data for AAPI subgroups, recognizing the importance of understanding the unique needs and experiences of each community. The chapter also discusses the barriers to data disaggregation, including concerns about sample sizes and opposition from some AAPI communities. Proponents of data disaggregation argue that oversampling and the proper use of disaggregated data would be beneficial in addressing inequities and acknowledging the differences among AAPI subgroups. Finally, the chapter concludes by emphasizing the imperative for data disaggregation in order to accurately assess the standing of all AAPI subgroups and develop targeted policies to improve the lives of AAPI community members. Despite the challenges and opposition, the chapter argues that the benefits of data disaggregation far outweigh the potential drawbacks, making it an essential tool for promoting equity and inclusivity within the diverse AAPI population.

Keywords *AAPI data disaggregation; model minority myth; health disparities; socioeconomic diversity; federal and state initiatives; sample size challenges; community opposition*

> *Priya, an Indian American software engineer, found herself lumped into the "model minority" stereotype, with her colleagues assuming she came from a wealthy background. In reality, Priya's parents struggled to make ends meet, and she had to work multiple jobs to pay for her education. The aggregated data on Asian American success stories masked the challenges faced by many Indian Americans like Priya.*

Achieving Health Equity: The Role of Law and Policy, First Edition. Y. Tony Yang.
© 2025 John Wiley & Sons Ltd. Published 2025 by John Wiley & Sons Ltd.

> *Kai, a Hmong American high school student, struggled to find mental health resources that catered to his community's unique needs. The lack of disaggregated data on the Hmong population made it difficult for policymakers to allocate resources effectively, leaving students like Kai without the support they needed to thrive.*
>
> *Leilani, a Native Hawaiian single mother, found herself struggling to access healthcare services due to language barriers and cultural differences. Despite the high rates of diabetes and heart disease among Native Hawaiians, the aggregated data on Asian American health outcomes painted a misleading picture of overall well-being, leaving communities like Leilani's underserved and overlooked.*

28.1 Diversity and Disparity: The Complexity of AAPI Data Aggregation

Before the 1960s, the term "Oriental" was used to describe all individuals of Asian descent. However, in 1968, a protest led by a Japanese-born student resulted in the adoption of the term "Asian American." Currently, the United States Census Bureau defines "Asian" as "persons having origins in any of the original peoples of the Far East, Southeast Asia, or the Indian subcontinent," while "Native Hawaiian or other Pacific Islander" refers to "persons having origins in any of the original peoples of Hawaii, Guam, Samoa, or other Pacific Islands." AAPI constitute the largest and fastest-growing racial group in the United States [1].

The Asian American population, which numbers approximately 20 million, originates from various countries and regions worldwide [2]. These include China (accounting for the largest percentage at 24%), the Philippines, India, Vietnam, Korea, Japan, and other countries in Asia. Additionally, the largely stateless Hmong people, primarily refugees from the Laos region, are also included. By 2065, the Asian American population is projected to nearly triple to 62 million people [3]. The AAPI community encompasses over 100 spoken languages and exhibits significant diversity in religious practices, languages, and healthcare beliefs, making it comprised of the most diverse of minoritized populations [4].

Despite the vast diversity within the AAPI population, data is often aggregated for collection and analysis purposes [5]. Aggregation involves "pooling together" data from different subgroups to generate summary findings for the overall group. While aggregation can be necessary, it requires a certain level of homogeneity among the aggregated subgroups. If subgroups differ substantially, data aggregation can obscure important differences [6]. Examining median annual household income reveals that the AAPI population lacks the necessary homogeneity for accurate data aggregation.

In 2015, the median annual AAPI household income was $73,060, which appears to suggest that the AAPI population is economically well-off compared to the median annual income for all United States households ($53,600) [7]. However, median annual household incomes for Bangladeshi ($49,800), Hmong ($48,000), Nepalese ($43,500), and Burmese ($36,000) populations were all below the national average. The disparity is so significant that the highest-paid AAPI worker earns six times as much as the lowest-paid AAPI worker, a ratio greater than any other racial or ethnic group in the United States [8]. Relying on aggregated data, such as median annual household income, can lead to the

"Model Minority Myth," which will be discussed later. This example demonstrates how aggregated data can provide a significantly narrowed and potentially misleading picture of the AAPI population's economic reality.

> *"Asian American communities and populations experience a wide range of different health disparities. We must unpack them with disaggregated granular data that can guide us with meaningful policy recommendations and practices."*
>
> Grace Ma, PhD, Founding Director, Center for Asian Health, Katz School of Medicine, Temple University

28.2 Model Minority Myth: Masking AAPI Health Disparities Through Aggregation

The term "model minority" refers to a minority group perceived as particularly successful, especially in a manner that contrasts with other minority groups [9]. The AAPI population is often seen as a model minority due to their apparent success in various aspects of life, such as academics and socioeconomics. However, as discussed below, data aggregation practices contribute to the perception of AAPI persons as the model minority, obscuring the more complex reality. The Model Minority Myth also poses other dangers, including the creation of rifts among minority groups [10].

Notably, the Model Minority Myth has been used to praise the AAPI population and its "success" in the United States while simultaneously denigrating Black Americans for their "failures." Proponents of the myth argue that the AAPI population succeeds through hard work, strong familial relationships, and adherence to rules [6]. They then claim that if Black Americans followed the same path, they too could succeed like the AAPI population. However, this perspective ignores the more pervasive and systematic discrimination faced by Black Americans [11]. Some critics argue that the myth can be used to avoid any responsibility for addressing racism or the damage it continues to inflict. Commentators also note that the Model Minority Myth erases the long history of racism that the AAPI community has faced for centuries [6], such as the 1871 Chinese Massacre in California, the Chinese Exclusion Act of 1882, and the internment of Japanese Americans during World War II [12].

Most importantly, data aggregation drives the Model Minority Myth, which significantly impacts the health of the AAPI population. Despite the myth, Asian Americans experience the highest language barriers compared to other racial groups, with Limited English Proficiency (LEP) highly correlated with medication noncompliance and inconsistent healthcare access [13]. Racial profiling of AAPI community members is also associated with poorer health outcomes [14]. Within the AAPI community, there are significant disparities in education and income, with Indian Americans generally being more educated and earning higher salaries than Laotian or Cambodian Americans [15]. This is crucial, as low socioeconomic status leads to greater instances of poor-quality healthcare. Additionally, the uninsured rate of Korean Americans (27%) is more than triple that of Japanese Americans (8%).

Disaggregating AAPI health data reveals clear differences in chronic diseases and conditions within the community [16]. While 8% of the US population has diabetes, compared to 10% of the AAPI community, a closer look reveals that 47% of American Samoans and 20% of Native Hawaiians have diabetes [17]. Similarly, while 3.5% of the general population suffers from post-traumatic stress disorder (PTSD) and 6.7% from depression, a study found that 62% of Cambodian refugees suffered PTSD and 51% had suffered major depression in the previous year [18]. Furthermore, Vietnamese women have the highest rates of cervical cancer among women of all racial and ethnic categories [19]. These examples demonstrate that aggregating health data among all AAPI community members perpetuates the Model Minority Myth and obscures significant health disparities within the population.

28.3 State-Led Initiatives: Advancing AAPI Data Disaggregation Amid Federal Inconsistency

At the national level, only the American Community Survey (ACS) and the US Census Bureau currently produce disaggregated data on subsets of the AAPI population [20]. The ACS, a part of the Census Bureau, provides crucial yearly information that helps determine the distribution of over $675 billion in federal and state funds. However, other surveys conducted and relied upon by federal agencies, including some by the Census Bureau, such as the Annual Social and Economic Supplement of its Current Population Survey, do not disaggregate data. Similarly, the Bureau of Labor Statistics and the Federal Reserve's Survey of Consumer Finances also fail to disaggregate data. The reasons behind federal agencies' reluctance to disaggregate AAPI data will be discussed later.

While the federal government's approach to data disaggregation is inconsistent at best, state and local governments are taking the lead. California is the most progressive state in collecting disaggregated data by AAPI ethnic community. Since the mid-1990s, California has mandated that state agencies, boards, and commissions collect and disaggregate data by race and ethnicity, with a specific focus on AAPI community members. In 2016, the state assembly passed AB-1726 to further strengthen California's original requirements [21]. Under AB-1726, state agencies, boards, or commissions that collect demographic data on the ancestry or ethnic origin of Californians must use separate collection categories and tabulations for specified Asian and Pacific Islander groups. Additionally, specified agencies must use separate collection categories and tabulations for major Asian groups and Native Hawaiian and other Pacific Islander groups, post the collected demographic data on their websites, and update it annually.

Other states have also taken steps toward increased data disaggregation. In 2019, the New York state legislature passed a similar bill, but it was vetoed by then-Governor Andrew Cuomo. In 2016, a proposed bill in Massachusetts aimed to increase data disaggregation by requiring all state agencies, quasi-state agencies, entities created by state statute, and subdivisions of state agencies to identify AAPI community members as defined by the US Census Bureau [22]. The bill would have applied to all types of data collection, reporting, or verification, and the entities would have been required to individually report data on Massachusetts' five largest AAPI ethnic groups. However, the bill did not pass, largely due to opposition from Chinese Americans, which will be discussed later.

In 2017, Rhode Island enacted a bill requiring the Department of Elementary and Secondary Education to use separate collection categories and tabulations for specified Asian ethnic groups according to the latest decennial census and to post the data on its website annually [23]. Similarly, Washington enacted a bill in 2016 mandating the disaggregation of student data collected and submitted using US Department of Education race and ethnicity guidelines [24].

28.4 Barriers to Disaggregation: Sample Sizes and Community Opposition

Two main barriers or arguments against data disaggregation for the AAPI population have emerged. The first argument contends that disaggregating data would result in sample sizes too small for extrapolating national data. A recent study of national survey leaders revealed that "it is small" was a common comment when asked about the size of the AAPI population represented in their data sets [25]. For example, one survey noted that only 53 out of 2500 respondents identified as AAPI community members, while another survey initially attempted to collect data on racial subgroups but had to revert to more standard ethnic categories when samples were insufficient [26]. If disaggregated data provides inadequate sample sizes, any potential benefits to the AAPI community from such data may be lost.

Oversampling, an intentional sampling process designed to include more members of a specific community in a sample could be a solution to the sample size problem [27]. In this context, data collectors would need to target specific AAPI sub-ethnic groups to ensure adequate representation. However, oversampling for data disaggregation purposes has its challenges. One survey leader noted that many AAPI subethnic groups live in geographically clustered areas, making oversampling relatively easy in those locations. However, national surveys cannot rely solely on geographically clustered samples.

The second argument against data disaggregation comes from within the AAPI population, particularly some Chinese communities [28]. They argue that disaggregated data could be used to implement policies like affirmative action, which they perceive as harmful. These communities are concerned that affirmative action policies might disadvantage them in areas such as school admissions and employment, by imposing quotas or other measures that could limit opportunities for individuals from their subgroup [29]. They fear that disaggregated data could highlight disparities and lead to targeted policies that might not be in their favor, thereby creating an unfair competitive environment. When Massachusetts proposed its bill, opponents labeled it an "Asian registry" and described it as singularly targeting Asian Americans by a fundamentally flawed categorizing system, which is not applied to any other identified ethnic groups. This opposition led to the bill's failure and prompted the legislature to consider drafting a new bill that would require detailed data collection on all racial groups.

Proponents of data disaggregation argue that such data should not be used to "target" other AAPI groups but rather to address inequities and acknowledge the clear differences among AAPI subgroups. Some believe that the benefits of social parity outweigh the fears expressed by opponents. Proponents maintain that the same disaggregated data would reveal other disparities among AAPI subgroups, leading governments to enact new and helpful policies.

28.5 Conclusion: Disaggregation Imperative

The AAPI population, the most diverse of all minority populations in the United States, is also the largest and fastest-growing racial group [30]. However, AAPIs exhibit some of the highest statistical variations among the population. For instance, the ratio between the highest and lowest-paid AAPI subgroups is the highest among all ethnic groups in the United States. Relying solely on general AAPI data leads to incomplete information, which can result in harmful outcomes like the Model Minority Myth.

To address this issue, governments at all levels should require agencies to disaggregate AAPI data. Disaggregation would lead to a greater recognition of the differences among the AAPI population and provide authorities with targets for improving the lives of all citizens. For example, if a local government disaggregates AAPI data and notices disparities in access to English language acquisition between Indian and Filipino Americans, it could use that information to fund a community learning center staffed by bilingual speakers of Tagalog and English.

Data disaggregation is crucial for accurately assessing the standing of all AAPI subgroups [31]. The AAPI population is too diverse for aggregated data to reliably inform policy decisions. Disaggregating data would put an end to the harmful Model Minority Myth and demonstrate that not all AAPIs are "doing better" than other minority racial groups. While more state and local governments have attempted to enact requirements for data disaggregation, opponents argue that it can lead to insufficient sample sizes and potentially harm the AAPI community. However, proponents maintain that oversampling and the proper use of disaggregated data would be far more beneficial than harmful.

In conclusion, the diversity within the AAPI population necessitates the disaggregation of data to ensure that the unique needs and challenges of each subgroup are recognized and addressed. By implementing data disaggregation policies, governments can develop targeted solutions to improve the lives of all AAPI community members and dismantle harmful stereotypes like the Model Minority Myth. Despite the challenges and opposition, the benefits of data disaggregation far outweigh the potential drawbacks, making it an essential tool for promoting equity and inclusivity.

Policy Recommendations for Improving Health Equity and Data Disaggregation

Category	Recommendations	Details
Legislative Changes	Enact legislation modeled after California AB 1726	Amend and expand applicability for uniform disaggregation of Asian and Pacific Islander subgroups
	Standardize race and ethnicity categories	Require uniform categories across state public health data systems and provide adequate appropriations
	Mandate enhanced data collection	Health systems must collect, analyze, and report enhanced race and ethnicity data
	Establish a Task Force on Health Equity	Study racial disparities in COVID-19 and recommend actions
	Fund information system upgrades	Ensure implementation of enhanced data collection and reporting
	Tie data collection to healthcare outcomes	Build accountability to improve health outcomes among diverse communities
	Require explanations for non-disaggregated data	Provide statements explaining why data was not disaggregated further
Regulatory Changes	Standardize race and ethnicity categories	Require health systems to collect, analyze, and report enhanced disaggregated data
	Tie data collection to healthcare outcomes	Create accountability for data collection and reporting

Category	Recommendations	Details
Policy Guidance	Adopt Data De-Identification Guidelines (DDG)	Assess data for identification risk before public release and update guidelines regularly
	Support innovations in data methods	Encourage advancements in balancing data granularity and privacy/security
Policy Actions	Establish a task force on racial disparities	Advisory body to study and address racial disparities in COVID-19
	Update state surveillance systems	Advocate for additional race and ethnicity categories and ensure federal compliance
	Partner with health systems	Collaborate to enhance data collection tools
	Support enhanced staff and resources	Ensure adequate staffing and resources for timely data analysis and reporting
	Standardize racial and ethnic categories	Implement consistent data collection tools across all state health agencies
	Implement privacy protections for disaggregated data	Use methods like pooling data to protect privacy while releasing small sample sizes
	Convene diverse stakeholders and coalitions	Discuss priorities for further data disaggregation
	Consult with tribal nations on data collection	Develop data-sharing agreements for tribal data

References

1 U.S. Census Bureau (2021). Asian American and Pacific islander heritage month: May 2021. https://www.census.gov/newsroom/facts-for-features/2021/asian-american-pacific-islander.html (accessed 24 August 2024).

2 Budiman, A. and Ruiz, N.G. (2021). *Key Facts About Asian Americans, A Diverse and Growing Population.* Pew Research Center. https://www.pewresearch.org/fact-tank/2021/04/29/key-facts-about-asian-americans/.

3 López, G., Ruiz, N.G., and Patten, E. (2017). *Key Facts About Asian Americans.* Pew Research Center. https://www.pewresearch.org/fact-tank/2017/09/08/key-facts-about-asian-americans/.

4 Ramakrishnan, K. and Ahmad, F.Z. (2014). *State of Asian Americans and Pacific Islanders Series: A Multifaceted Portrait of a Growing Population.* Center for American Progress. https://americanprogress.org/article/state-of-asian-americans-and-pacific-islanders-series/.

5 Holland, A.T. and Palaniappan, L.P. (2012). Problems with the collection and interpretation of Asian-American health data: omission, aggregation, and extrapolation. *Annals of Epidemiology* 22 (6): 397–405. https://doi.org/10.1016/j.annepidem.2012.04.001.

6 Chow, K. (2017). *'Model Minority' Myth Again Used as a Racial Wedge Between Asians and Blacks.* NPR. https://www.npr.org/sections/codeswitch/2017/04/19/524571669/model-minority-myth-again-used-as-a-racial-wedge-between-asians-and-blacks.

7 U.S. Census Bureau (2019). Income and poverty in the United States: 2018. https://www.census.gov/data/tables/2019/demo/income-poverty/p60-266.html (accessed 24 August 2024).

8 Kochhar, R. and Cilluffo, A. (2018). *Income Inequality in the U.S. Is Rising Most Rapidly Among Asians.* Pew Research Center. https://www.pewresearch.org/social-trends/2018/07/12/income-inequality-in-the-u-s-is-rising-most-rapidly-among-asians/.

9 Yi, S.S., Kwon, S.C., Sacks, R., and Trinh-Shevrin, C. (2020). Commentary: persistence and health-related consequences of the model minority stereotype for Asian Americans. *Ethnicity & Disease* 26 (1): 133–138. https://doi.org/10.18865/ed.26.1.133.

10 Poon, O., Squire, D., Kodama, C. et al. (2016). A critical review of the model minority myth in selected literature on Asian Americans and Pacific Islanders in higher education. *Review of Educational Research* 86 (2): 469–502. https://doi.org/10.3102/0034654315612205.

11 Kim, C.J. (1999). The racial triangulation of Asian Americans. *Politics and Society* 27 (1): 105–138. https://doi.org/10.1177/0032329299027001005.

12 Lee, E. (2015). *The Making of Asian America: A History.* Simon & Schuster.

13 Jang, D. (2018). Challenges in health equity for Asian American, Native Hawaiian, and Pacific Islander communities. *Health Equity* 2 (1): 177–179. https://doi.org/10.1089/heq.2018.0015.

14 Gee, G.C., Spencer, M., Chen, J. et al. (2007). The association between self-reported racial discrimination and 12-month DSM-IV mental disorders among Asian Americans nationwide. *Social Science & Medicine* 64 (10): 1984–1996. https://doi.org/10.1016/j.socscimed.2007.02.013.

15 Cook, W.K., Weir, R.C., Ro, M. et al. (2012). Improving Asian American, Native Hawaiian, and Pacific Islander health: national organizations leading community research initiatives. *Progress in Community Health Partnerships : Research, Education, and Action* 6 (1): 33–41.

16 Ancheta, A.N. (2006). *Race, Rights, and the Asian American Experience.* Rutgers University Press.

17 Karter, A.J., Schillinger, D., Adams, A.S. et al. (2013). Elevated rates of diabetes in Pacific Islanders and Asian subgroups. *Diabetes Care* 36 (3): 574–579. https://doi.org/10.2337/dc12-0722.

18 Marshall, G.N., Schell, T.L., Elliott, M.N. et al. (2005). Mental health of Cambodian refugees 2 decades after resettlement in the United States. *JAMA* 294 (5): 571–579. https://doi.org/10.1001/jama.294.5.571.

19 Miller, B.A., Chu, K.C., Hankey, B.F., and Ries, L.A. (2008). Cancer incidence and mortality patterns among specific Asian and Pacific Islander populations in the U.S. *Cancer Causes & Control* 19 (3): 227–256. https://doi.org/10.1007/s10552-007-9088-3.

20 Revankar, S. and Agarwala, A. (2024). Stepping away from the monolith: the disaggregation of asian cardiovascular data. *The American Journal of Cardiology* 219: 120–122.

21 California Assembly Bill 1726 (2016). An act to amend Section 8310.7 of the Government Code, relating to data. https://leginfo.legislature.ca.gov/faces/billTextClient.xhtml?bill_id=201520160AB1726.

22 The Commonwealth of Massachusetts (2016). An act relative to Asian American data. https://malegislature.gov/Bills/189/S2245 (accessed 24 August 2024).

23 State of Rhode Island General Assembly (2017). An act relating to education – all students count act. http://webserver.rilin.state.ri.us/BillText/BillText17/SenateText17/S0439.pdf.

24 Washington State Legislature (2016). HB 1541 – implementing strategies to close the educational opportunity gap, based on the recommendations of the educational opportunity gap oversight and accountability committee. https://app.leg.wa.gov/billsummary?BillNumber=1541&Year=2015 (accessed 24 August 2024).

25 Nguyen, T.T., Nguyen, M.H., Nguyen, T. et al. (2018). Oversampling Asian American and Native Hawaiian/Other Pacific Islanders (AANHPIs) in health surveys. *Journal of Racial and Ethnic Health Disparities* 5 (3): 502–509. https://doi.org/10.1007/s40615-017-0398-1.

26 Shimkhada, R., Scheitler, A.J., and Ponce, N.A. (2021). Capturing racial/ethnic diversity in population-based surveys: data disaggregation of health data for Asian American, Native Hawaiian, and Pacific Islanders (AANHPIs). *Population Research and Policy Review* 40 (1): 81–102.

27 Kauh, T.J., Read, J.G., and Scheitler, A.J. (2019). The critical role of racial/ethnic data disaggregation for health equity. *Population Research and Policy Review* 1–7. https://doi.org/10.1007/s11113-020-09631-6.

28 Wong, F. and Halgin, R. (2006). The "model minority": bane or blessing for Asian Americans? *Journal of Multicultural Counseling and Development* 34 (1): 38–49. https://doi.org/10.1002/j.2161-1912.2006.tb00025.x.

29 Dong, S. (1995). "Too Many Asians": the challenge of fighting discrimination against Asian-Americans and preserving affirmative action. *Stanford Law Review* 1027–1057.

30 Museus, S.D. (2013). Asian Americans and Pacific Islanders: a national portrait of growth, diversity, and inequality. In: *The Misrepresented Minority*, 11–41. Routledge.

31 Teranishi, R.T., Nguyen, T.L., and Alcantar, C.M. (2015). The data quality movement for the Asian American and Pacific Islander community: an unresolved civil rights issue. In: *The Misrepresented Minority: New Insights on Asian Americans and Pacific Islanders, and the Implications for Higher Education* (ed. R.T. Teranishi and L.B. Pazich), 67–84. Stylus Publishing.

Part IV

Physical Environment: The Role of Housing, Transit, Water, and Climate Change

This part explores the crucial role of the physical environment in health equity, focusing on housing, transportation, water access, and climate change. Chapter 29 discusses achieving health equity through housing laws and policies, examining how residential segregation and inadequate housing impact health and proposing legal interventions to create inclusive and healthy communities. Chapter 30 addresses advancing transportation for health equity, highlighting the need for equitable transportation systems that provide safe, reliable, and affordable access to essential services, particularly for marginalized populations. Chapter 31 focuses on providing access to clean water for health equity, emphasizing the importance of modernizing infrastructure, ensuring affordability, and protecting water quality to safeguard public health. Chapter 32 examines addressing climate change-induced health disparities, stressing the need for policies that prioritize frontline communities, enhance public health responses, and integrate health equity into climate planning. Collectively, these chapters provide a roadmap for creating a healthier and more equitable physical environment by addressing the systemic issues in housing, transportation, water access, and climate resilience, and advocating for comprehensive policies that center the needs of vulnerable populations.

29

Achieving Health Equity Through Housing Laws and Policies

Abstract

This chapter explores the complex relationship between housing and health, with a specific focus on the impact of residential segregation in the United States. It begins by establishing the connection between an individual's neighborhood and their overall well-being, highlighting how segregated neighborhoods often suffer from various disadvantages that contribute to poor health outcomes. This chapter then delves into how certain laws and policies, such as the Low-Income Housing Tax Credit (LIHTC), nuisance ordinances, rent control, the Housing Choice Voucher Program (HCVP), and zoning laws, have unintentionally furthered residential segregation despite their intended purposes. It also discusses positive legal interventions, including land banks, inclusionary zoning, the Earned Income Tax Credit (EITC), and initiatives like the "Moving to Opportunity for Fair Housing" (MTO) program. This chapter concludes by emphasizing the need for a comprehensive, multilevel approach involving federal, state, and local authorities, as well as private stakeholders, to effectively address and reduce residential segregation, thereby fostering more inclusive communities that promote improved health, safety, and equality for all residents.

Keywords *residential segregation; housing policies; health equity; Low-Income Housing Tax Credit (LIHTC); nuisance ordinances; Housing Choice Voucher Program (HCVP); inclusionary zoning; social determinants of health*

> *Rosa, a single mother of three living in a marginalized neighborhood in South Chicago, says "Every morning, I worry about my children playing outside because of the pollution. We don't have access to parks, and fresh food markets are miles away. Is this the American dream we were promised?"*
>
> *Mr. Jones, an elderly African American man who grew up during the era of redlining, witnessed firsthand the decline of his neighborhood due to divestments. He represents the generation that felt the direct brunt of segregationist policies.*
>
> *Carmen, a young Latina mother and beneficiary of the Housing Choice Voucher Program, struggles to find housing in a neighborhood that offers better opportunities for her children due to existing racial and economic barriers.*

29.1 Housing and Health: The Impact of Segregation

Housing is an integral part of public health infrastructure and the social determinants of health. Research and expert findings emphasize that geography plays a pivotal role in determining the quality of life [1]. The phrase "place matters" encapsulates the notion that an individual's neighborhood significantly influences their overall health. A mere "decent dwelling" does not guarantee health and well-being. Instead, the broader community's ability to cater to an individual's fundamental needs is imperative for ensuring a healthy lifestyle. While most Americans desire healthy homes in diverse communities, historical and current data reveals a disconnect [2]. Legislative efforts over the past half-century, at both federal and state levels, aimed to foster community integration. But these efforts stand in contrast to additional forces that perpetuate neighborhood segregation in the United States, such as White flight and divestment in non-White communities. Scholars have also documented how individual and collective interests in preserving White spaces, stigma of non-White cultural practices, as well as minorities own fears of the dangers of inhabiting predominately White spaces also interfere with legal effort to integrate [3].

Residential segregation, defined as the separation of different groups within a geographic area, has been and remains closely associated with persistent racial health disparities [4]. From 1950 to 2018, the White population in the United States declined from 90% to 60%. Yet, in 2018, neighborhoods inhabited by an average White resident were 71% White. Conversely, neighborhoods of an average Black resident comprised 45% Black residents, and those of Latino or Hispanic residents were 47% Latino or Hispanic. Such segregated neighborhoods often suffer from lower home values, environmental hazards, limited access to nutritious food, and inadequate spaces for physical activity. These factors do not exist because of the individuals who live here, but rather are a byproduct of historical redlining and perceptions of non-White neighborhoods [5]. This inequality contributes to severe health outcomes that are correlated with poor housing, including asthma, heart diseases, depression, reduced lifespan, and increased infant mortality rates [6]. Compounding the issue, healthcare access in these segregated neighborhoods mirrors the patterns of residential segregation. Particularly in predominantly Black residential areas, there's limited access to primary care and specialists. Hospital flight and outdated healthcare facilities are well-documented phenomena in minority neighborhoods [7]. It's noted that residential segregation accounts for about half of the racial disparity in hospital admissions [8]. Even when racial minorities from segregated neighborhoods access healthcare, they often receive care of a lower quality compared to Whites. Despite the establishment of anti-discrimination laws at both federal and state levels, residential segregation persists as a pressing challenge [9].

> *"Your zip code is a more powerful predictor of your health than your genetic code."*
> David R. Williams, Ph.D., Professor and Chair of the Department of Social and Behavioral Sciences at the Harvard T.H. Chan School of Public Health

29.2 How Laws and Policies Post-fair Housing Act Have Furthered Residential Segregation

29.2.1 The Low-Income Housing Tax Credit

The LIHTC was introduced by the Tax Reform Act of 1986 [10]. Its primary objective is to incentivize private investors, through federal income tax credits, to invest in affordable rental housing. Between 1987 and 2015, this initiative facilitated the construction of over three million housing units, thanks to federal subsidies. Theoretically, the LIHTC is supposed to promote fair and integrated housing patterns. However, that has not been the case.

Concerns arise when analyzing the impact of the LIHTC on racial segregation and poverty concentration. To start, the legacy of discriminatory mortgage practices consistently pushed racial minorities into the rental market. Additionally, White and wealthy politicians used their social capital to disallow public housing construction in their neighborhoods [11]. This pattern encouraged a vacuum once the LIHTC was established. A significant portion of LIHTC-funded developments ended up situated in low-income neighborhoods, predominately minority communities [11]. That pattern has persisted until today. Consequently, most affordable rental units under this program are found in areas that are largely non-White, job-deficient, and marred by higher pollution rates and subpar schools.

The allocation of the LIHTC is determined by a Qualified Application Plan (QAP). The Internal Revenue Code mandates that the QAP prioritizes developments in high-poverty regions. Moreover, developers venturing into such areas are entitled to tax credits of up to 30%. This naturally steers more developers toward impoverished neighborhoods. Given these patterns, some critics argue that the LIHTC might exacerbate residential segregation rather than alleviate it. While there isn't conclusive evidence that the LIHTC intensifies segregation, it's evident that the program doesn't significantly advance racial and socioeconomic integration [12].

29.2.2 Nuisance Ordinances

Nuisance and crime-free property ordinances, enacted by local municipalities, are the next policies under scrutiny [13]. These ordinances cover a broad spectrum of behaviors deemed to be nuisances. However, research indicates that these ordinances often obstruct access to secure housing. A case in point is Milwaukee, Wisconsin, where, between 2008 and 2009, one-third of all nuisance citations resulted from domestic violence incidents. Often, these citations led property owners to evict the abused tenants, predominantly women. Furthermore, properties in primarily Black neighborhoods were most likely to receive such citations. The implications of these findings are severe: such policies potentially force abused women to make a distressing choice between reporting their abusers, risking eviction, or enduring further abuse without seeking help.

Beyond jeopardizing access to emergency aid, critics argue that nuisance ordinances also deplete the availability of rental housing. This depletion occurs either by revoking property rental licenses or by deterring homeowners from offering rental spaces due to concerns over potential nuisance-related complications.

29.2.3 Rent Control

Rent control programs, similar to nuisance ordinances, are established at the municipal level [14]. These programs cap the amount landlords can charge for renting or renewing a lease on a property. While some programs implement stringent price ceilings, others lean toward rent stabilization models. However, reviews of these programs suggest that they often result in more issues than they resolve. The consensus among American economists is that rent control initiatives tend to diminish both the number and the quality of available housing.

29.2.4 Housing Choice Voucher Program

The US Department of Housing and Urban Development (HUD) oversees the HCVP [15]. This program stands as the federal government's primary initiative to aid very low-income families, the elderly, and the disabled in securing decent, safe, and sanitary housing within the private market. Local public housing agencies (PHAs), funded by HUD, are responsible for managing the HCVP. In this system, PHAs directly pay landlords a subsidy, and the tenant covers the remaining balance between the subsidy and the actual rent. Furthermore, for a rental unit to qualify, it must satisfy the health and safety standards set by the PHA.

While the HCVP plays a crucial role in addressing housing challenges, its relationship with residential segregation is complex. On the positive side, housing vouchers have consistently demonstrated effectiveness in diminishing homelessness and housing instability, marking the HCVP as an essential resource for low-income renters. However, its role in fostering racial integration remains ambiguous. One study indicated that while HCVP participants could secure housing, it wasn't necessarily in their preferred locations [16]. Another research highlighted that a mere 18% of HCVP-using families resided in areas with poverty rates below 20% [17].

A potential hurdle to integration through HCVP is its geographical tethering to specific housing authorities or PHAs. This structure can hinder a voucher recipient living in a high-poverty zone from relocating to a low-poverty area. Although possible, such a move is logistically challenging and often not feasible for the working poor who utilize the vouchers. Another concern stems from the reported harassment of voucher holders by community members, who might escalate concerns about these individuals to housing authorities or the police. Lastly, constrained resources and funding for the HCVP can make the housing hunt arduous for those with vouchers.

29.2.5 Zoning Laws

Modern zoning laws, especially those that limit population density, aim to mitigate potential issues such as traffic congestion and environmental degradation [18]. However, these laws have not always been purely utilitarian. Historically, following the Supreme Court's ruling against racial covenants and racial zoning in the early twentieth century, cities shifted their strategies. They began implementing zoning laws ostensibly focused on curbing neighborhood density. Yet, in practice, these laws often served as tools to deter Black Americans from settling in predominantly White neighborhoods.

Studies underscore the segregative implications of these zoning laws [19]. One such research illustrates this through a concept called the "chain of exclusion." This chain begins with land use controls hindering housing growth. It then leads to a decrease in multifamily housing. This reduction, in turn, diminishes the availability of rental units. The subsequent effect is a decline in housing affordability, culminating in a reduced minority population in the area.

Further evidence emphasizes the significant role of density-based zoning laws in perpetuating both class and racial segregation in the United States. In essence, while zoning laws might be grounded in valid concerns like managing the adverse impacts of overpopulation, they often result in undesirable side effects, whether unintended or deliberately designed.

29.3 Positive Legal Interventions

Challenges in housing integration arise from deep-rooted social dynamics shaped by historical prejudices, socioeconomic disparities, and cultural divides. Historical practices like redlining fostered divisions in communities, impacting infrastructure, education, and amenities across racial lines. This history, combined with tendencies to live near those with similar backgrounds and the effects of gentrification, has solidified racial enclaves and heightened tensions. To combat this, legal measures aim to promote racial diversity in housing. However, achieving genuine integration requires not just legal frameworks but a profound understanding and resolution of underlying social issues.

29.3.1 Land Banks

In 2017, a staggering 9.3% of US housing units remained vacant throughout the year [20]. This presents a significant concern, as vacant properties often correlate with increased neighborhood crime, illicit drug activities, and diminished perceptions of safety. When properties are declared vacant, municipalities are tasked with their acquisition and subsequent disposal.

One solution is the utilization of land banks [21]. Defined by HUD, land banks are either governmental or nonprofit organizations created with the intent to manage, repurpose, and stabilize neighborhoods by addressing vacant urban properties.

Evidence indicates that land banks effectively transform vacant properties into beneficial assets, fostering positive community uses. However, a challenge arises due to the limited number of land banks available relative to the vast number of vacant properties, especially in larger cities.

The logical step would be to expand the number of local land banks, given their proven impact in enhancing urban living conditions. Land banks are governmental entities or nonprofit corporations that focus on the conversion of vacant, abandoned, and tax-delinquent properties into productive use. These organizations acquire troubled properties and repurpose them in ways that support community goals, such as developing affordable housing or creating green spaces.

But the path to expansion isn't without its hurdles. One of the primary challenges is the complexity and diversity of real estate markets and property laws across different jurisdictions. Expanding land banks requires navigating through legal intricacies, differing tax foreclosure processes, and property rights issues that may vary from one location to another.

Increasing the reach of land banks brings along added administrative costs. Managing a large inventory of properties necessitates substantial funding and administrative capacity. Land banks require adequate staffing, technical resources, and expertise to ensure the proper maintenance, redevelopment, and eventual resale or repurposing of acquired properties.

Additionally, while the idea of expanding land banks is attractive, it's uncertain whether they can be scaled efficiently to confront the pervasive issue of vacancy, particularly in cities where the housing conditions are already strained. In places with acute housing crises, the demand for solutions may far outstrip the capacity of a land bank to acquire and rehabilitate properties in a timely manner.

Land banks also need to be cognizant of community needs and economic realities. Expansion efforts may face resistance from local stakeholders who may have differing views on property usage or who may be concerned about gentrification and its impact on existing residents.

In summary, while land banks offer a promising avenue for urban revitalization, understanding the intricacies and challenges associated with their expansion is crucial for stakeholders and policymakers aiming to leverage their potential benefits.

29.3.2 Inclusionary Zoning

Density zoning (where ordinances and regulations limit the development of housing based on land use intensity) has been linked to increased segregation, but an alternative approach – known as inclusionary zoning – can counteract this trend. Inclusionary zoning policies typically have several components [22]:

1) A mandate for developers to allocate a certain percentage of a development for affordable housing.
2) Defined income levels to determine eligibility for affordable housing.
3) A specified time frame for which the affordability criteria must be met.
4) Provisions for exemptions or buyouts, allowing developers certain flexibilities.

Research indicates that while inclusionary zoning can bolster both the production of affordable housing and integration, achieving both outcomes simultaneously can present challenges [23].

Another proposed strategy involves "upzoning," or revising zoning regulations to permit the construction of taller or denser buildings. When combined with more substantial subsidies for low-income residents, upzoning in affluent areas can diminish segregation. This is because such policies make housing in wealthier areas accessible to groups that have been historically marginalized.

29.3.3 Earned Income Tax Credit

The EITC is a tax benefit provided by the Internal Revenue Service for low- to moderate-income workers and their families [24]. It serves to lower the tax liability for eligible individuals, potentially resulting in a refund. Research indicates that the EITC plays a dual role: it not only alleviates poverty but also contributes to improved health outcomes. In terms of housing, recipients of the EITC can allocate their refund toward significant expenses. For example, if not utilized for debt settlement, the refund could serve as a down payment on a home. Similarly, renting families can use the refund to cover their monthly rent obligations.

29.3.4 Other Policy and Legal Interventions

The MTO was a decade-long research project spearheaded by HUD [25]. This initiative blended rental assistance with personalized housing counseling, aiming to assist extremely low-income families in relocating from impoverished urban sectors to neighborhoods with lower poverty rates [26].

Key findings from the MTO study revealed that families who benefited from this program were more likely than their counterparts in a control group to:

1) Reside in areas with lower poverty.
2) Inhabit higher-quality homes.
3) Live in less racially segregated communities.
4) Foster social connections with more affluent individuals.
5) Feel a heightened sense of safety in their surroundings.

Moreover, families that transitioned out of public housing noted positive health outcomes, such as reduced weight gain, enhanced diabetes management, and better mental well-being, compared to those who remained in public housing or low-income areas.

To further these gains, the Health in All Policies (HiAP) strategy can be integrated alongside fair housing solutions [27]. HiAP is a method where health implications are factored into the formation and execution of public policies. This approach, when applied to "place-based community development programs," has the potential to significantly diminish neighborhood segregation through bolstered economic growth.

29.4 Conclusion: Addressing Residential Segregation for Better Health

The negative repercussions of residential segregation are unequivocally evident and profoundly impactful, leading to suboptimal health outcomes, escalated poverty rates, and diminished neighborhood safety. Though efforts have been made to mitigate this through various legal measures and policies, the progress toward meaningful integration has been limited.

A significant challenge in addressing residential segregation lies in the unintended consequences of certain policies. For instance, while zoning laws intend to enhance public health by controlling population density, they sometimes inadvertently deepen class and racial segregation in the United States.

At the federal level, policymakers can champion nationwide policies and legislations aimed at dismantling structural barriers contributing to segregation. For example, amending HUD policies to incentivize integration and ensuring fair allocation of resources can be crucial steps.

State and local authorities have the power to enforce and adapt policies to their specific contexts. This can include revisiting and revising zoning laws. Inclusionary zoning policies, such as upzoning, have shown promise in counteracting segregation by providing marginalized groups access to affluent neighborhoods. Policymakers at this level should actively explore and expand such initiatives while collecting empirical evidence to gauge their impact.

Private actors, including real estate developers and housing corporations, can also contribute significantly by adopting inclusive practices and collaborating with government bodies to ensure diverse and equitable residential spaces.

It is imperative for policymakers and legislators across all levels to pursue a persistent and concerted effort toward fostering residential integration. In doing so, they must exercise caution to ensure that policies, even if well-intentioned, do not inadvertently exacerbate segregation. This necessitates a careful, data-driven evaluation of the policies before implementation and regular assessments of their impact thereafter.

A comprehensive, multilevel approach involving federal, state, and local authorities, as well as private stakeholders, is crucial to make substantial strides toward reducing residential segregation. Policymakers must establish clear, actionable steps that delineate the responsibilities and capacities of each stakeholder, thereby ensuring coordinated and effective efforts. By adopting such a strategic approach, we can move closer toward creating inclusive communities that foster improved health, safety, and equality for all residents.

Key Policies and Equity Considerations in Housing and Health

Category	Policy/Lever	Description	Key Points and Considerations
Prevent Structural Racism	Redlining	Systematic denial of services to neighborhoods based on racial/ethnic composition	Historical practice with lingering effects; impacts access to jobs and services
	Exclusionary Zoning	Local ordinances that prevent affordable housing development	Increases housing costs and segregates communities
	Racist Restrictive Covenants	Legal obligations in property deeds preventing sales to certain races	Outlawed but still present; deters buyers
	Gentrification	Renovation of neighborhoods leading to displacement of low-income residents	Causes housing instability and displacement, affecting health
	Discriminatory lending practices	Higher rates of loan denial and higher interest rates for communities of color	Reinforces segregation and economic disparities
Increase Affordability	Affordable Housing Programs	Public housing, Section 8 vouchers, and subsidized housing options	Limited reach; long wait times; insufficient to meet demand
	Funding Protection	Support for Affirmatively Furthering Fair Housing Act and National Housing Trust Fund	Advocates for increased and protected funding
	Fair Lending Oversight	Federal oversight of lending standards	Ensures equitable access to mortgages and loans
Advance Quality and Safety	Healthy Housing Standards	Tools and standards for maintaining healthy housing conditions	Adoption improves housing quality
	Proactive Inspections	Regular checks to ensure safety and quality	Reduces fear of reporting issues among vulnerable communities
Support Neighborhoods	Infrastructure Improvements	Development of transportation, green spaces, and healthy food markets	Enhances community health and equity
	Community-Led Development	Community land trusts and participatory planning	Empowers residents and ensures development meets community needs
Ensure Stability	Tenant Protections	Just-cause eviction laws, free legal assistance, rent control policies	Provides security for renters and prevents unjust evictions
	Cross-Sector Partnerships	Models like Support and Services at Home (SASH) in Vermont	Holistic support through coordination among services
	Disaster Recovery	Equitable deployment of federal disaster recovery funds	Ensures vulnerable populations receive necessary support post-disasters

Category	Policy/Lever	Description	Key Points and Considerations
Community Engagement	Implicit Bias Training	Educating community partners and decision-makers	Promotes understanding and mitigation of biases in housing development
	Community-Based Partnerships	Collaborations with faith-based organizations, schools, and local groups	Strengthens community engagement and resource distribution
	Health in All Policies (HiAP) and Health Impact Assessment (HIA)	Decision-making tools to integrate health and equity considerations	Encourages comprehensive consideration of health impacts in housing policy and program decisions

References

1 Helburn, N. (1982). Geography and the quality of life. *Annals of the Association of American Geographers* 72 (4): 445–456.

2 Woods, L.L. 2nd, Shaw-Ridley, M., and Woods, C.A. (2014). Can health equity coexist with housing inequalities? A contemporary issue in historical context. *Health Promotion Practice* 15 (4): 476–482.

3 Harris, C.I. (1992). Whiteness as property. *Harvard Law Review* 106: 1707. Brown, D.A. (2021). The Whiteness of Wealth: How the Tax System Impoverishes Black Americans – And How We Can Fix It. http://ebookcentral.proquest.com/lib/harvard-ebooks/detail.action?docID=6507628 (last visited November 8, 2021).

4 Hernández, D. and Swope, C.B. (2019). Housing as a platform for health and equity: evidence and future directions. *American Journal of Public Health* 109 (10): 1363–1366.

5 Lynch, E.E., Malcoe, L.H., Laurent, S.E. et al. (2021). The legacy of structural racism: Associations between historic redlining, current mortgage lending, and health. *SSM Population Health* 14: 100793.

6 Bryant-Stephens, T.C., Strane, D., Robinson, E.K. et al. (2021). Housing and asthma disparities. *The Journal of Allergy and Clinical Immunology* 148 (5): 1121–1129.

7 Clark, B. (2005). Hospital flight from minority communities: how our existing civil rights framework fosters racial inequality in healthcare. *DePaul Journal of Health Care Law* 9: 1023. Eberth, J.M. et al. (2022). The problem of the color line: spatial access to hospital services for minoritized racial and ethnic groups. *Health Affairs (Millwood)* 41: 237.

8 Sarrazin, M.S., Campbell, M.E., Richardson, K.K., and Rosenthal, G.E. (2009). Racial segregation and disparities in health care delivery: conceptual model and empirical assessment. *Health Services Research* 44 (4): 1424–1444.

9 Moran-McCabe, K., Waimberg, J., and Ghorashi, A. (2020). Mapping housing laws in the United States: a resource for evaluating housing policies' impacts on health. *Journal of Public Health Management and Practice* 26 (Suppl 2) Advancing Legal Epidemiology: S29–S36.

10 Gold, S. (2020). Does public housing reduce housing cost burden among low-income families with children? *Journal of Children & Poverty* 26 (1): 1–21.

11 Anderson, C.L. Affirmative action for affordable housing. *Howard Law Journal* 60: 105.

12 Ports, K.A., Rostad, W.L., Luo, F. et al. (2018). The impact of the low-income housing tax credit on children's health and wellbeing in Georgia. *Children and Youth Services Review* 93: 390–396.

13 Moran-McCabe, K., Gutman, A., and Burris, S. (2018). Public health implications of housing laws: nuisance evictions. *Public Health Reports (Washington, DC : 1974)* 133 (5): 606–609.

14 Diamond, R., McQuade, T., and Qian, F. (2019). The effects of rent control expansion on tenants, landlords, and inequality: evidence from San Francisco. *American Economic Review* 109 (9): 3365–3394.

15 Camacho-Rivera, M., Rosenbaum, E., Yama, C., and Chambers, E. (2017). Low-income housing rental assistance, perceptions of neighborhood food environment, and dietary patterns among Latino adults: the AHOME study. *Journal of Racial and Ethnic Health Disparities* 4 (3): 346–353.

16 Hexter, K., Keating, W.D., Jones, M.D. et al. (2015). *Understanding the Location Decisions of the Cuyahoga Metropolitan Housing Authority's Housing Choice Voucher Holders: Pilot Study.* All Maxine Goodman Levin School of Urban Affairs Publications.

17 Sard, B. and Rice, D. (2016). *Realizing the Housing Voucher Program's Potential to Enable Families to Move to Better Neighborhoods.* Washington, DC: Center on Budget and Policy Priorities.

18 Alexander, E.R. (2007). Zoned out: regulation, markets and choices in transportation and metropolitan land-use, by Jonathan Levine. *Journal of Urban Affairs* 29 (3): 331–332.

19 Resseger, M. (2022). *The Impact of Land Use Regulation on Racial Segregation: Evidence from Massachusetts Zoning Borders.* Mercatus Research Paper. https://ssrn.com/abstract=4244120.

20 Bollwahn, B. (2019). *Property Disposition Matters: The Current Status of Land Bank Programs in the United States.* San Marcos, TX: Masters of Public Administration, Texas State University.

21 Whitaker, S. and Fitzpatrick, T.J. (2014). Land bank 2.0: an empirical evaluation. FRB of Cleveland Working Paper No. 12-30r. https://ssrn.com/abstract=2182175.

22 Rothwell, J.T. and Massey, D.S. (2010). Density zoning and class segregation in U.S. metropolitan areas. *Social Science Quarterly* 91 (5): 1123–1143.

23 Iglesias, T. (2015). Maximizing inclusionary Zoning's contributions to both affordable housing and residential integration. *Washburn Law Journal* 54 (4): https://ssrn.com/abstract=2587413.

24 Das, V. (2023). The effect of state Earned Income Tax Credit (EITC) eligibility on food insufficiency during the COVID-19 pandemic. *Review of Economics of the Household* 21 (2): 485–518.

25 Lens, M.C. and Gabbe, C.J. (2017). Employment proximity and outcomes for moving to opportunity families. *Journal of Urban Affairs* 39 (4): 547–562.

26 Antonakos, C.L., Coulton, C.J., Kaestner, R. et al. (2020). Built environment exposures of adults in the moving to opportunity experiment. *Housing Studies* 35 (4): 703–719.

27 Khayatzadeh-Mahani, A., Ruckert, A., Labonté, R. et al. (2019). Health in all policies (HiAP) governance: lessons from network governance. *Health Promotion International* 34 (4): 779–791.

30

Advancing Transportation for Health Equity Through Policies

Abstract

This chapter explores the current state of transportation inequity and its impact on health disparities, particularly for communities of color, low-income populations, people with disabilities, and older adults. This chapter highlights the systemic disinvestment and discriminatory policies that have led to inadequate public transportation, unsafe active commuting conditions, and exposure to air pollution in marginalized communities. To address these inequities, this chapter proposes an agenda for transportation justice policy, which includes participatory community planning, equitable transportation funding, antiracist mobility policies, accessible and resilient mobility ecosystems, data-driven and community-defined metrics, capacity building, narrative shift, and cross-sector collaboration. The health sector is identified as having a significant role in advocating for and supporting transportation equity as a social determinant of health. This chapter emphasizes the need for a long-term, multisector approach that centers on the lived experiences and self-determined solutions of impacted communities. It calls for a paradigm shift in how the health sector engages with transportation justice, moving beyond transactional solutions to address the structural roots of inequity and build community power. This chapter concludes by emphasizing the critical importance of transportation justice as a pathway to eliminating health disparities and creating thriving, just communities for all.

Keywords   *transportation inequity; health disparities; public transit access; participatory community planning; antiracist mobility policies; equitable funding; data-driven metrics; cross-sector collaboration*

> *Jamal, a Black man in his early 30s, relied on public transit to commute to his job at a grocery store. Despite living only five miles away, Jamal's commute often took over an hour due to infrequent bus service and multiple transfers. The long commute left him exhausted and with little time for his family or personal health, contributing to his high blood pressure and diabetes.*
>
> *Lila, an elderly Asian woman, lived in a neighborhood with poorly maintained sidewalks and no accessible crosswalks. Fearing for her safety, Lila rarely left her home, leading to social isolation and depression. The lack of safe, accessible transportation infrastructure in her community prevented Lila from accessing essential services and social connections vital for her physical and mental well-being.*

Achieving Health Equity: The Role of Law and Policy, First Edition. Y. Tony Yang.
© 2025 John Wiley & Sons Ltd. Published 2025 by John Wiley & Sons Ltd.

> *The Jackson family, living in a low-income, predominantly Black neighborhood, suffered from higher rates of asthma and respiratory illnesses compared to residents in wealthier, white neighborhoods. The Jacksons' community was exposed to disproportionate levels of air pollution due to the nearby highway and industrial facilities, a result of racist planning policies that concentrated environmental hazards in communities of color.*

30.1 The State of Transportation Inequity

The disparities in our transportation systems are stark [1]. Communities of color, low-income populations, people with disabilities, and older adults are more likely to depend on walking, biking, and public transportation to meet daily needs [2]. Yet these same groups often live in areas with the sparsest access to safe active transportation infrastructure and affordable, reliable transit – a legacy of structural racism and regressive funding policies.

Consider public transportation, a lifeline for many disadvantaged groups. Over 60% of public transit riders are people of color [3]. Black workers are most likely to commute by public transit at 11%, compared to 5% of white workers [4]. The lowest-earning 20% of households are nearly six times less likely to have a vehicle than their higher-earning counterparts [5]. For many, public transit makes the difference between accessing healthcare, groceries, and employment or being cut off from these essential needs.

However, minority and low-income neighborhoods have long faced systemic disinvestment in public transportation by government agencies. A study of transit access in 52 major metro areas found that residents of color can reach 23–34% fewer jobs within 45 minutes by transit compared to white residents [6]. This gap in access has grown even as service has expanded, indicating ongoing inequities in transit siting and frequency decisions.

Lack of transit forces many disadvantaged individuals to rely on costly and inefficient alternatives like borrowing vehicles or using ride-hailing services, further straining budgets. These barriers are compounded for people with disabilities who require accessible transportation, and rural residents who often have no public transit options at all. Tribal communities are particularly underserved, with a quarter of reservation residents lacking access to a vehicle [7].

The disproportionate lack of adequate public transportation in marginalized communities is mirrored by hazardous conditions for active commuting. Low-income census tracts have half as many sidewalks as high-income tracts and are more than twice as likely to lack street lighting and marked crosswalks [8]. Meanwhile, African-Americans make up 12% of the population but account for 20% of pedestrian deaths [9].

These dangerous conditions reflect discriminatory patterns of underinvestment and neglect that have made walking and biking in communities of color unsafe. A study found that the majority of Black census tracts are 82% more likely than white tracts to have at least one pedestrian death per year [10]. In the majority of Latinx communities, that figure jumps to 97%. Tribal lands are also drastically overrepresented in pedestrian and cyclist fatalities.

Racism further puts communities of color at risk through systemic overpolicing of streets and public spaces. Black cyclists are 3.3 times more likely to be stopped by police than white cyclists [11]. In several cities, 100% of cycling citations are issued to Black and Latinx individuals, for minor infractions like biking on the sidewalk that stem from lack of safe infrastructure. This pervasive criminalization reinforces barriers to mobility and health.

The burden of transportation inequities extends beyond lack of physical access and safety to include exposure to noise and air pollution. Nationally, people of color are exposed to 63% more particulate matter pollution (PM2.5) pollution from vehicles than white residents, with larger disparities in Black and Asian communities [12]. This unjust concentration of traffic pollution, due to racist policies like highway siting through minority neighborhoods, increases risks of asthma, diabetes, low birth weight, and cognitive decline.

Cumulatively, transportation barriers and harms severely undermine health for marginalized groups. Lack of transportation is a leading cause of missed medical appointments, delayed care, and poor management of chronic diseases [13]. Food insecurity is higher among families with transportation difficulties who cannot reliably access grocery stores [14]. Social isolation and depression are more prevalent among older adults and people with disabilities who lack transportation to engage in community activities [15]. Pedestrian injuries and deaths are endemic in low-income communities of color with substandard infrastructure [16].

These intersecting transportation inequities are deeply entangled with broader structures of injustice that create and perpetuate health disparities [17]. Residential segregation, displacement, environmental racism, unequal school funding, and mass incarceration – the fundamental causes of health inequities – are inextricable from transportation policy decisions that disadvantage communities of color and concentrate poverty. As such, advancing transportation justice is an essential strategy to dismantle structural racism and promote health equity.

> *"In the US, an estimated 5.8 million individuals delay medical care every year due to transportation barriers, including lack of a private vehicle; inconvenient, unreliable, and expensive transportation; and poor road infrastructure. Racially minoritized populations, patients with lower socioeconomic status, and patients with comorbidities are more likely to face transportation barriers and longer travel times for medical care."*
>
> American Journal of Public Health (2020)

30.2 An Agenda for Transportation Justice Policy

To operationalize transportation justice [18], this chapter outlines an organizing, policy, and investment agenda spanning multiple sectors and levels of governance. This agenda includes several key components.

30.2.1 Participatory Community Planning

Authentic community engagement, where residents have the power to drive decisions and not just provide token input, must be mandatory and robustly funded in all transportation planning processes. Models like participatory budgeting, community coalitions, and citizen advisory boards can help institutionalize accountability and ensure that the voices of marginalized groups are centered [19].

Planning processes should incorporate inclusive outreach strategies, language access, and compensation for participation, recognizing the barriers that often exclude low-income communities and communities of color. Explicit anti-displacement protections must be built into all transportation plans and projects to prevent the harmful gentrification that can occur when new infrastructure increases property values and pushes out long-term residents [20].

30.2.2 Equitable Transportation Funding

Transportation funding streams and allocation formulas must be overhauled to prioritize the communities with the highest mobility needs and the least resources. We recommend increasing funding for public transit, walking, and biking infrastructure to at least 50% of overall transportation spending, ensuring that these modes receive a fair share relative to their importance for health equity [21].

Funds should be targeted directly to low-income communities and communities of color using metrics that capture mobility equity gaps, not just raw population numbers [22]. This targeted universalism approach recognizes that these communities have faced historic disinvestment and require additional resources to achieve equitable access.

Highway expansion projects that worsen air pollution, destroy neighborhoods, and perpetuate segregation should be prohibited from receiving funding [23]. The savings from these canceled projects should be redirected toward public transit improvements and community-identified reparations efforts to address past harms.

Equity and access for marginalized groups should be the primary criteria for all transportation project selection and prioritization, rather than vehicle speed or traditional measures of mobility. Funded projects should be linked to affordable housing production and anti-displacement measures to ensure that low-income residents can remain in newly transit-accessible areas.

30.2.3 Antiracist Mobility Policies

Discriminatory policies and practices that criminalize the mobility of communities of color and restrict their access to public spaces must be reformed. This includes ending racially biased police enforcement of walking, biking, and presence in public spaces, and redirecting those funds to infrastructure improvements in high-need areas.

Punitive policies that criminalize poverty, such as fare evasion penalties and minor violations like jaywalking tickets, should be eliminated [24]. These policies disproportionately target low-income communities of color and fail to recognize the structural inequities that make transportation unaffordable and inaccessible for many.

Exclusionary zoning laws that prohibit multifamily housing and restrict affordable transit-oriented development in high-opportunity neighborhoods should be overturned [25]. These laws maintain race and class segregation and limit access to transportation, jobs, education, and other key determinants of health.

Civil rights protections and Title VI regulations that prohibit discrimination in transportation programs must be robustly enforced [26]. Strengthened guidance, monitoring, and oversight can hold transportation agencies accountable for delivering equitable services and benefits to marginalized groups.

30.2.4 Accessible and Resilient Mobility Ecosystems

Holistic investments are needed to create complete, multimodal transportation networks that equitably serve all people and their needs across the lifespan. In underserved low-income communities and communities of color, this requires building out frequent, affordable, and reliable public transit systems, including 24-hour service, bus rapid transit, demand response options for seniors and people with disabilities, and accessibility features throughout. A Complete Streets approach to planning, designing, and building streets enables safe access for all users, including pedestrians, bicyclists, motorists, and transit riders of all ages and abilities [27]. This approach also emphasizes the needs of those who have experienced systemic underinvestment or whose needs have not been met through traditional transportation methods. A Complete Streets policy specifies how a community will plan, design, and maintain streets to ensure they are safe for all users [28]. Implementing a strong policy begins transforming a community's practices, processes, and plans [29].

Comprehensive networks of safe walking and biking facilities should be prioritized in low-income neighborhoods that have been marginalized by past infrastructure decisions. These networks should be intentionally designed for connectivity to transit stops and essential destinations like schools, health centers, grocery stores, and parks.

To further increase access and affordability, fare-free public transit should be instituted for low-income groups, people with disabilities, and youth [30]. Eliminating cost as a barrier to mobility can open up new opportunities for health and well-being.

Culturally relevant outreach, education, and signage about transportation options and safety are essential to support use among populations with limited English proficiency or low literacy levels. Multilingual travel training programs, community mobility ambassadors, and real-time translated transit information can make systems more inclusive and welcoming [31].

As climate disasters and disruptions disproportionately impact marginalized communities, transportation resilience planning must center their mobility needs. Emergency evacuation plans should incorporate low-income and transit-dependent populations and ensure that transit restarts quickly to enable an equitable recovery. Investments should also prioritize zero-emission transit vehicles to reduce traffic pollution, especially in communities experiencing cumulative environmental health burdens.

The transportation workforce itself must also reflect the diversity of the communities being served. Transit agencies and transportation departments should implement inclusive hiring pathways and representation goals to recruit women, people of color, and other underrepresented groups into quality career opportunities in the sector [32].

30.2.5 Data-Driven and Community-Defined Metrics

To guide transportation equity efforts and hold agencies accountable, metrics and evaluation strategies must evolve to center equity and meaningfully reflect community experiences. Quantitative data should include mobility equity indices that capture disparities in access to destinations and opportunities by race, income, language, age, and ability [33]. Affordability measures that reveal the cumulative cost burden of transportation relative to household incomes in low-income neighborhoods should be standard practice.

Performance monitoring should go beyond congestion and traditional commute measures to look at travel time, frequency, and reliability for the essential trips that enable health and well-being. This means assessing access to healthcare, education, food, social connections, and recreation, with data disaggregated by relevant demographic and geographic equity dimensions.

Critically, community members should have the power in defining the transportation indicators and outcomes that matter to them. Participatory processes can elevate priorities around connectedness, safety, cultural vibrancy, and other goals that reflect local values and visions. Community narratives and experiential knowledge should be valued equally to quantitative data in decision-making.

Collecting both quantitative and qualitative transportation equity data will require building new community-engaged data infrastructures. Participatory action research methods like storytelling, photovoice, community mapping, and citizen science can contextualize lived experiences and empower residents as experts [34]. Academic and agency partnerships with neighborhood-based organizations can build capacity for ongoing data collection guided by community interests.

Ultimately, data is only as valuable as its translation into accountability. Transportation agencies should adopt equity performance measures and link them to staff and leadership evaluations, compensation, and future funding to create incentives for progress. Benchmarks should be co-created with the community and reflect ambitious targets around eliminating racial gaps and advancing equity.

30.2.6 Capacity Building and Narrative Shift

Achieving durable shifts in transportation planning, policy, and resource allocation will require long-term capacity and power building in historically marginalized communities. Sustained funding is needed for community-based organizations leading intersectional organizing around transportation justice, affordable housing, environmental justice, and related issues in low-income neighborhoods and communities of color. Multiyear general operating support can enable them to be proactive and responsive to evolving opportunities.

Recruitment and leadership development programs focused on diversifying the transportation profession are also essential. Paid internships, mentorship initiatives, and career pipelines that target women and people of color for positions in planning, engineering, policy, and advocacy can help transform the faces and perspectives shaping transportation decisions.

These workforce diversity efforts should be complemented by required antiracism, mobility justice, and cultural humility training for all transportation professionals and decision-makers. Building a shared understanding of the historical and present-day manifestations of transportation inequity, and cultivating the skills to work effectively in partnership with impacted communities, is critical for institutional transformation.

Narrative change campaigns are another way to build political will for transportation justice. Effective messaging can articulate public transit, walking, and biking as core to racial equity, public health, climate resilience, and community well-being. Storytelling that humanizes mobility injustices and community-driven solutions is vital for persuading policymakers and the public.

Arts and culture strategies offer creative avenues for communities to envision and advocate for equitable transportation futures. Youth-led projects like murals, videos, and interactive installations can engage the next generation in imagining new possibilities for mobility justice. Using data visualization, mapping, and technology tools in compelling ways can also illuminate transportation inequities and build support for action.

Across all of these capacity-building approaches, the goal should be to enable and amplify the collective power of marginalized communities to drive their own transportation futures. Advocates and funders must take a backseat to community leadership, while contributing resources and technical support to build sustainability.

30.2.7 Cross-Sector Collaboration

Advancing transportation justice is not the job of transportation agencies alone. It will require other sectors, from housing to economic development to public health, to break down silos and recognize how their decisions and resource allocations impact mobility equity. Government, philanthropy, academia, and community-based organizations all have roles to play in aligning efforts through an equity lens.

The health sector in particular has a significant stake and potential impact. Hospitals and health systems can utilize community health needs assessments and allocate community benefit dollars to identify and support neighborhood transportation solutions [35]. They can leverage their role as anchor institutions and major employers to support equitable transit-oriented development and affordable housing near their facilities. And they can use their purchasing and investment power to contract with transportation providers that demonstrate equitable practices.

Public health departments and Medicaid programs can be powerful advocates for transportation equity as a social determinant of health. Pushing for the expansion of Medicaid funding for active transportation and public transit access initiatives is a promising opportunity [13]. Providing data on the links between transportation and health outcomes, and incorporating mobility justice into professional training and research agendas, can also build evidence and urgency.

Most importantly, health leaders should show up as collaborative partners in community-led transportation equity coalitions. Contributing time, connections, and resources to support grassroots organizing, while amplifying community voices in decision-making spaces, is vital for solidarity and impact. Recognizing community members as experts and centering their lived experiences in defining problems and solutions is a necessary paradigm shift.

Realizing equitable transportation systems that truly promote health and opportunity for all is a long-term, multisector endeavor. It will require deep community partnerships, a commitment to antiracist policy and systems change, and sustained investment targeting the communities that have been systematically harmed and neglected. The public health field has a key role to play in this ecosystemic approach, but how we show up matters immensely. Transportation justice must be understood as a process of building power, agency, and self-determination in marginalized communities, not simply a transactional exchange of resources.

30.3 Conclusion: Transportation Justice Drives Health Equity

Transportation is a fundamental determinant of health equity. Where we live, and the opportunities or barriers we face in accessing health-promoting resources, are inextricably linked to transportation. But our current transportation systems – shaped by a legacy of racist policies and planning decisions – are rife with inequities that concentrate harms and limit access for low-income communities and communities of color. These disparities in transportation mirror and perpetuate health disparities.

Advancing health equity demands that we adopt a transportation justice approach. This means moving beyond band-aid solutions to address the structural and systemic roots of transportation inequity. It requires confronting transportation injustice as a manifestation of racism and centering the lived experiences and self-determined solutions of impacted communities in policy and planning decisions.

The evidence-based recommendations presented here – from overhauling funding streams and planning practices to be accountable to equity, to building community power and capacity – offer an actionable policy agenda for transportation justice. But this is only a starting point. Ultimately, the specific strategies must be tailored to local contexts and arise from authentic partnerships with communities most harmed by transportation inequities and committed to leading change.

For the health sector, embracing transportation justice will require new ways of operating. Hospitals and health departments must see championing equitable transportation access as mission-critical to improving community health, not an optional side project. We must show up humbly to learn from and take direction from grassroots leaders. We must leverage our data, expertise, and influence to change institutional practices and hold decision-makers accountable for transportation equity impacts. And we must be willing to share and shift power and resources to communities to drive solutions.

This is challenging but essential work for all those committed to eliminating health disparities. Transportation justice is a pathway to build healthy, thriving, and just communities for all. The road ahead is long, but the destination is worth the journey. It is time to mobilize a movement at the intersection of transportation equity and health justice. Our collective future depends on it.

Key Policy Strategies for Advancing Transportation and Health Equity

Key Areas	Policy Strategies
Reframe the Transportation Conversation	Connect messages to issues people care about. Educate the press. Use trusted messengers. Share case studies and fact sheets.
Allocate Funding and Resources Equitably	Create a national vision for transportation. Set safety performance targets. Pass a binding, federal Complete Streets policy. Promote multimodal agency culture. Ensure budget transparency. Prioritize disenfranchised populations. Fund inclusive projects.
Improve Transportation Leadership	Invest in future leaders. Hire diverse decision-makers. Redefine expertise. Link health and transportation in education.
Prioritize Underrepresented Communities	Give power to disenfranchised communities. Remove participation barriers. Hire community-reflective staff. Build shared capacity.
Provide People-Focused Infrastructure	Build cross-disciplinary partnerships. Gain political support. Simplify decision-making processes. Share resources. Use demonstration projects.
Invest Without Displacement	Measure and reward non-displacing projects. Strengthen investment safeguards. Coordinate transportation, housing, and land use. Update zoning for walkable development. Invest in equitable transit development. Build shared prosperity.

References

1 Bullard, R.D. and Johnson, G.S. Environmental justice: grassroots activism and its impact on public policy decision making. *Journal of Social Issues* 56 (3): 555–578. https://doi.org/10.1111/0022-4537.00184.

2 Heaps, W., Abramsohn, E., and Skillen, E. (2021). *Public Transportation in the US: A Driver of Health and Equity*. Health Affairs Health Policy Brief.

3 American Public Transportation Association (2017). Who rides public transportation. https://www.apta.com/wp-content/uploads/Resources/resources/reportsandpublications/Documents/APTA-Who-Rides-Public-Transportation-2017.pdf (accessed 24 August 2024).

4 U.S. Bureau of Labor Statistics (2021). Labor force statistics from the current population survey. https://www.bls.gov/cps/tables.htm (accessed 24 August 2024).

5 Federal Highway Administration (2018). National household travel survey. https://nhts.ornl.gov/ (accessed 24 August 2024).

6 Stacy, C., Su, Y., Noble, E., Stern, A., Blagg, K., Rainer, M., & Ezike, R. (2020). How can Cities Create More Equitable Transportation Systems? Urban Institute. https://www.urban.org/sites/default/files/publication/102991/how-can-cities-create-more-equitable-transportation-systems.pdf

7 National Congress of American Indians. (2019). Transportation infrastructure in Indian country. https://www.ncai.org/policy-issues/economic-development-commerce/transportation-infrastructure (accessed 24 August 2024).

8 Gibbs, K., Slater, S. J., Nicholson, N., Barker, D. C., & Chaloupka, F. J. (2012). Income Disparities in Street Features That Encourage Walking. Bridging the Gap Program, University of Illinois at Chicago. https://muscatineiowa.gov/DocumentCenter/View/26373/Study-on-Income-Disparities-in-Street-Features-that-Encourage-Walking-PDF.

9 Dangerous by Design 2021 (2021). Smart growth America. https://smartgrowthamerica.org/dangerous-by-design/ (accessed 24 August 2024).

10 Maciag, M. (2014). *Pedestrians Dying at Disproportionate Rates in America's Poorer Neighborhoods*. Governing. https://www.governing.com/topics/public-justice-safety/gov-pedestrian-deaths-analysis.html.

11 Barajas, J.M. (2021). Biking where Black: connecting transportation planning and infrastructure to disproportionate policing. *Transportation Research Part D: Transport and Environment* 99: 103027. https://doi.org/10.1016/j.trd.2021.103027.

12 Union of Concerned Scientists (2019). Inequitable exposure to air pollution from vehicles in the northeast and mid-Atlantic. https://www.ucsusa.org/resources/inequitable-exposure-air-pollution-vehicles (accessed 24 August 2024).

13 Syed, S.T., Gerber, B.S., and Sharp, L.K. (2013). Traveling towards disease: transportation barriers to health care access. *Journal of Community Health* 38 (5): 976–993. https://doi.org/10.1007/s10900-013-9681-1.

14 Ver Ploeg, M., Larimore, E., and Wilde, P. (2017). *The Influence of Foodstore Access on Grocery Shopping and Food Spending*. Economic Research Service, U.S. Department of Agriculture https://www.ers.usda.gov/webdocs/publications/85442/eib-180.pdf.

15 Reinhard, E., Courtin, E., van Lenthe, F.J., and Avendano, M. (2018). Public transport policy, social engagement and mental health in older age: a quasi-experimental evaluation of free bus passes in England. *Journal of Epidemiology and Community Health* 72 (5): 361–368. https://doi.org/10.1136/jech-2017-210038.

16 Loukaitou-Sideris, A. and Sideris, A. (2009). What brings children to the park? Analysis and measurement of the variables affecting children's use of parks. *Journal of the American Planning Association* 76 (1): 89–107. https://doi.org/10.1080/01944360903418338.

17 Williams, D.R. and Collins, C. (2001). Racial residential segregation: a fundamental cause of racial disparities in health. *Public Health Reports* 116 (5): 404–416. https://doi.org/10.1093/phr/116.5.404.

18 Hansmann, K.J. and Razon, N. (2024). Transportation justice and health. *The Milbank Quarterly* 102 (1): 11–27. https://doi.org/10.1111/1468-0009.12676.

19 Participatory Budgeting Project. (2021). What is PB? https://www.participatorybudgeting.org/what-is-pb/ (accessed 24 August 2024).

20 Chapple, K. and Loukaitou-Sideris, A. (2019). *Transit-Oriented Displacement or Community Dividends? Understanding the Effects of Smarter Growth on Communities.* MIT Press https://doi.org/10.7551/mitpress/11652.001.0001.

21 TransitCenter (2021). Invest in transit: a case for expanding federal funding for public transportation. https://transitcenter.org/invest-in-transit-a-case-for-expanding-federal-funding-for-public-transportation/ (accessed 24 August 2024).

22 Creger, H., Espino, J., and Sanchez, A.S. (2018). *Mobility Equity Framework: How to Make Transportation Work for People.* The Greenlining Institute https://greenlining.org/publications/2018/mobility-equity-framework/.

23 Brown, J.R., Morris, E.A., and Taylor, B.D. (2009). Planning for cars in cities: planners, engineers, and freeways in the 20th century. *Journal of the American Planning Association* 75 (2): 161–177. https://doi.org/10.1080/01944360802640016.

24 Schweitzer, L. and Valenzuela, A. (2004). Environmental injustice and transportation: the claims and the evidence. *Journal of Planning Literature* 18 (4): 383–398. https://doi.org/10.1177/0885412204262958.

25 Rothstein, R. (2017). *The Color of Law: A Forgotten History of How Our Government Segregated America.* Liveright Publishing.

26 Federal Transit Administration (2012). Circular FTA C 4702.1B: Title VI requirements and guidelines for federal transit administration recipients. https://www.transit.dot.gov/sites/fta.dot.gov/files/docs/FTA_Title_VI_FINAL.pdf.

27 Babb, A. and Watkins, K.E. (2016). Complete streets policies and public transit. *Transportation Research Record* 2543 (1): 14–24.

28 Hui, N., Saxe, S., Roorda, M. et al. (2018). Measuring the completeness of complete streets. *Transport Reviews* 38 (1): 73–95.

29 Gregg, K. and Hess, P. (2019). Complete streets at the municipal level: a review of American municipal complete street policy. *International Journal of Sustainable Transportation* 13 (6): 407–418.

30 Perone, J.S. (2002). *Advantages and Disadvantages of Fare-free Transit Policy.* National Center for Transportation Research, University of South Florida https://www.nctr.usf.edu/pdf/473-133.pdf.

31 Blumenberg, E. and Agrawal, A.W. (2014). Getting around when you're just getting by: transportation survival strategies of the poor. *Journal of Poverty* 18 (4): 355–378. https://doi.org/10.1080/10875549.2014.951905.

32 TransitCenter (2018). From sorry to superb: everything you need to know about great bus stops. https://transitcenter.org/wp-content/uploads/2018/10/Sorry_To_Superb.pdf (accessed 24 August 2024).

33 Corburn, J., Curl, S., and Arredondo, G. (2015). A health-in-all-policies approach addresses many of Richmond, California's place-based hazards, stressors. *Health Affairs* 34 (11): 1905–1913. https://doi.org/10.1377/hlthaff.2015.0634.

34 Wang, C. and Burris, M.A. (1997). Photovoice: concept, methodology, and use for participatory needs assessment. *Health Education & Behavior* 24 (3): 369–387.

35 James, C.V., Moonesinghe, R., Wilson-Frederick, S.M. et al. (2017). Racial/ethnic health disparities among rural adults – United States, 2012-2015. *Morbidity and Mortality Weekly Report. Surveillance Summaries* 66 (23): 1–9. https://doi.org/10.15585/mmwr.ss6623a1.

31

Providing Access to Clean Water for Health Equity Through Policies

Abstract

This chapter discusses the pressing issue of water insecurity in the United States and its disproportionate impact on low-income communities and communities of color. This chapter begins by introducing the concept of water insecurity and its significance as a public health issue, particularly in light of the COVID-19 pandemic. It then delves into the root causes of water access inequities, including aging and inadequate infrastructure, discriminatory policies, underinvestment, regulatory failures, and the emerging threats posed by climate change. This chapter highlights how these challenges are not distributed equally, with marginalized populations bearing the brunt of the consequences. The health implications of water insecurity are explored in detail, ranging from waterborne illnesses and chemical contamination to the adverse effects of droughts, flooding, and water shutoffs on physical and mental well-being. This chapter emphasizes the urgent need for comprehensive policy solutions to address this multifaceted crisis. It outlines key policy priorities, such as increasing infrastructure investment, ensuring affordable water service, strengthening water quality protections, supporting household-level solutions, reforming water governance, and building climate resilience with a focus on water equity. This chapter underscores the importance of recognizing water as a human right and the critical role of community-driven solutions in achieving universal access to clean, safe, and affordable water. It concludes by emphasizing the transformative potential of equitable water policies in advancing health equity and social justice and the need for bold, collective action to make the human right to water a reality for all.

Keywords   *water insecurity; health equity; aging infrastructure; discriminatory policies; climate change impact; affordable water access; water governance reform; community-driven solutions*

> *When the water supply to their mobile home park was cutoff due to the owner's failure to pay the bill, the Hernandez family was left without running water for weeks. They were forced to rely on bottled water for drinking and cooking and to use buckets of water from a neighbor's hose for bathing and flushing toilets. The stress and hardship took a toll on the family's physical and mental health.*

Achieving Health Equity: The Role of Law and Policy, First Edition. Y. Tony Yang.
© 2025 John Wiley & Sons Ltd. Published 2025 by John Wiley & Sons Ltd.

> *In the small rural town of Millfield, the water system had not been upgraded in decades. When the old pipes finally failed, the predominantly low-income and African American residents were left without access to clean water. Many couldn't afford to buy bottled water and had to choose between paying for water or other essentials like food and medicine. The lack of safe water led to a surge in waterborne illnesses, exacerbating existing health disparities in the community.*
>
> *As the drought worsened, the wells serving the Smith family's farmhouse ran dry. With no connection to the municipal water system and no money to drill a deeper well, they had to haul water from a nearby town for their daily needs. The time and effort spent securing water took away from work and school, putting the family under immense strain. They worried about the long-term impacts on their livelihood and their children's future.*

31.1 Water Insecurity in America

Water is life. Access to clean, safe, and affordable water is a basic human need and should be a guaranteed human right [1]. Yet in the United States, the wealthiest country in the world, millions of people lack access to this essential resource [2]. Water insecurity – the lack of sufficient quantity or quality of water, or unaffordable water costs – disproportionately impacts low-income communities and communities of color [3]. The adverse health consequences are substantial, far-reaching, and entirely preventable [4].

The COVID-19 pandemic underscored that access to clean water for drinking and hygiene is a critical public health issue. But water insecurity is not a new problem. It is the product of a long history of discriminatory policies, underinvestment in aging infrastructure, and persistent social and environmental inequities [5]. Climate change threatens to exacerbate water access challenges in the coming years [6]. Urgent policy action is needed to confront the root causes of water insecurity and enact comprehensive solutions. We must leverage this moment to transform our approach to water access and center health equity in infrastructure investments and water governance reforms.

> *"The tragedy in Flint, Michigan, riveted the public health community to the problem of water access, highlighting its pernicious influence on low-income, minority families. Nearly one-third of US adults were inadequately hydrated, with African Americans, Hispanics, and individuals at lower incomes at significantly higher risk for inadequate hydration than Whites and those with higher incomes."*
>
> American Journal of Public Health (2017)

31.2 Causes of Water Insecurity and Access Inequities

Water insecurity in the United States is not due to an absolute scarcity of water. While certain regions like the Southwest face increasing water constraints, the country as a whole has ample water resources. Rather, lack of access to clean, affordable water for many communities is the result of aging and deteriorating infrastructure, inequitable policies and underinvestment, regulatory failures, and the emerging threats of climate change. Marginalized populations bear the brunt of these challenges.

31.2.1 Aging and Inadequate Infrastructure

The majority of the country's water systems were built over 50 years ago [7]. Much of this infrastructure is now reaching the end of its lifespan and requires upgrading or replacement. Outdated pipes are vulnerable to leaks and contamination. Old lead service lines threaten water safety. Sewage and stormwater systems are overwhelmed, resulting in overflows that harm water quality.

An estimated 2 million people in the United States, primarily low-income and communities of color, live without access to running water and basic indoor plumbing [8]. Native American households are 19 times more likely than white households to lack indoor plumbing [9]. In the Navajo Nation, nearly a third of the population does not have a tap or toilet at home. This lack of water and sanitation infrastructure is the legacy of decades of federal underinvestment and neglect of tribal communities.

Racial discrimination in housing and development policies has also resulted in Black, Hispanic, and other communities of color being denied access to municipal services, including water and sewer connections [10]. Practices like redlining and exclusionary zoning have relegated these communities to underserved unincorporated areas on the fringes of cities. The population of these urbanized areas without city services has grown to over 5 million [10]. Some regions, so-called "colonias" along the US-Mexico border, and rural areas lack access to safe drinking water and waste disposal [11].

Failing and fragmented water infrastructure puts communities at risk. Systems serving predominantly low-income areas and populations of color are more likely to have water quality violations [12]. Small systems – which serve 40% of the population but account for over 70% of quality violations – struggle with technical, managerial, and financial barriers to providing reliable service [13]. Hundreds of small rural systems serving low-income communities have recently been unable to provide any water at all due to aging infrastructure and contaminated sources.

31.2.2 Inequitable Water Policies and Underinvestment

The federal government's retreat from funding water infrastructure has exacerbated access disparities [14]. Adjusted for inflation, federal spending on water utilities decreased by 77% between 1977 and 2017. This has shifted the burden to local utilities, who have had to raise rates to make up revenue. The result is a water affordability crisis.

The average water bill has increased by over 30% since 2012, rising far faster than incomes [15]. For low-income households, water costs can account for over 12% of disposable income. Atleast 13.8 million low-income households struggle to pay for basic water and sanitation access [16]. Millions have experienced the threat or reality of disconnection from these essential services due to inability to pay. Water shutoffs disproportionately impact Black and Latinx households [17].

Declining federal resources have also reduced assistance to disadvantaged communities. Funding has not been adequately targeted to the areas with the greatest water infrastructure needs. In California's agricultural Central Valley, low-income Latinx farmworker communities rely on groundwater contaminated with agricultural pollutants, while nearby cities receive clean surface water [18]. Distance from urban centers, lack of financial and technical resources, language barriers, and political disenfranchisement limit small, low-income communities' ability to access infrastructure funding and maintain robust water systems.

31.2.3   Climate-Related Threats

The impacts of climate change, including sea-level rise, extreme storms, flooding, and drought, are putting further stress on deteriorating water infrastructure and diminishing already scarce water resources in some regions [19]. Tens of millions of Americans are expected to face declining water availability in the coming years. Competition for limited supplies is growing.

Disadvantaged communities are on the front lines of climate impacts on water [20]. Tribal communities, low-income households, and communities of color are more likely to be located in flood-prone areas. Extreme weather events and flooding can overwhelm and contaminate water supplies, causing service disruptions. These communities are also less likely to have the resources to quickly recover from disasters.

In coastal areas, rising seas cause sewer systems to back up and contaminate surface waters. Saltwater intrusion into aquifers can render groundwater unusable. Prolonged droughts, like the ongoing megadrought in the West, deplete surface water sources and groundwater basins. Shallow domestic wells serving rural households are especially vulnerable to going dry during drought [21].

Again, access to alternative water sources when primary supplies are threatened is not equal. During droughts in California's Central Valley, many small community water systems were forced to provide bottled water to residents or truck in water at high cost. Meanwhile, large agricultural interests continue to deplete groundwater for irrigation. Much more needs to be done to equitably allocate scarce water resources and protect access for the most vulnerable during climate shocks.

31.3   Health Disparities of Water Insecurity

The lack of access to adequate water quantity and quality or affordable water service in the United States has profound health implications. Water insecurity affects health through numerous pathways:

Waterborne illness: Contamination of drinking water supplies with pathogens like bacteria, viruses, and protozoa can cause gastrointestinal illnesses [22]. Risks are especially high for children, the elderly, pregnant women, and those with weakened immune systems. Water system deficiencies and disease outbreaks are more common in low-income communities and communities of color.

Chemical contamination: Pollutants in drinking water, such as lead, arsenic, nitrates, pesticides, and industrial chemicals, are linked to a range of chronic health impacts [23]. These include various cancers, reproductive harm, adverse birth outcomes, cardiovascular and kidney disease, and impaired brain development in children. An estimated 63 million Americans have been exposed to potentially unsafe water in the last decade.

Drought-related health impacts: Droughts can increase exposure to contaminated water as pollutants become concentrated in shrinking water supplies [24]. Low water levels can cause toxic algal blooms. Dry conditions also increase the risk of West Nile virus and Valley fever as habitats for mosquitos and soil pathogens expand. Water shortages are linked with higher rates of water-washed diseases, dehydration, and heat-related illness. The mental health consequences of drought for rural communities can be severe.

Flooding-related health impacts: Extreme rainfall and flooding can introduce pathogens and contamination into water systems [25]. Contact with flood waters is associated with increased rates of gastrointestinal illnesses and wound infections. Mold growth in water-damaged homes contributes to asthma and respiratory problems. The trauma of flooding events and displacement results in lasting mental health impacts.

Unaffordability and shutoffs: As water bills rise beyond what low-income households can pay, families face wrenching trade-offs that undermine their health and well-being [26]. To afford water, people cut back on other essentials like food and medicine. When faced with shutoffs for nonpayment, families lose access to water for cooking, cleaning, and hygiene. Shutoffs are associated with higher risks of water-related illness and other health problems like elevated blood pressure and mental distress.

The health impacts of water insecurity are not distributed equally. They fall most heavily on populations already burdened by poverty, discrimination, pre-existing health disparities, and other environmental injustices. Children in low-income communities and communities of color have the highest risk of elevated blood lead levels from contaminated water [27]. Water service shutoffs for inability to pay disproportionately affect Black and Latinx households [28]. The Navajo Nation, lacking adequate water and sanitation infrastructure, experienced one of the highest rates of COVID-19 infection in the country [29].

31.4 Comprehensive Policy Solutions

Achieving universal access to clean, safe, affordable water demands transformative policy change. A siloed, fragmented approach will not suffice. Ensuring water security and advancing health equity requires a cohesive strategy that addresses the multifaceted causes of the water access crisis. Key policy priorities include

Massively increase infrastructure investment: The federal government must significantly scale-up investment in water infrastructure, with an emphasis on underserved and disinvested communities. It is estimated that the United States needs to spend nearly $1 trillion over the next 20 years just to bring systems into a state of good repair [30]. Targeted funding is needed for disadvantaged communities to upgrade treatment facilities, replace lead service lines, and prevent sewage overflows and contamination. Resources should support not just capital projects but also operations and maintenance to ensure sustained water access.

Ensure affordable water service: A comprehensive federal water affordability program, akin to the Low Income Home Energy Assistance Program, should be established [31]. This should include bill payment assistance, percentage-of-income payment plans, debt relief, and shutoff prevention for low-income households. Consumer protections should cap rates and ban punitive practices like property liens for unpaid water bills. Funding mechanisms for water systems should be reformed so that costs are not disproportionately borne by those least able to pay.

Strengthen water quality protections: Health-based standards for contaminants in drinking water must be updated to reflect the latest science [32]. The capacity of water systems to monitor for regulated and unregulated contaminants should be enhanced. Increased funding is needed for treatment upgrades, especially for small systems. Policies to prevent water pollution at its source, like restricting toxic chemicals, managing agricultural runoff, and protecting source water, can reduce public exposure and water treatment costs.

Support household-level solutions: While fixing centralized water systems is essential, distributed approaches are also needed. Flexible funding should be available to households for premise plumbing repairs, private well testing and treatment, and decentralized water and sanitation solutions. This is particularly important for remote areas where connecting to a central system is not feasible. Assistance programs should address barriers like eligibility restrictions and complex application processes.

Reform water governance: Governance and financing models for water systems are highly fragmented and localized. This leaves small, under-resourced communities ill-equipped to address water challenges on their own. Consolidation and regionalization of water systems can help achieve economies of scale while ensuring local accountability. Statewide initiatives should identify at-risk water systems and support solutions like shared services and capacity development. Representation of impacted communities in decision-making is critical.

Climate resilience and water equity: Adapting to climate impacts on water resources is imperative [33]. Integrated planning across climate mitigation, water management, land use, and public health is needed to build resilience, especially for vulnerable populations. Funding should prioritize nature-based solutions that provide multiple community benefits in addition to water security. Equitable policies for water shortage contingency plans and demand management are needed to protect access for essential needs during droughts. Flood mitigation investments and insurance affordability programs should target at-risk communities.

Recognize the human right to water: Establishing safe, clean, affordable, and accessible water as a legally protected human right can catalyze and guide equitable policymaking. Defining core elements of the right and setting standards of adequacy provides a framework for progressive realization and accountability. A national water access plan should set targets, timelines, and metrics. Ultimately, a federal funding guarantee for water and sanitation access may be needed to ensure no one is left behind, just as we ensure access to basic education.

Community-driven solutions: Most essentially, directly impacted communities must be at the forefront of developing and implementing water access solutions. Outreach and collaborative planning with disadvantaged communities is critical to understanding lived experiences of water insecurity and to direct resources where they are most needed. Community organizations are vital partners in advancing policies and projects and ensuring accountability. Participatory budgeting and decision-making can help drive equitable investment. Building long-term capacity and community self-determination should be the goal.

Policy Solutions and Equity Aspects for Water Infrastructure Improvement

Policy Solution	Description	Equity Aspect
Increase Federal Investment	Significantly boost federal funding for water infrastructure through existing and new sources	Ensure funding prioritizes communities with critical needs and historically underinvested areas
Support Natural Infrastructure	Promote nature-based solutions like green roofs, rain gardens, and wetland restoration over traditional infrastructure	Focus implementation on low-income communities and communities of color that lack green space
Ensure Affordability for All	Develop local customer assistance programs, equitable rate structures, and comprehensive federal bill assistance programs	Address affordability crisis affecting low-income households and prevent water shutoffs in vulnerable communities
Maintain Environmental Safeguards	Enforce existing environmental laws and ensure infrastructure projects do not harm water quality or public health	Protect low-income communities and communities of color from increased pollution and environmental hazards
Target Disadvantaged Communities	Direct new funding under principles of equity to areas with the most serious water quality problems	Set aside funds for tribal and historically marginalized communities that struggle with water infrastructure

31.5 Conclusion: Achieving Water Equity Through Policy

Water is the basis for health, well-being, and human potential [34]. But the human right to safe, affordable water remains unrealized for far too many people in the United States, particularly in low-income communities and communities of color. Aging, inadequate infrastructure, underinvestment, inequitable policies, and climate change threats have created a water access crisis with far-reaching consequences for public health.

Ambitious, transformative action is urgently needed to resolve this crisis. We must dramatically increase public investment in water infrastructure, target resources to close equity gaps, keep water affordable, strengthen contamination prevention and response, and build climate resilience. Reforming our splintered systems of water governance and finance is critical. The communities facing the greatest water insecurity must be engaged as full partners in developing community-driven solutions.

By enacting equitable water policies, we can ensure that everyone has access to this most basic and vital resource, regardless of race, income, or geography. Doing so will allow individuals and communities to not just survive, but to thrive. The benefits of universal water security for health equity and social justice would be transformational.

We have the knowledge, wealth, and technology to make the human right to water a reality. What has been lacking until now is the political will. We must seize the current moment of heightened awareness and momentum for change. It is time for bold action commensurate with the magnitude of the challenge. No policy goal could have a more profound impact in creating the conditions for health equity. Clean, safe, affordable water for all must be our North Star. With concerted, collective effort – led by impacted communities themselves – we can achieve it.

References

1 United Nations (2010). Resolution 64/292: The Human Right to Water and Sanitation. https://digitallibrary.un.org/record/687002?ln=en&v=pdf.

2 Dig Deep & US Water Alliance (2019). Closing the water access gap in the United States: a national action plan. http://uswateralliance.org/sites/uswateralliance.org/files/publications/Closing%20the%20Water%20Access%20Gap%20in%20the%20United%20States_DIGITAL.pdf (accessed 23 August 2024).

3 Meehan, K., Jurjevich, J.R., Chun, N.M., and Sherrill, J. (2020). Geographies of insecure water access and the housing–water nexus in US cities. *Proceedings of the National Academy of Sciences* 117 (46): I 28700–28707. https://doi.org/10.1073/pnas.2007361117.

4 Switzer, D. and Teodoro, M.P. (2018). Class, race, ethnicity, and justice in safe drinking water compliance. *Social Science Quarterly* 99 (2): 524–535. https://doi.org/10.1111/ssqu.12397.

5 Balazs, C.L. and Ray, I. (2014). The drinking water disparities framework: on the origins and persistence of inequities in exposure. *American Journal of Public Health* 104 (4): 603–611. https://doi.org/10.2105/AJPH.2013.301664.

6 Lall, U., Josset, L., and Russo, T. (2020). A snapshot of the world's groundwater challenges. *Annual Review of Environment and Resources* 45: 171–194. https://doi.org/10.1146/annurev-environ-102017-025800.

7 American Society of Civil Engineers (2021). 2021 report card for America's infrastructure: drinking water. https://infrastructurereportcard.org/cat-item/drinking-water-infrastructure/.

8 Roller, Z., Gasteyer, S., Nelson, N. et al. (2019). *Closing the Water Access Gap in the United States: An Action Plan*. DigDeep. https://www.digdeep.org/close-the-water-gap.

9 DigDeep & US Water Alliance. (2019). Closing the water access gap in the United States: a national action plan. http://uswateralliance.org/sites/uswateralliance.org/files/publications/Closing%20the%20Water%20Access%20Gap%20in%20the%20United%20States_DIGITAL.pdf (accessed 24 August 2023).

10 McDonald, Y.J. and Grineski, S.E. (2012). Disparities in access to residential plumbing: a binational comparison of environmental injustice in El Paso and Ciudad Juárez. *Population and Environment* 34 (2): 194–216. https://doi.org/10.1007/s11111-012-0154-8.

11 Jepson, W. and Vandewalle, E. (2016). Household water insecurity in the global north: a study of rural and periurban settlements on the Texas–Mexico border. *The Professional Geographer* 68 (1): 66–81. https://doi.org/10.1080/00330124.2015.1028324.

12 Allaire, M., Wu, H., and Lall, U. (2018). National trends in drinking water quality violations. *Proceedings of the National Academy of Sciences* 115 (9): 2078–2083. https://doi.org/10.1073/pnas.1719805115.

13 Fedinick, K.P., Taylor, S., and Roberts, M. (2019). *Watered Down Justice*. Natural Resources Defense Council (NRDC). https://www.nrdc.org/resources/watered-down-justice.

14 US Water Alliance (2017). An equitable water future: a national briefing paper. http://uswateralliance.org/sites/uswateralliance.org/files/publications/uswa_waterequity_FINAL.pdf (accessed 24 August 2024).

15 Mack, E.A. and Wrase, S. (2017). A burgeoning crisis? A nationwide assessment of the geography of water affordability in the United States. *PLoS One* 12 (1): e0169488. https://doi.org/10.1371/journal.pone.0169488.

16 Rockowitz, D., Askew-Merwin, C., Sahai, M. et al. (2018). *Household Water Security in Metropolitan Detroit: Measuring the Affordability Gap*. University of Michigan Poverty Solutions. https://poverty.umich.edu/files/2018/08/PovertySolutions-PolicyBrief-0818-r2.pdf.

17 Swain, M., McKinney, E., and Susskind, L. (2020). Water shutoffs in older American cities: causes, extent, and remedies. *Journal of Planning Education and Research* 0739456X20904431. https://doi.org/10.1177/0739456X20904431.

18 Balazs, C., Morello-Frosch, R., Hubbard, A., and Ray, I. (2012). Environmental justice implications of arsenic contamination in California's San Joaquin Valley: a cross-sectional, cluster-design examining exposure and compliance in community drinking water systems. *Environmental Health* 11 (1): 1–12. https://doi.org/10.1186/1476-069X-11-84.

19 Kates, R.W., Colten, C.E., Laska, S., and Leatherman, S.P. (2006). Reconstruction of New Orleans after Hurricane Katrina: a research perspective. *Proceedings of the National Academy of Sciences* 103 (40): 14653–14660. https://doi.org/10.1073/pnas.0605726103.

20 Bautista, E., Hansel, W., Osorio, J.C., and Dwyer, G. (2019). New perspectives on community-based collaboration for water equity and sustainability: a case study of the Salinas Valley. *Local Environment* 24 (3): 215–230. https://doi.org/10.1080/13549839.2018.1558074.

21 Feinstein, L., Phurisamban, R., Ford, A. et al. (2017). *Drought and Equity in California*. Pacific Institute https://pacinst.org/publication/drought-equity-california/.

22 Exum, N.G., Betanzo, E., Schwab, K.J. et al. (2018). Extreme precipitation, public health emergencies, and safe drinking water in the USA. *Current Environmental Health Reports* 5 (2): 305–315. https://doi.org/10.1007/s40572-018-0200-5.

23 Chappells, H. and Campbell, N. (Eds.). (2021). *Water, Technology and the Nation-State*. Routledge https://doi.org/10.4324/9780367816407.

24 Stanke, C., Kerac, M., Prudhomme, C. et al. (2013). Health effects of drought: a systematic review of the evidence. *PLoS Currents* 5: https://doi.org/10.1371/currents.dis.7a2cee9e980f91ad7697b570bcc4b004.

25 Du, W., FitzGerald, G.J., Clark, M., and Hou, X.Y. (2010). Health impacts of floods. *Prehospital and Disaster Medicine* 25 (3): 265–272. https://doi.org/10.1017/S1049023X00008141.

26 Gaber, N., Vaughn, L., and Schwartz, S. (2013). Water insecurity and psychosocial distress in Detroit. *Geoforum* 53: 169–179. https://doi.org/10.1016/j.geoforum.2013.06.001.

27 Yeter, D., Banks, E.C., and Aschner, M. (2020). Disparity in risk factor severity for early childhood blood lead among predominantly African-American Black children: the 1999 to 2010 US NHANES. *International Journal of Environmental Research and Public Health* 17 (5): 1552. https://doi.org/10.3390/ijerph17051552.

28 Gonzalez, S., Ong, P., Pierce, G., and Hernandez, A. (2021). Keeping the Lights and Water on: COVID-19 and Utility Debt in Los Angeles' Communities of Color. https://escholarship.org/uc/item/3317w1fb

29 Cory, S. (2024). Assessing SARS-CoV-2 disease morbidity within the Navajo Tribal Nation in relation to the reduced access to equitable water infrastructure and health policy. Doctoral dissertation. University of Pittsburgh.

30 American Society of Civil Engineers (2019). 2017 infrastructure report card: drinking water. https://www.infrastructurereportcard.org/wp-content/uploads/2017/01/Drinking-Water-Final.pdf (accessed 24 August 2024).

31 Teodoro, M.P. (2019). Water and sewer affordability in the United States. *AWWA Water Science* 1 (2): e1129. https://doi.org/10.1002/aws2.1129.

32 Vanderwarker, A. (2012). Water and environmental justice. In: *A Twenty-First Century US Water Policy* (ed. J. Christian-Smith and P.H. Gleick), 52–89. Oxford University Press. https://doi.org/10.1093/acprof:osobl/9780199859443.003.0003.

33 Butler, L.J., Scammell, M.K., and Benson, E.B. (2016). The Flint, Michigan, water crisis: a case study in regulatory failure and environmental injustice. *Environmental Justice* 9 (4): 93–97. https://doi.org/10.1089/env.2016.0014.

34 Connor, R. (2015). *The United Nations World Water Development Report 2015: Water for a Sustainable World*, vol. vol. 1. UNESCO publishing.

32

Addressing Climate Change-Induced Health Disparities Through Policy and Planning

Abstract

This chapter examines the disproportionate impact of climate change on frontline communities, which are predominantly low-income and Black, Indigenous, and people of color (BIPOC) populations. These communities face heightened risks due to increased exposure to climate hazards, limited access to resources, and government neglect. The chapter emphasizes the need for equitable climate policies that prioritize the needs of frontline communities and addresses the health inequities exacerbated by climate change. This chapter discusses the challenges faced by frontline communities, the limitations of existing laws and regulations in addressing climate inequity, and the potential role of the Office of Climate Change and Health Equity (OCCHE) in shaping US climate policy. It also presents examples of states that have successfully integrated health equity into climate statutes. This chapter proposes three key policy approaches to reduce health inequity: involving frontline community advocates in climate policy development, strengthening public health responses, and increasing focus on the relationship between climate and health equity through public education, research, and targeted funding. This chapter concludes by emphasizing the importance of embracing health equity as a cornerstone of climate policy, recognizing climate change and environmental justice as social determinants of health, and dedicating public health resources to support frontline communities.

Keywords   *climate change; health disparities; frontline communities; environmental justice; public health responses; equitable climate policies; community advocacy; policy and planning*

> *In the aftermath of Hurricane Maria, Carmen, a 65-year-old Puerto Rican woman, struggled to access healthcare for her diabetes. With the island's power grid devastated and medical supplies running low, Carmen's health deteriorated rapidly. The slow and insufficient government response left her community without the resources needed to rebuild and recover, exacerbating existing health disparities.*
>
> *Tyrone, a young African American man from a low-income neighborhood in Louisiana, suffered from severe anxiety and depression following the destruction caused by Hurricane Katrina. Despite*

> *his worsening mental health, Tyrone found it nearly impossible to access affordable mental health-care in his community, which lacked the resources and infrastructure to address the long-term psychological impacts of the disaster.*
>
> *Malia, a Native American mother living on tribal lands, feared for her children's health as extreme heatwaves became more frequent. With limited access to air conditioning and healthcare services, Malia watched helplessly as her children suffered from heat exhaustion and respiratory issues. The lack of government support and resources left her community vulnerable to the growing threats of climate change.*

32.1 Climate Change: A Threat Multiplier Exacerbating Health Inequities

Climate change poses a significant and immediate threat to public health [1]. Beyond causing acute death and injury, climate disasters contribute to a wide range of health issues, including respiratory illnesses, allergies, food-, insect-, and water-borne diseases, cancer, heart disease, and mental health problems [2]. The impact of climate change is often described as a "threat multiplier" due to its propensity to aggravate existing economic and social disparities [3]. Consequently, American communities that have historically faced and continue to face disenfranchisement and discrimination are disproportionately affected by the consequences of climate change, experiencing them earlier and more severely than others [4].

Recognizing the link between climate change and health equity, the Biden administration acknowledges the necessity of addressing both issues in any comprehensive climate change and environmental justice policy [5]. The administration has committed to allocating 40% of all benefits from climate change investments to communities that have been unduly burdened by pollution and disinvestment. To achieve this goal, the US government must be willing to enact laws and regulations that directly tackle climate change-related health inequities and dedicate substantial resources to frontline communities. Only through such targeted and proactive measures can the administration effectively mitigate the disproportionate impact of climate change on vulnerable populations and promote health equity in the face of this global crisis.

> *"The impact of climate change will fall disproportionately upon developing countries and the poor persons within all countries. It will therefore exacerbate inequalities in health status and access to adequate food, clean water and other resources."*
>
> Former chairman of the Intergovernmental Panel on Climate Change, Rajendra Pachauri

32.2 Frontline Communities: Disproportionate Climate Impacts and Inadequate Support

Frontline communities, primarily consisting of low-income and BIPOC populations, bear a disproportionate burden of climate change impacts [6]. These heightened risks can stem from increased exposure to climate hazards, limited access to resources, government neglect, or a combination of these factors. For instance, economically disadvantaged communities often settle on coastal or heavily polluted land due to its affordability [7]. Consequently, these communities are more vulnerable to the effects of climate change compared to the general population as they already face a higher "baseline" of environmental degradation.

The concentration of BIPOC and low-income populations in frontline communities can be attributed to historical and cultural factors [8]. Native Americans, for example, often remain on tribal lands despite lacking essential services, such as healthcare and disaster response resources. Moreover, inadequate government support exacerbates the climate-related challenges faced by frontline communities. Prior to Hurricane Maria, up to half of Puerto Rico's population lived in poverty, and the island's power grid was at risk of collapse [9]. The hurricane devastated the power grid and destroyed 80% of Puerto Rico's crop value. The US government's response was slow and insufficient, with congressionally approved funds taking years to disburse, ongoing power grid issues, and tens of thousands of Puerto Ricans still unable to rebuild their homes despite enduring additional severe storms. Similarly, minority and low-income populations in Louisiana suffered the greatest losses from Hurricane Katrina [10]. Frontline communities often lack the political influence needed to direct resources to their neighborhoods in the aftermath of a climate catastrophe. While natural disasters may destroy homes, schools, and public utilities across socioeconomic lines, marginalized communities are significantly less likely to receive government assistance for rebuilding, perpetuating a cycle of disasters even as wealthier neighbors who experienced the same event resume their normal lives.

Furthermore, existing climate policies fail to adequately address the mental trauma experienced by frontline communities in the wake of climate disasters [11]. Up to 25% of a population may exhibit PTSD symptoms following a disaster, and the mental health impact of major climate and public health catastrophes, such as Hurricane Katrina and COVID-19, is well-documented [12]. However, despite being disproportionately affected by these disasters, minorities, including Latinos and Black women, have less access to mental healthcare compared to white individuals [13]. Psychiatrists and social workers have advocated for the development of programs that monitor and treat mental health issues in the immediate aftermath of an environmental disaster, as well as proactive efforts to integrate social services into disaster relief plans [14]. To effectively support frontline communities, these programs must include procedures for identifying vulnerable individuals and prioritizing their access to mental health resources.

32.3 Addressing Climate Inequity: Challenges and Progress in Policy and Legislation

Advocates for frontline communities often emphasize that current climate change adaptation plans are not feasible for poor and vulnerable populations [15]. These plans typically require communities to allocate significant resources to climate preparedness disregarding the fact that most frontline communities lack the necessary assets. Moreover, systemic inequities in policymaking have repeatedly led to the exclusion and disenfranchisement of marginalized people in government responses to the climate crisis.

Existing laws and regulations designed to prevent discrimination against marginalized communities in the distribution of federal resources have proven ineffective in addressing systemic inequity in climate policy. For instance, while Title VI of the Civil Rights Act prohibits discrimination based on race and national origin in the allocation of federal financial resources, the Supreme Court ruled that the Act does not establish a private right of action [16]. In 2020, the Trump administration rolled back provisions of the National Environmental Policy Act (NEPA) that required federal agencies to conduct environmental impact reviews for federal projects [17]. This rollback disproportionately affects low-income and minority neighborhoods as environmentally hazardous projects are often concentrated in these communities.

Since 1994, Executive Order 12898 has encouraged environmental justice by directing federal agencies to consider the "disproportionately high and adverse human health or environmental effects of [their] programs, policies, and activities on minority populations and low-income populations" [18]. However, executive orders lack the force of true legislation because they are only enforceable by the president, and citizens cannot challenge compliance with an executive order.

On a positive note, the Biden administration has acknowledged health disparities in climate policy and developed a playbook aimed at bridging the gap between health and social services [19]. The White House has stated that "action on climate change and environmental justice is a health equity imperative" and has set an ambitious goal to improve health equity through climate initiatives. To support this goal, the administration established the Office of Climate Change and Health Equity (OCCHE) under the Department of Health and Human Services (HHS) [20]. Although OCCHE has the potential to play a crucial role in shaping US climate policy, it has faced budget constraints due to Congress's reluctance to allocate requested funding. Despite these challenges, OCCHE has made progress, such as releasing guidance in 2023 on leveraging the 2022 Inflation Reduction Act (IRA), which provides funding for climate-resilient and renewable infrastructure. In the future, OCCHE could develop similar funding guidance specifically for organizations serving frontline communities.

Much of the day-to-day implementation of climate change policy occurs at the state level. Notably, states have successfully reduced health disparities by directly integrating health equity into climate statutes. For example, New York's 2019 Climate Leadership and Community Protection Act mandates that the state invest at least 35% (with a goal of 40%) of clean energy and energy efficiency resources in disadvantaged communities [21]. New York has also established an air quality monitoring program that identifies communities with disproportionately high air pollution burdens, targeting these areas for mobile air screening and data collection. Washington state requires its utilities to seek public feedback and assess operational impacts on frontline communities, and the state is currently working on identifying communities overburdened by pollution [22]. California has increased penalties for polluters who harm the state's frontline populations [23]. Lastly, Illinois passed the Climate and Equitable Jobs Act, which aims to assist individuals who worked in fossil fuels in finding new employment [24]. The Act established "hubs" that connect these individuals, many of whom are members of frontline communities, with workforce development programs and new jobs in clean energy.

Policy and Equity Considerations in Addressing Climate-Related Health Impacts

Policy Area	Challenges and Issues	Equity Considerations	Proposed Actions
Health System Resilience	Climate threats disrupting healthcare operations; increased demand for health services during crises.	Marginalized communities suffer more due to inadequate healthcare infrastructure.	Strengthen healthcare and public health sectors' resilience; develop contingency plans for resource availability during emergencies; encourage local collaboration for resilient community strategies.
Decarbonization of Healthcare	Health sector contributes significantly to greenhouse gas emissions.	Low-income communities disproportionately affected by pollution.	Support health sector in reducing carbon emissions through guidance, incentives, and investments; require public reporting of sustainability activities; integrate decarbonization into healthcare standards.

Policy Area	Challenges and Issues	Equity Considerations	Proposed Actions
Data Synthesis and Application	Information gaps in climate and health data.	Data needed on the impact of climate change on vulnerable populations.	Orchestrate efforts to close information gaps, synthesize data, and identify practical applications; develop evaluation tools and guidelines for preparedness and adaptation strategies.
Communication and Education	Need for effective climate-related health communication.	Disproportionate health impacts on marginalized groups due to climate change.	Develop and coordinate climate and health communication efforts; educate health professionals and the public on climate-related health threats; link climate change to clinical outcomes in health screenings.

32.4 Equitable Climate Policies: Engaging Communities, Strengthening Health Responses, and Prioritizing Research

To reduce health inequity, future climate policies must specifically address the needs of frontline communities. The following paragraphs outline three policy approaches to develop tailored strategies. First, frontline community advocates must be involved in the development and enforcement of climate policy. Second, public health responses must be strengthened to safeguard vulnerable communities. Finally, an increased focus must be put on the relationship between climate and health equity. Each strategy plays a role in ensuring that climate policies are comprehensive and equitable, addressing the unique needs of those most impacted by climate events.

First, effective climate policy should always be informed by the needs of frontline communities due to their particular vulnerability to the climate crisis. This requires multifaceted strategies. Fundamentally, frontline community advocates should be involved in drafting laws and regulations and should sit on advisory councils or committees overseeing the enactment of climate policy. Their vocal involvement ensures that climate adaptation projects will be tailored to their specific needs, such as the relative lack of mental health support for minorities. States already have a "growing trend toward participatory process," as evidenced by New York's 22-member Climate Action Council and Washington's Environmental Justice Council. Relatedly, financial incentives and support mechanisms should be written into laws and regulations to encourage care for frontline communities. As discussed above, such solutions have been deployed at both the federal (e.g. the IRA) and state levels, but more should be done to ensure that frontline communities are prioritized for climate resiliency projects funded by general laws.

Climate policy should also integrate continuous monitoring and evaluation frameworks for frontline communities. This involves collecting data on environmental, health, and economic indicators to ensure that policies are effectively reducing the disparities faced by these communities. Other states should mirror Washington in requiring public utilities to accept public feedback and analyze their environmental footprints, particularly in frontline communities. By tethering operational success to environmental impact, policymakers could effectively encourage monitoring of climate impacts and ensure that policies are flexible and adaptable to new discoveries about climate change.

A second critical policy approach to mitigating the impact of climate change on frontline communities is to enhance public health responses. While healthcare system disruptions can negatively impact any population, they are catastrophic for frontline communities. These communities are already less likely to have access to healthcare and mental health resources and rely on public assistance. Simultaneously, their increased chance of experiencing a climate disaster makes it more likely they will need robust and prepared public health resources.

The Center for American Progress recommends that OCCHE spearhead efforts to improve health providers' preparedness for climate disasters. OCCHE can encourage hospitals to analyze their supply chains for vulnerabilities, particularly those affecting key resources like food, water, and medicine. Coordinating with HHS agencies like the NIH and the Agency for Healthcare Research and Quality, OCCHE can push for examinations of hospital infrastructure, leading to the proactive design or retrofitting of facilities that will enable them to withstand likely weather events. OCCHE is also well-positioned to coordinate climate response plans that integrate medical, public health, and social services. The CDC's Climate and Health Program and the Administration for Strategic Preparedness and Response's Hospital Preparedness Program and Regional Disaster Health Response System Pilot could serve as models for federally led climate responses that also include community engagement.

Third, climate laws should be drafted with a focus on the connection between climate and health equity. This approach requires an integrated effort to educate the public, dedicate research, and allocate funding specifically to understand and address the intersection of health and climate change, especially as it pertains to frontline communities.

Many people still do not understand that climate change can significantly impact human health as well as the environment [25]. Educating the public about this relationship is essential to gathering the public buy-in necessary to create laws that address systemic health inequities in climate policy. Federal agencies can launch public awareness campaigns about the health impacts of climate change, such as exacerbated respiratory problems, heat-related illnesses, and the spread of infectious diseases [26]. The fact that these negative impacts are unevenly distributed should also become public knowledge.

Climate policy should dedicate research and funding specifically to the study of climate impacts on minorities, low-income, and other marginalized communities [27]. Much like other health problems, these groups remain underrepresented in climate and health research. One simple way to jump-start information gathering would be to undo the repeal of the NEPA provisions requiring environmental impact reviews for public works projects in frontline communities. Also, OCCHE can be mobilized to synthesize information on the effect of climate change on the health of vulnerable communities that is currently discreetly collected by agencies such as the EPA, CDC, and NIH. A centralized repository of this data can inform future climate law and policy. For instance, studying the impact of heatwaves in urban low-income areas can lead to targeted actions like setting up cooling centers or greening projects [28].

Finally, laws must allocate funding aimed at improving our general understanding of the relationship between health and climate. The Biden administration has already made efforts to secure OCCHE the funding it needs for some of the projects outlined above; however, Congress continues to oppose expanding the agency's budget. Meaningful improvements for frontline communities can only occur if the government is willing to dedicate the necessary resources.

32.5 Conclusion: Embracing Health Equity as a Cornerstone of Climate Policy

Frontline communities bear a disproportionate burden of the health impacts of climate change, despite ongoing government indifference. To effectively address these inequities, it is crucial to recognize that climate change and environmental justice are social determinants of health and to dedicate public health resources to support these populations [29]. At its core, this approach involves prioritizing frontline communities at every stage of the climate policy-making process, strengthening public health resources, and explicitly incorporating provisions that promote health equity into climate laws and policies.

References

1 Haines, A., Kovats, R.S., Campbell-Lendrum, D., and Corvalán, C. (2006). Climate change and human health: impacts, vulnerability and public health. *Public Health* 120 (7): 585–596.

2 Ebi, K.L. and Hess, J.J. (2020). Health risks due to climate change: inequity in causes and consequences: study examines health risks due to climate change. *Health Affairs* 39 (12): 2056–2062.

3 Huntjens, P. and Nachbar, K. (2015). Climate change as a threat multiplier for human disaster and conflict. *The Hague Institute for Global Justice* 1–24.

4 Bullard, R.D. (2021). Environmental justice-once a footnote, now a headline. *Harvard Environmental Law Review* 45: 243.

5 Cha, J.M., Farrell, C., and Stevis, D. (2022). Climate and environmental justice policies in the first year of the Biden administration. *Publius: The Journal of Federalism* 52 (3): 408–427.

6 Fernandez-Bou, A.S., Ortiz-Partida, J.P., Classen-Rodriguez, L.M. et al. (2021). 3 challenges, 3 errors, and 3 solutions to integrate frontline communities in climate change policy and research: lessons from California. *Frontiers in Climate* 3: 717554.

7 Bullard, R.D. (ed.) (2007). *Growing Smarter: Achieving livable Communities, Environmental Justice, and Regional Equity*. MIT Press.

8 Jantarasami, L.C. et al. (2018). Tribes and Indigenous peoples. In: *Impacts, Risks, and Adaptation in the United States: Fourth National Climate Assessment*, vol. vol. II. Washington, DC: U.S. Global Change Research Program.

9 Rivera, F.I. (2020). Puerto Rico's population before and after Hurricane Maria. *Population and Environment* 42 (1): 1–3.

10 Aune, K.T., Gesch, D., and Smith, G.S. (2020). A spatial analysis of climate gentrification in Orleans Parish, Louisiana post-Hurricane Katrina. *Environmental Research* 185: 109384.

11 Lawrance, E., Thompson, R., Fontana, G., and Jennings, N. (2021). The impact of climate change on mental health and emotional wellbeing: current evidence and implications for policy and practice. Grantham Institute briefing paper 36.

12 Gawrych, M. (2022). Climate change and mental health: a review of current literature. *Psychiatria Polska* 56 (4): 903–915.

13 Cianconi, P., Betrò, S., and Janiri, L. (2020). The impact of climate change on mental health: a systematic descriptive review. *Frontiers in Psychiatry* 11: 490206.

14 Palinkas, L.A., O'Donnell, M.L., Lau, W., and Wong, M. (2020). Strategies for delivering mental health services in response to global climate change: a narrative review. *International Journal of Environmental Research and Public Health* 17 (22): 8562.

15 Krigel, K., Benjamin, O., Cohen, N., and Tchetchik, A. (2023). Municipal authorities' climate change adaptation plans: barriers to the inclusion of intensified needs of vulnerable populations. *Urban Climate* 49: 101433.

16 Williams, K. (2021). The impact of foresight: reframing discriminatory intent to properly remedy environmental racism. *Houston Law Review* 59: 1231.

17 Yozwiak, M., Abell, H., and Carley, S. (2021). Energy policy reversal during the Trump administration: examination of its legacy and implications for federalism. *Publius: The Journal of Federalism* 51 (3): 429–458.

18 Brower, S. (2021). Environmental [in] Justice: why executive order 12898 falls short of creating environmental equity for vulnerable communities. *Minnesota Journal of Law & Inequality* 4 (1): 1–30.

19 Elder, M. (2021). Optimistic prospects for US climate policy in the Biden Administration. *Institute for Global Environmental Strategies* 1–25.

20 Stephenson, J. (2021). New federal office will tackle climate change as health threat borne unequally by vulnerable groups. *JAMA Health Forum* 2 (9), e213351. American Medical Association.

21 Shi, L. and Moser, S. (2021). Transformative climate adaptation in the United States: trends and prospects. *Science* 372 (6549): eabc8054.

22 Grodnik-Nagle, A., Sukhdev, A., Vogel, J., and Herrick, C. (2023). Beyond climate ready? A history of Seattle public utilities' ongoing evolution from environmental and climate risk management to integrated sustainability. *Sustainability* 15 (6): 4977.

23 Fowlie, M., Walker, R., and Wooley, D. (2020). *Climate Policy, Environmental Justice, and Local Air Pollution*. Berkeley: University of California.

24 Lee, C. (2020). A game changer in the making? Lessons from states advancing environmental justice through mapping and cumulative impact strategies. *Environmental Law Reporter* 50: 10203.

25 Reidmiller, D., Hayhoe, K., Easterling, D. R. et al. (2018). Climate Science in the Fourth US National Climate Assessment. AGU Fall Meeting Abstracts 2018, U24A-01.

26 Climate Leadership Initiative. (2010). Ready for Change: Preparing Public Health Agencies for the Impacts of Climate Change. https://scholarsbank.uoregon.edu/xmlui/handle/1794/10741

27 Shi, L., Chu, E., Anguelovski, I. et al. (2016). Roadmap towards justice in urban climate adaptation research. *Nature Climate Change* 6 (2): 131–137.

28 Palinkas, L.A., Hurlburt, M.S., Fernandez, C. et al. (2022). Vulnerable, resilient, or both? A qualitative study of adaptation resources and behaviors to heat waves and health outcomes of low-income residents of urban heat islands. *International Journal of Environmental Research and Public Health* 19 (17): 11090.

29 Balbus, J.M., McCannon, C.J., Mataka, A., and Levine, R.L. (2022). After COP26 – putting health and equity at the center of the climate movement. *New England Journal of Medicine* 386 (14): 1295–1297.

Index

Printed and bound by CPI Group (UK) Ltd, Croydon, CR0 4YY

12/11/2024

14591148-0001